AF837688

AI-driven Medical Image Analysis in Precision Radiation Therapy

AI-driven Medical Image Analysis in Precision Radiation Therapy provides a comprehensive overview of the latest developments in artificial intelligence for medical imaging, focusing on applications in precision radiation therapy. Written by a team of experts, it offers an accessible perspective on how AI is transforming cancer treatment for a broad audience, from computer science and engineering to the medical sector. The text covers key techniques such as image synthesis, segmentation, and registration, but its primary focus is on practical clinical applications. It showcases recent studies in image-guided and adaptive radiation therapy, real-time tumor motion tracking, and treatment response assessment for both photon and proton therapies. Furthermore, this book addresses the real-world challenges of implementing these AI techniques in a clinical setting, equipping readers with the practical knowledge needed for successful integration. It is an essential guide for students and newcomers, as well as a valuable reference for experienced medical physicists and radiation oncologists.

Key Features:

- Provides in-depth coverage of cutting-edge AI applications in medical image processing, including image synthesis, segmentation, and registration techniques specifically designed for radiation therapy contexts.
- Discusses real-world implementations of AI-driven technologies in precision radiation therapy.
- Addresses the practical challenges of integrating AI systems into clinical workflows.

Xiaofeng Yang, PhD, DABR, is the Paul W. Doetsch Professor and Vice Chair for Medical Physics Research in the Department of Radiation Oncology at Emory University School of Medicine. He directs the Deep Biomedical Imaging Lab, where he develops innovative AI-enabled analytical and computational methods to advance quantitative imaging in cancer diagnosis and treatment, with the goal of improving the accuracy and precision of cancer radiotherapy. Dr. Yang also holds adjunct faculty appointments in the Medical Physics and Machine Learning programs at the Georgia Institute of Technology, the Department of Biomedical Informatics at Emory University, and the Wallace H. Coulter Department of Biomedical Engineering at Emory University and Georgia Tech. He is a Fellow of SPIE.

Tonghe Wang, PhD, DABR, is an assistant attending physicist in the Department of Medical Physics at the Memorial Sloan Kettering at the main campus. Dr. Wang received his BS in physics from Peking University in China in 2013 and a PhD in medical physics from Georgia Institute of Technology in 2017, with research experience in iterative Computed tomography (CT) reconstruction. Dr. Wang completed a medical physics residency at Emory University in 2019 and stayed at Emory as an assistant professor and board-certified medical physicist before joining Memorial Sloan Kettering in 2022.

Imaging in Medical Diagnosis and Therapy
Series Editors: Bruce R. Thomadsen, David W. Jordan

Role and Applications in Radiation Dosimetry
Indra J. Das

Clinical 3D Dosimetry in Modern Radiation Therapy
Ben Mijnheer

Hybrid Imaging in Cardiovascular Medicine
Yi-Hwa Liu, Albert J. Sinusas

Observer Performance Methods for Diagnostic Imaging: Foundations, Modeling, and Applications with R-Based Examples
Dev P. Chakraborty

Ultrasound Imaging and Therapy
Aaron Fenster, James C. Lacefield

Dose, Benefit, and Risk in Medical Imaging
Lawrence T. Dauer, Bae P. Chu, Pat B. Zanzonico

Big Data in Radiation Oncology
Jun Deng, Lei Xing

Monte Carlo Techniques in Radiation Therapy: Introduction, Source Modelling, and Patient Dose Calculations, Second Edition
Frank Verhaegen, Joao Seco

Monte Carlo Techniques in Radiation Therapy: Applications to Dosimetry, Imaging, and Preclinical Radiotherapy, Second Edition
Joao Seco, Frank Verhaegen

Introductory Biomedical Imaging: Principles and Practice from Microscopy to MRI
Bethe A. Scalettar, James R. Abney

Medical Image Synthesis: Methods and Clinical Applications
Xiaofeng Yang

Artificial Intelligence in Radiation Oncology and Biomedical Physics
Gilmer Valdes, Lei Xing

3D Ultrasound:Devices, Applications, and Algorithms
Aaron Fenster

3D Printing in Radiation Therapy: A Handbook
James Robar

Handbook of Radiotherapy Planning: Core Skills and Practical Considerations
Minsun Kim and Mu-Han Lan

Comprehensive Brachytherapy: Physical and Clinical Aspects
Peter J. Hoskin, Dimos Baltas, Ali S. Meigooni and Christian Kiristis

AI-driven Medical Image Analysis in Precision Radiation Therapy
Xiaofeng Yang and Tonghe Wang

For more information about this series, please visit: https://www.routledge.com/Imaging-in-Medical-Diagnosis-and-Therapy/book-series/CRCIMAINMED

AI-driven Medical Image Analysis in Precision Radiation Therapy

Edited by

Xiaofeng Yang and Tonghe Wang

CRC Press
Taylor & Francis Group
Boca Raton London New York

CRC Press is an imprint of the
Taylor & Francis Group, an **informa** business

Designed cover image: Shutterstock

First edition published 2026
by CRC Press
2385 NW Executive Center Drive, Suite 320, Boca Raton FL 33431

and by CRC Press
4 Park Square, Milton Park, Abingdon, Oxon, OX14 4RN

CRC Press is an imprint of Taylor & Francis Group, LLC

© 2026 selection and editorial matter, Xiaofeng Yang and Tonghe Wang; individual chapters, the contributors

This book contains information obtained from authentic and highly regarded sources. While all reasonable efforts have been made to publish reliable data and information, neither the author[s] nor the publisher can accept any legal responsibility or liability for any errors or omissions that may be made. The publishers wish to make clear that any views or opinions expressed in this book by individual editors, authors or contributors are personal to them and do not necessarily reflect the views/opinions of the publishers. The information or guidance contained in this book is intended for use by medical, scientific or health-care professionals and is provided strictly as a supplement to the medical or other professional's own judgement, their knowledge of the patient's medical history, relevant manufacturer's instructions and the appropriate best practice guidelines. Because of the rapid advances in medical science, any information or advice on dosages, procedures or diagnoses should be independently verified. The reader is strongly urged to consult the relevant national drug formulary and the drug companies' and device or material manufacturers' printed instructions, and their websites, before administering or utilizing any of the drugs, devices or materials mentioned in this book. This book does not indicate whether a particular treatment is appropriate or suitable for a particular individual. Ultimately it is the sole responsibility of the medical professional to make his or her own professional judgements, so as to advise and treat patients appropriately. The authors and publishers have also attempted to trace the copyright holders of all material reproduced in this publication and apologize to copyright holders if permission to publish in this form has not been obtained. If any copyright material has not been acknowledged please write and let us know so we may rectify in any future reprint.

Except as permitted under U.S. Copyright Law, no part of this book may be reprinted, reproduced, transmitted, or utilized in any form by any electronic, mechanical, or other means, now known or hereafter invented, including photocopying, microfilming, and recording, or in any information storage or retrieval system, without written permission from the publishers.

For permission to photocopy or use material electronically from this work, access www.copyright.com or contact the Copyright Clearance Center, Inc. (CCC), 222 Rosewood Drive, Danvers, MA 01923, 978-750-8400. For works that are not available on CCC please contact mpkbookspermissions@tandf.co.uk

For Product Safety Concerns and Information please contact our EU representative GPSR@taylorandfrancis.com. Taylor & Francis Verlag GmbH, Kaufingerstraße 24, 80331 München, Germany.

Trademark notice: Product or corporate names may be trademarks or registered trademarks and are used only for identification and explanation without intent to infringe.

ISBN: 9781032716008 (hbk)
ISBN: 9781032769165 (pbk)
ISBN: 9781003480365 (ebk)

DOI: 10.1201/9781003480365

Typeset in Times
by codeMantra

Contents

Series Preface

Since their inception over a century ago, advances in the science and technology of medical imaging and radiation therapy are more profound and rapid than ever before. Further, the disciplines are increasingly cross-linked as imaging methods become more widely used to plan, guide, monitor, and assess treatments in radiation therapy. Today, the technologies of medical imaging and radiation therapy are so complex and computer-driven that it is difficult for the people (physicians and technologists) responsible for their clinical use to know exactly what is happening at the point of care, when a patient is being examined or treated. The people best equipped to understand the technologies and their applications are medical physicists, and these individuals are assuming greater responsibilities in the clinical arena to ensure that what is intended for the patient is actually delivered in a safe and effective manner.

The growing responsibilities of medical physicists in the clinical arenas of medical imaging and radiation therapy are not without their challenges, however. Most medical physicists are knowledgeable in either radiation therapy or medical imaging, and expert in one or a small number of areas within their disciplines. They sustain their expertise in these areas by reading scientific articles and attending scientific talks at meetings. In contrast, their responsibilities increasingly extend beyond their specific areas of expertise. To meet these responsibilities, medical physicists periodically must refresh their knowledge of advances in medical imaging or radiation therapy, and they must be prepared to function at the intersection of these two fields. How to accomplish these objectives is a challenge.

At the 2007 annual meeting of the American Association of Physicists in Medicine in Minneapolis, this challenge was the topic of conversation during a lunch hosted by Taylor & Francis Publishers and involving a group of senior medical physicists (Arthur L. Boyer, Joseph O. Deasy, C.-M. Charlie Ma, Todd A. Pawlicki, Ervin B. Podgorsak, Elke Reitzel, Anthony B. Wolbarst, and Ellen D. Yorke). The conclusion of this discussion was that a book series should be launched under the Taylor & Francis banner, with each volume in the series addressing a rapidly advancing area of medical imaging or radiation therapy of importance to medical physicists. The aim would be for each volume to provide medical physicists with the information needed to understand technologies driving a rapid advance and their applications to safe and effective delivery of patient care.

Each volume in this series is edited by one or more individuals with recognized expertise in the technological area encompassed by this book. The editors are responsible for selecting the authors of individual chapters and ensuring that the chapters are comprehensive and intelligible to someone without such expertise. The enthusiasm of volume editors and chapter authors has been gratifying and reinforces the conclusion of the Minneapolis luncheon that this series of books addresses a major need of medical physicists.

The series "Imaging in Medical Diagnosis and Therapy" would not have been possible without the encouragement and support of the series manager, Lou Chosen, Executive Editor at Taylor & Francis. The editors and authors, and most of all I, are indebted to his steady guidance of the entire project.

William R. Hendee
Founding Series Editor

Contributors

Stephen R. Bowen
Department of Radiation Oncology
University of Washington School of Medicine
Seattle, Washington
and
Department of Radiology
University of Washington School of Medicine
Seattle, Washington

Joe Y. Chang
Department of Radiation Oncology
The University of Texas MD Anderson Cancer Center
Houston, Texas

Serdar Charyyev
Department of Radiation Oncology
Stanford University
Stanford, California

Jingchu Chen
Department of Radiation Oncology, Winship Cancer Institute
Emory University
Atlanta, Georgia
and
School of Mechanical Engineering
Georgia Institute of Technology
Atlanta, Georgia

Xinru Chen
Radiation Physics
University of Texas MD Anderson Cancer Center
Houston, Texas

Sunan Cui
Department of Radiation Oncology
University of Washington School of Medicine
Seattle, Washington

Zach Eidex
Department of Radiation Oncology, Winship Cancer Institute, School of Medicine
Emory University
Atlanta, Georgia

Jie Fu
Department of Radiation Oncology
University of Washington School of Medicine
Seattle, Washington

Suwen Ge
Department of Computer Science
Columbia University
New York, New York

Clemens Grassberger
Department of Radiation Oncology
University of Washington School of Medicine
Seattle, Washington

Mingzhe Hu
Department of Computer Science and Informatics
Emory University
Atlanta, Georgia
and
Department of Radiation Oncology, Winship Cancer Institute, School of Medicine
Emory University
Atlanta, Georgia

Jue Jiang
Department of Medical Physics
Memorial Sloan Kettering Cancer Center
New York, New York

Yunxiang Li
Department of Radiation Oncology
University of Texas Southwestern Medical Center
Dallas, Texas

Yingzi Liu
Division of the Biological Sciences
The University of Chicago
Chicago, Illinois

Amgad Muneer
Department of Imaging Physics
The University of Texas MD Anderson Cancer Center
Houston, Texas

Dong Nie
Department of Computer Science
University of North Carolina
Chapel Hill, North Carolina

Hao Peng
Department of Radiation Oncology
Stanford University
Stanford, California

Dong Joo Rhee
Radiation Physics
University of Texas MD Anderson Cancer Center
Houston, Texas

Xinrui Song
Department of Biomedical Engineering
Rensselaer Polytechnic Institute
Troy, New York

Zhen Tian
Division of the Biological Sciences
The University of Chicago
Chicago, Illinois

Ruiyuan Wang
Department of Computer Science
University of Waterloo
Waterloo, Canada

Tonghe Wang
Department of Medical Physics
Memorial Sloan Kettering Cancer Center
New York, New York

Zhichao Wang
The George W. Woodruff School of Mechanical Engineering
Georgia Institute of Technology
Atlanta, Georgia

Jia Wu
Department of Imaging Physics
The University of Texas MD Anderson Cancer Center
Houston, Texas
and
Department of Thoracic/Head and Neck Medical Oncology
The University of Texas MD Anderson Cancer Center
Houston, Texas
and
Institute for Data Science in Oncology
The University of Texas MD Anderson Cancer Center
Houston, Texas

Jacob Wynne
Radiation Oncology
Altru Health System
Grand Forks, North Dakota

Qiuyu Xiao
Department of Computer Science
University of North Carolina
Chapel Hill, North Carolina

Jiacheng Xie
Department of Radiation Oncology
University of Texas Southwestern Medical Center
Dallas, Texas

Pingkun Yan
Department of Biomedical Engineering
Rensselaer Polytechnic Institute
Troy, New York

Jinzhong Yang
Radiation Physics
University of Texas MD Anderson Cancer Center
Houston, Texas

Xiaofeng Yang
Department of Radiation Oncology, Winship Cancer Institute, School of Medicine
Emory University
Atlanta, Georgia

Zi Yang
Department of Radiation Oncology
Stanford University
Stanford, California

Faisal Yaseen
Department of Bioinformatics and Medical Education
University of Washington School of Medicine
Seattle, Washington

You Zhang
Department of Radiation Oncology
University of Texas Southwestern Medical Center
Dallas, Texas

Feng Zhao
School of Computational Science and Engineering
Georgia Institute of Technology
Atlanta, Georgia

Yao Zhao
Radiation Physics
University of Texas MD Anderson Cancer Center
Houston, Texas

Introduction

Artificial intelligence (AI) has been an emerging technology in health care, and its impact on radiation oncology is particularly large. With its unprecedented ability to analyze large datasets, recognize subtle patterns, and generate clinically meaningful predictions, AI is redefining how we approach medical image analysis and patient-specific cancer care. As imaging technologies become increasingly sophisticated and data-rich, AI serves as a crucial role in enhancing efficiency, consistency, and precision across the radiation therapy workflow.

Radiation therapy is fundamentally reliant on imaging. Accurate tumor localization, treatment planning, dose delivery, and therapy monitoring all depend on high-quality image acquisition and interpretation. However, the growing complexity of imaging data has outpaced traditional manual processing, which is time-consuming and subject to interobserver variability. AI addresses these limitations by automating key tasks and helping clinical decision-making. Whether in external beam radiation therapy (EBRT), brachytherapy, proton therapy, or other treatment modalities, AI is developed to revolutionize the use of imaging to deliver highly personalized and adaptive treatments.

This book is structured into 12 chapters. The first five chapters introduces the technical groundwork for AI-based medical image analysis. Chapter 1 covers image synthesis techniques, including generative models that synthesize missing modalities, enhance image quality, or augment rare datasets. Chapter 2 focuses on image segmentation, a foundational task in treatment planning, highlighting how AI has achieved expert-level accuracy in delineating tumors and critical structures. Chapter 3 reviews image registration, an important step in aligning multimodal datasets for tasks such as dose accumulation, adaptive planning, and longitudinal assessment. Chapter 4 examines radiomics, which leverages quantitative imaging features to discover associations with treatment response and outcomes. Finally, Chapter 5 provides a comprehensive overview of vision-language models for medical image analysis, exploring how these multimodal AI systems integrate visual and textual information to enhance segmentation, classification, and reasoning in medical imaging tasks.

The next six chapters transitions from core techniques to clinical applications of AI in precision radiation therapy. Chapter 6 introduces AI's contributions to image-guided radiation therapy (IGRT), where real-time imaging and intelligent automation help reduce uncertainty. Chapter 7 discusses adaptive radiation therapy (ART), showcasing how AI enables dynamic plan adaptation in response to anatomical and physiological changes throughout the treatment course. Chapter 8 focuses on motion management, where AI-driven models help predict, track, and compensate for organ and patient motion. In Chapter 9, we explore AI's role in proton and flash therapy, particularly in optimizing beam delivery and developing novel planning strategies. Chapter 10 focuses on brachytherapy, emphasizing AI's role in automating segmentation, applicator reconstruction, and dose prediction. Chapter 11 addresses treatment response assessment, demonstrating how AI can extract prognostic information from longitudinal imaging to inform personalized care.

While the potential of AI in radiation oncology is vast, its integration into clinical practice introduces important considerations around transparency, trust, and safety. Chapter 12 critically examines these dimensions, discussing ethical challenges, regulatory frameworks, and the need for explainable AI in high-stakes decision-making from the perspective of physician.

By combining technical foundations, practical implementations, and ethical reflections, this book aims to equip researchers, clinicians, and students with a comprehensive understanding of AI's role in advancing medical image analysis in radiation oncology. Our hope is to foster innovation, encourage responsible adoption, and ultimately improve outcomes for patients around the world.

DOI: 10.1201/9781003480365-1

1 Medical Image Synthesis

Ruiyuan Wang, Suwen Ge, Zhichao Wang, Qiuyu Xiao, and Dong Nie

1.1 INTRODUCTION

1.1.1 The Role of Medical Imaging in Precision Radiation Therapy

Medical imaging is fundamental to modern clinical practice, playing a critical role in diagnosis, treatment planning, and monitoring of diseases. In precision radiation therapy, accurate and timely acquisition of patient-specific anatomical and functional information through imaging is essential for optimizing treatment efficacy while minimizing toxicity to healthy tissues. Modalities such as computed tomography (CT), magnetic resonance imaging (MRI), and positron emission tomography (PET) are routinely used, each providing unique insights into the patient's condition. These modalities offer complementary information vital for informed clinical decision-making.

For instance, CT is indispensable in radiation therapy, providing electron density information necessary for accurate dose calculations and heterogeneity corrections. However, CT often lacks sufficient soft-tissue contrast, complicating the precise delineation of tumors and adjacent organs at risk (OARs), particularly in complex regions like the brain and abdomen. In contrast, MRI offers superior soft-tissue differentiation, critical for accurately defining target volumes and sparing critical structures. This advantage is particularly evident in prostate stereotactic body radiation therapy (SBRT), where high-precision delineation is required, and for visualizing structures like the urethra, which are often indistinct on CT scans. Modern diagnostic modalities like MRI and CT inherently produce three-dimensional (3D) volumetric data, essential for comprehensive treatment planning.

Despite their individual strengths, each modality also presents limitations. Beyond its contrast limitations, CT exposes patients to ionizing radiation. MRI, while radiation-free and excellent for soft-tissue detail, is more expensive, requires longer acquisition times, and does not directly provide electron density information needed for conventional radiotherapy planning or PET attenuation correction. Additionally, MRI can be susceptible to geometric distortions, though studies suggest that for sites like the pelvis, these distortions have minimal impact on dosimetric accuracy.

1.1.2 Medical Image Synthesis: Definition and Clinical Needs

The constraints of acquiring all desired imaging modalities for every patient—due to cost, radiation dose, patient comfort, or scanner availability—have driven interest in medical image synthesis. This process involves computationally generating a target imaging modality from available ones, enabling clinicians to access critical information without additional imaging. Medical image synthesis can be of immense benefit in various clinical scenarios, particularly within precision radiation therapy.

Key clinical needs addressed by image synthesis in this context include:

- Enabling MR-Only Radiotherapy Workflows: A prominent application is the generation of synthetic CT (sCT) images from MRI data. This allows for dose calculation directly using MRI as the primary imaging modality, thereby eliminating the need for a separate CT scan.

DOI: 10.1201/9781003480365-2

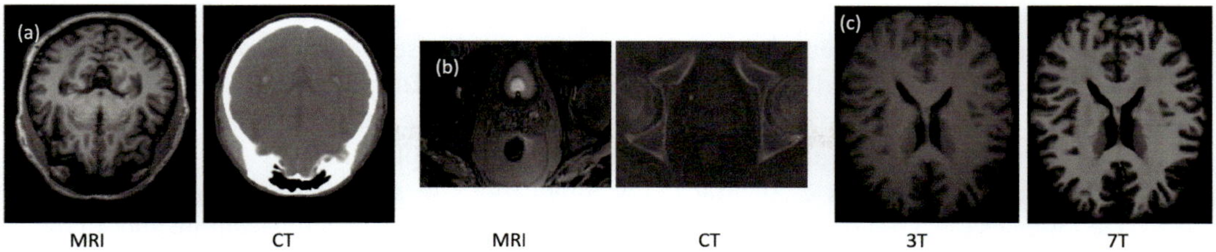

FIGURE 1.1 Examples of medical image synthesis tasks. (a) Corresponding MRI (left) and CT (right) brain images. (b) Corresponding MRI (left) and CT (right) pelvic images. (c) Corresponding 3T MRI (left) and 7T MRI (right) brain images. These pairs illustrate the significant appearance differences that synthesis methods aim to bridge.

This not only streamlines the clinical workflow and reduces patient burden but also mitigates geometric uncertainties arising from imperfect CT–MRI registration, as shown in Figure 1.1a and b.

- Improved Visualization and Target Delineation: Synthesis can generate images that enhance the visibility of specific anatomical structures or implanted fiducial markers, which are crucial for accurate target localization and image-guided radiation therapy (IGRT). For example, synthesizing 7T-like MRI quality from more commonly available 3T MRI scans can provide finer anatomical details for planning, or synthesizing T2-weighted MRI from T1-weighted MRI can aid in brain tumor assessment, as shown in Figure 1.1c.
- Data Augmentation for Artificial Intelligence (AI) Model Training: The performance of deep learning models in medical imaging heavily relies on large, diverse datasets. Synthetic images can be used to augment existing datasets, particularly for rare conditions or underrepresented patient populations, thereby improving the robustness and generalization of AI tools for tasks like segmentation or outcome prediction.
- Facilitating Advanced Treatment Techniques: Synthesized images can aid in deformable image registration for adaptive radiotherapy (ART) by bridging the appearance gap between different modalities or imaging time points.
- Privacy-Preserving Data Sharing and Collaboration: Synthetic medical images hold the potential to facilitate the sharing of realistic medical data for research, education, and AI development without exposing sensitive patient information, thereby addressing critical privacy concerns.
- Predictive Imaging and Education: Emerging applications include predicting disease progression or future anatomical changes from baseline images and creating diverse datasets for educational purposes.

Essentially, medical image synthesis strives to provide clinically valuable imaging information that might otherwise be infeasible to acquire, without imposing additional costs, radiation risks, or logistical burdens on the patient and health care system.

1.1.3 Challenges in Medical Image Synthesis

Medical image synthesis is a complex task with several inherent challenges:

- Complex Inter-Modality Mappings: The relationship between the image intensities and tissue characteristics across different modalities is often highly complex, nonlinear, and ill-posed. For instance, the visual appearance of tissues in an MRI scan can be vastly different from their appearance in a CT scan due to the distinct physical principles underlying each imaging technique.

- Synthesizing Pathological Regions: A significant hurdle is the accurate synthesis of abnormal or pathological tissues, such as tumors or lesions. These regions often exhibit heterogeneous appearances and contrast characteristics that differ substantially from healthy tissues, making them particularly hard to model and synthesize accurately. Yet, these are often the most critical regions for diagnosis and treatment planning.
- Geometric and Dosimetric Accuracy: For applications in radiation therapy, the synthesized images must not only be visually realistic but also geometrically accurate and, in the case of sCT, possess reliable Hounsfield unit (HU) values for accurate dose calculation. Any inaccuracies can have direct consequences on the planned treatment delivery.
- Feature Engineering in Traditional Methods: Conventional machine learning approaches often necessitated the manual design of features to capture inter-modality relationships, a labor-intensive and potentially suboptimal process.
- Model Generalization and Robustness: Synthesized image quality can vary depending on the anatomical region, the specific imaging protocols of the source data, and interpatient variability. Ensuring that synthesis models generalize well across different scanners, sites, and patient populations remains a challenge.
- Evaluation of Synthetic Images: Quantifying the "realism" and clinical utility of synthetic images is difficult. While pixel-wise metrics exist, they may not always correlate with perceptual quality or clinical acceptability.
- Diversity and Mode Collapse: Some generative models, particularly earlier generative adversarial network (GAN) architectures, can suffer from issues like mode collapse, where the model produces a limited variety of samples, failing to capture the full spectrum of the target data distribution.

1.1.4 Overview of AI-Based Synthesis Techniques

The advent of AI, particularly deep learning, has revolutionized the field of medical image synthesis by providing powerful tools to address many of the aforementioned challenges. Unlike traditional machine learning methods that rely on predefined feature extraction, deep learning models can automatically learn hierarchical feature representations directly from the data in an end-to-end manner.

- Convolutional Neural Networks (CNNs): CNNs have become the workhorse for many image analysis tasks, including synthesis. Architectures like fully convolutional networks (FCNs) and U-Net are particularly well suited for image-to-image translation tasks, capable of producing structured outputs while preserving spatial information. These networks learn intricate nonlinear mappings by combining feature representation learning with the mapping process itself.
- Generative Adversarial Networks (GANs): GANs have emerged as a powerful paradigm for generating highly realistic images. They employ a unique training strategy involving two competing networks: a generator that creates synthetic images and a discriminator that tries to distinguish synthetic images from real ones. This adversarial process often leads to perceptually superior results compared to models trained solely with pixel-wise loss functions.
- Diffusion Probabilistic Models: More recently, diffusion models have demonstrated state-of-the-art performance in image generation, often surpassing GANs in terms of image quality and sample diversity. These models learn to reverse a carefully designed noising process, gradually transforming random noise into coherent, high-fidelity images. Their application to 3D medical image synthesis is a rapidly advancing area of research.

These AI-driven approaches, with their ability to model highly complex relationships and generate realistic outputs, form the core of modern medical image synthesis research and are the central focus of this chapter.

1.2 FUNDAMENTALS OF DEEP LEARNING FOR IMAGE SYNTHESIS

Deep learning, a subfield of machine learning, has become the predominant approach for tackling complex tasks in medical image analysis, including image synthesis. These models, characterized by their multilayered architectures, can automatically learn hierarchical representations of data, enabling them to model highly nonlinear relationships between input and output images. This section provides an overview of the fundamental deep learning concepts and architectures that form the bedrock of modern AI-driven medical image synthesis.

1.2.1 Basic Neural Network Concepts

At its core, a neural network is composed of interconnected processing units called neurons (or nodes), organized in layers. Each neuron receives inputs, performs a weighted sum of these inputs (a dot product), adds a bias, and then typically applies a nonlinear activation function to produce an output. The weights and biases are parameters that the network learns during the training process. Convolution (which will be introduced in later sections) and self-attention are widely used operation units.

Activation functions are crucial components, as they introduce nonlinearity into the network, allowing it to learn complex patterns that go beyond simple linear transformations. Without nonlinearity, a deep stack of layers would behave like a single linear layer. Common activation functions include sigmoid, hyperbolic tangent (tanh), rectified linear unit (ReLU), and their variants like leaky ReLU, parametric ReLU (PReLU), and exponential linear unit (ELU). ReLU, in particular, has gained popularity in deep CNNs because it can alleviate the vanishing gradient problem and accelerate training compared to sigmoid or tanh functions (Figure 1.2).

$$\text{sigmoid}(x) = 1/(1+e-x) \tag{1.1}$$

$$\text{ReLU}(x) = \max(0, x) \tag{1.2}$$

$$\tanh(x) = \frac{2}{1+e^{-2x}} - 1 \tag{1.3}$$

$$\text{LeakyReLU}(x) = \begin{cases} \alpha x, & x < 0 \\ x, & x \geq 0 \end{cases} \tag{1.4}$$

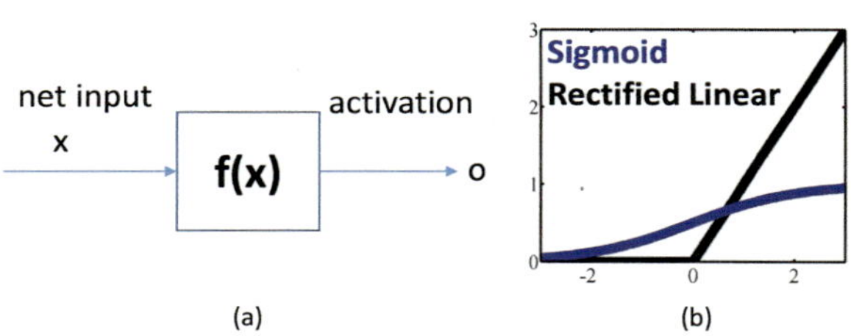

FIGURE 1.2 (a) Activation function in neural networks and (b) typical activation functions.

$$\mathrm{RPeLU}(x)=\begin{cases}\theta x, & x<0\\ x, & x\geq 0\end{cases} \tag{1.5}$$

$$\mathrm{eLU}(x)=\begin{cases}\alpha\left(e^{x}-1\right), & x<0\\ x, & x\geq 0\end{cases} \tag{1.6}$$

1.2.2 Convolutional Neural Networks (CNNs)

CNNs are a specialized class of deep learning models that have demonstrated exceptional performance on visual data, making them highly suitable for medical image processing. They are designed to automatically and adaptively learn spatial hierarchies of features from input images. Key characteristics and operations in CNNs include:

- Convolutional Layers: These layers apply trainable filters (also known as kernels) to the input image (or feature maps from previous layers). Each filter is convolved across the spatial dimensions of the input, computing dot products between the filter entries and the input at each position. This operation allows the network to learn to detect various features like edges, textures, and more complex patterns. In the context of medical image synthesis, the 3D convolution operation is particularly important for volumetric data, as defined in Equation 1.7:

$$a_{ij}(x,y,z)=f\left(\sum_{c=1}^{C}\sum_{p=0}^{P_i-1}\sum_{q=0}^{Q_i-1}\sum_{r=0}^{R_i-1}W_{ijc}(p,q,r)\,a_{(i-1)c}(x-p-\delta_p,y-q-\delta_q,z-r-\delta_r\right) \tag{1.7}$$

where x, y, z denotes the 3D voxel position, W is a 3D filter, and a is a 3D feature map from the previous $(i-1)$th layer.

- Local Receptive Fields: Neurons in a convolutional layer are connected only to a local region of the input, known as the receptive field. This property allows the network to learn local patterns efficiently.
- Parameter Sharing: The same filter (set of weights) is used across all spatial locations in the input feature map. This significantly reduces the number of parameters in the model compared to fully connected networks, making CNNs more efficient to train and less prone to overfitting.
- Pooling Layers: These layers are often inserted periodically between successive convolutional layers to progressively reduce the spatial dimensions (downsample) of the feature maps. Common pooling operations include max pooling and average pooling. Pooling helps to reduce the number of parameters and computational cost, and also provides a degree of translation invariance, contributing to overfitting control, as in Equation 1.8:

$$x_j^l=f\left(\beta_j^l\,\mathrm{down}\left(x_i^{l-1}\right)+b_j^l\right) \tag{1.8}$$

where $down(\cdot)$ denotes a subsampling function. The most commonly used pooling methods are max pooling and average pooling.

- Batch Normalization (BN): Often used after convolutional layers and before activation functions, BN normalizes the output of the previous layer by re-centering and rescaling. This helps to stabilize and accelerate the training process, reduce internal covariate shift, and can act as a regularizer.
- Hierarchical Feature Learning: CNNs learn a hierarchy of features; early layers learn low-level features (e.g., edges, corners), and deeper layers build upon these to detect more complex, high-level features or abstract concepts.

2D vs. 3D CNNs in Medical Imaging: While most early CNNs were designed for 2D natural images, medical imaging modalities like MRI, CT, and PET predominantly generate 3D volumetric data. Applying 2D CNNs slice by slice to such data can lead to a loss of inter-slice contextual information and may suffer from discontinuity problems across slices. 3D CNNs inherently address this by using 3D convolution operations and 3D pooling. A 3D convolution applies a 3D filter to a volume, preserving the spatial neighborhood of the 3D image. This allows 3D CNNs to better model the 3D spatial information crucial for accurate analysis and synthesis of volumetric medical images. CNNs can be adapted for various tasks, such as classification and regression, by changing the architecture of the final layers and the choice of loss function. In a typical classification/regression setup, a CNN might take an image (or an image patch) as input and output a single value representing a class label or a regressed value. However, for image synthesis, a structured output with spatial dimensions (i.e., an image) is required.

1.2.3 Key Architectures for Image-to-Image Tasks

For image synthesis, where the goal is to transform an input image into an output image, specialized CNN architectures [1,2] that can produce dense, structured predictions are necessary.

1.2.3.1 Fully Convolutional Networks (FCNs)

Conventional CNNs often use fully connected layers toward the end of the network to produce a final output, such as a class score. However, these fully connected layers discard spatial information and produce a nonspatial output (e.g., a single vector). FCNs overcome this limitation by exclusively using convolutional layers (and pooling/upsampling layers), enabling them to take an input of arbitrary size and produce an output map of corresponding spatial dimensions.

In medical image synthesis, FCNs are used to estimate target images, typically in a patch-by-patch manner. An input source image patch is fed into the FCN, which then generates a corresponding target image patch. This approach offers several advantages over predicting each voxel independently with a separate CNN:

- Preservation of Neighborhood Information: FCNs can preserve neighborhood information within each predicted patch, leading to more coherent and spatially consistent outputs.
- Prediction Efficiency: Predicting an entire patch in a single forward pass through the network is significantly more efficient than voxel-wise prediction.

A typical FCN architecture for image synthesis, as illustrated in Figure 1.3, consists of a stack of layers that may include (dilated) convolutions, BN, and activation functions (like ReLU). To preserve spatial resolution, which is crucial for image synthesis, pooling layers are often avoided or used sparingly. To compensate for the limited receptive field that results from not using pooling, techniques like using larger filter sizes or dilated convolutions are employed. Dilated convolutions "inflate" the kernel by inserting holes, effectively increasing the receptive field without increasing the number of parameters or computational cost, allowing the network to capture more contextual information.

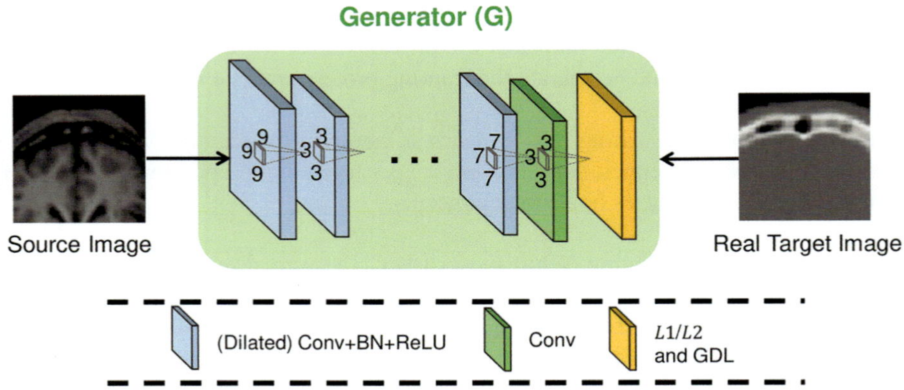

FIGURE 1.3 The 3D FCN architecture for estimating a target image from a source image.

1.2.3.2 U-Net Architecture

While avoiding pooling layers in FCNs helps maintain spatial resolution, pooling is an efficient way to increase the receptive field and reduce computational load. The U-Net architecture, originally proposed for biomedical image segmentation, elegantly addresses this trade-off and has become highly popular for various medical image synthesis tasks. The U-Net has a characteristic "U-shaped" encoder–decoder structure:

- Contracting Path (Encoder): This part follows a typical CNN structure, consisting of repeated blocks of convolutional layers followed by max pooling operations. The encoder progressively downsamples the input, capturing contextual information and learning increasingly abstract feature representations at lower spatial resolutions.
- Expanding Path (Decoder): This part symmetrically mirrors the encoder. It consists of upsampling layers (e.g., transposed convolutions) that increase the resolution of the feature maps, followed by convolutional layers.
- Skip Connections: The key innovation of U-Net is the introduction of long-range skip connections that concatenate feature maps from the encoder path with the corresponding, spatially aligned feature maps in the decoder path. These connections allow the decoder to directly access high-resolution features from the encoder, which helps in recovering fine-grained details and precise localization that might have been lost during the downsampling operations in the encoder. This mechanism effectively combines semantic information (from deeper layers) with spatial information (from shallower layers).

A typical 3D U-Net architecture used for medical image synthesis is shown in Figure 1.4. The network usually produces an output image of the same size as the input. Due to its ability to effectively learn complex mappings while preserving spatial details, U-Net and its many variants are frequently employed as generator networks in more advanced synthesis frameworks like GANs. These foundational architectures, FCNs and U-Nets provide the structural basis for many of the AI-driven image synthesis techniques discussed in the subsequent sections of this chapter.

Their adaptability to 3D medical data and their capacity for dense prediction make them indispensable tools in the pursuit of generating high-fidelity synthetic medical images.

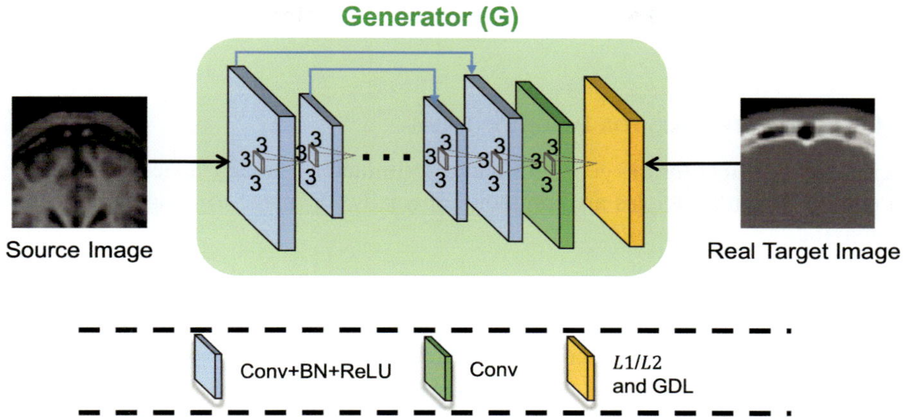

FIGURE 1.4 The 3D U-Net architecture for estimating a target image from a source image.

1.3 GENERATIVE ADVERSARIAL NETWORKS FOR MEDICAL IMAGE SYNTHESIS

GANs, first introduced by Goodfellow et al. [3,4], represent a significant paradigm shift in generative modeling and have achieved remarkable success in synthesizing realistic images. Their unique adversarial training process allows them to learn complex data distributions and generate high-fidelity outputs, making them a popular choice for medical image synthesis tasks where realism and preservation of fine details are crucial.

1.3.1 Principles of Adversarial Learning

The core idea behind GANs is an adversarial process involving two neural networks: a Generator (G) and a Discriminator (D), which are trained simultaneously in a competitive manner.

- The Generator (G): The generator's role is to learn the underlying distribution of the real data and produce synthetic (fake) data samples that are indistinguishable from real samples. In the context of image synthesis, G typically takes a source image (or random noise in some GAN variants) as input and outputs a synthetic target image.
- The Discriminator (D): The discriminator acts as a binary classifier. Its task is to evaluate an input image and determine whether it is a real image from the true data distribution or a synthetic image produced by the generator.

The Adversarial Game: The training process can be conceptualized as a zero-sum game. The generator G strives to produce increasingly realistic images to "fool" the discriminator D into classifying them as real. Concurrently, the discriminator D learns to become better at distinguishing real images from the synthetic ones created by G. This dynamic competition drives both networks to improve over time. Ideally, at convergence, the generator produces samples that are so realistic that the discriminator can no longer differentiate them from real images (i.e., D's accuracy is around 50% for a binary classification).

Training Process: The training of G and D is typically performed in an alternating fashion. In each training iteration:

- The discriminator D is updated by training it on a mini-batch of real target images (labeled as "real") and a mini-batch of synthetic images generated by G (labeled as "fake").
- The generator G is then updated. Its objective is to produce images that the discriminator D misclassifies as "real." During this phase, the discriminator's weights are typically kept fixed.

This iterative process allows G to progressively learn the complex patterns and distributions of the target medical images.

1.3.2 GAN Architectures for Image Synthesis

The specific architectures for the generator and discriminator can vary depending on the application, but certain design principles are common, especially for image-to-image translation tasks in medical imaging.

1.3.2.1 Generator (G) Architectures

The generator network is responsible for transforming an input (e.g., a source modality image) into a synthetic target modality image. Due to the requirement of producing spatially structured outputs (images), generator architectures in medical image synthesis often leverage designs from semantic segmentation or image reconstruction:

- Fully Convolutional Networks (FCNs): As discussed in Section 1.2.3.1, FCNs are well suited for dense prediction tasks. In GANs for medical image synthesis, a 3D FCN is often adopted as the generator. A typical 3D FCN generator (as shown in Figure 1.3) consists of a series of convolutional layers, often combined with BN and ReLU activation functions. To preserve spatial resolution, which is critical in image synthesis, pooling layers are frequently avoided within the generator.
- U-Net Architecture: The U-Net architecture (Section 1.2.3.2) is also a popular choice for generators in medical image GANs. Its encoder–decoder structure with skip connections is effective in capturing both contextual information and fine-grained details, leading to high-quality synthetic images.

1.3.2.2 Discriminator (D) Architectures

The discriminator's role is to classify an input image as either real or synthetic. It is typically implemented as a standard CNN designed for binary classification.

A common discriminator architecture includes several stages of convolutional layers, BN, ReLU activations, and max pooling layers to extract features and reduce dimensionality, followed by one or more fully connected layers that culminate in a single output node with a sigmoid activation function. This sigmoid output represents the probability that the input image is real.

1.3.3 Essential Loss Functions for High-Fidelity Synthesis

The success of GAN training hinges on appropriately defined loss functions for both the generator and the discriminator. These often combine adversarial losses with content-matching (reconstruction) losses.

1.3.3.1 Adversarial Loss

The adversarial loss quantifies how well the generator and discriminator are performing in their competitive game.

- Discriminator's Adversarial Loss (L_D): The discriminator aims to maximize its ability to correctly classify real images as real (e.g., label 1) and synthetic images as fake (e.g., label 0). A common choice is the binary cross-entropy (BCE) loss:

$$L_D(X,Y) = L_{\text{BCE}}\big(D(Y),1\big) + L_{\text{BCE}}\Big(D\big(G(X)\big),0\Big) \tag{1.9}$$

  where X is the source input, Y is the real target, $G(X)$ is the generated image, and $D(.)$ is the discriminator's output probability.

- Generator's Adversarial Loss (L_{ADV}). The generator aims to produce images (X) that the discriminator classifies as real (label 1). Its adversarial loss is often formulated as

$$L_{ADV}(X) = L_{BCE}\left(D\left(G(X)\right),1\right) \tag{1.10}$$

- Wasserstein GAN with Gradient Penalty (WGAN-GP) Loss: For improved training stability and to mitigate issues like mode collapse, WGAN-GP loss is sometimes used, particularly for global discriminators. The discriminator (critic) loss is

$$L_{D1}(X,Y) = E_x\left[D1\left(G(X)\right)\right] - E_Y\left[D1(Y)\right] + \lambda E_{\hat{X}}\left[\left(\left\|\nabla_{\hat{X}} D1\left(\hat{X}\right)\right\|_2 - 1\right)^2\right] \tag{1.11}$$

1.3.3.2 Reconstruction Loss (Content Loss)

While the adversarial loss encourages realism, it does not explicitly ensure that the generated image $G(X)$ is a meaningful and accurate transformation of the source image X corresponding to the ground-truth target Y. To enforce content similarity, a reconstruction loss is added to the generator's objective function.

This is typically an L_1 or L_2 norm between the generated image and the real target image (Equation 1.12):

$$L_G(X,Y) = \left\|Y - G(X)\right\|_p^p \tag{1.12}$$

where Y is the ground-truth target image, $G(X)$ is the generated target image from the source image X by the Generator network G, and $p=1$ for $L1$ loss and $p=2$ for $L2$ loss. $L1$ is often preferred as it tends to produce less blurry images and is more robust to outliers compared to L_2 loss. L_2 loss, while sometimes leading to blurrier results, can offer faster convergence and more stable reconstruction in some cases.

1.3.3.3 Image Gradient Difference Loss (GDL)

To specifically address the issue of blurriness in generated images, particularly when $L2$ reconstruction loss is used, an image gradient difference loss (GDL) can be incorporated. GDL aims to preserve the sharpness of edges by minimizing the difference in the magnitudes of image gradients between the ground-truth target image$Y$and the synthetic image $L_{GDL}\left(\hat{Y}\right)$. A common formulation is

$$L_{GDL}\left(Y,\hat{Y}\right) = \left\|\left|\nabla Y_x\right| - \left|\nabla \hat{Y}_x\right|\right\|^2 + \left\|\left|\nabla Y_y\right| - \left|\nabla \hat{Y}_y\right|\right\|^2 + \left\|\left|\nabla Y_z\right| - \left|\nabla \hat{Y}_z\right|\right\|^2 \tag{1.13}$$

This encourages the synthetic image to maintain regions with strong gradients, effectively compensating for the smoothing tendencies of other loss terms.

1.3.3.4 Total Generator Loss

The final loss function for training the generator is usually a weighted sum of the adversarial loss, the reconstruction loss, and potentially other regularization terms like GDL. For example,

$$L_{G\_total}(X,Y) = \lambda_1 L_{ADV}(X) + \lambda_2 L_G(X,Y) + \lambda_3 L_{GDL}\left(Y, G(X)\right) \tag{1.14}$$

where the hyperparameters λ_1, λ_2, and λ_3 balance the contribution of each term.

1.3.4 Advanced GAN Techniques for Enhanced Performance

Several advanced techniques have been developed to improve the stability, quality, and applicability of GANs in medical image synthesis.

1.3.4.1 Dilated Convolutions in Generators

When pooling layers are avoided in the generator to preserve spatial resolution, the effective receptive field of the convolutional filters can become limited. Dilated convolutions (also known as atrous convolutions) address this by "inflating" the filter kernel with zeros between its elements. This expands the receptive field, allowing the network to capture broader contextual information without increasing the number of parameters or computational cost, and without downsampling the feature maps.

1.3.4.2 Residual Learning in Generators

Inspired by the success of residual networks (ResNets) in training very deep architectures, residual learning principles can be applied to GAN generators:

- Long-Term Residual Units: Instead of learning a direct mapping from source X to target Y, the generator can be formulated to learn a residual mapping, $(X) = Y - X$.

  The final output is then $G(X) = X + R_{\text{learned}}(X)$. This is particularly useful when the source and target images are highly correlated (e.g., in 3T-to-7T MRI synthesis or image denoising). The network essentially learns the difference, which can be an easier task if the difference is sparse or small. Figure 1.5 illustrates such a long-term residual connection where the source image is added to the network's output.

1.3.4.3 Auto-Context Model (ACM) for Refinement

The auto-context model (ACM) is an iterative refinement strategy that can enhance the output of GANs by incorporating broader contextual information. In this approach,

1. A first GAN is trained to produce an initial synthetic target image.
2. Subsequent GANs are trained iteratively, where the input to each new GAN includes not only the original source image patch but also the synthetic target patch generated by the GAN from the previous iteration. These are often concatenated as multiple input channels. This iterative process allows the network to progressively refine the synthesis, leveraging the context from the entire previously estimated target image, thereby overcoming limitations imposed by the restricted receptive field of a single patch-based prediction. Figure 1.6 shows this scheme.

1.3.4.4 Dual-Discriminator Architectures

To provide more comprehensive adversarial feedback, some approaches employ multiple discriminators:

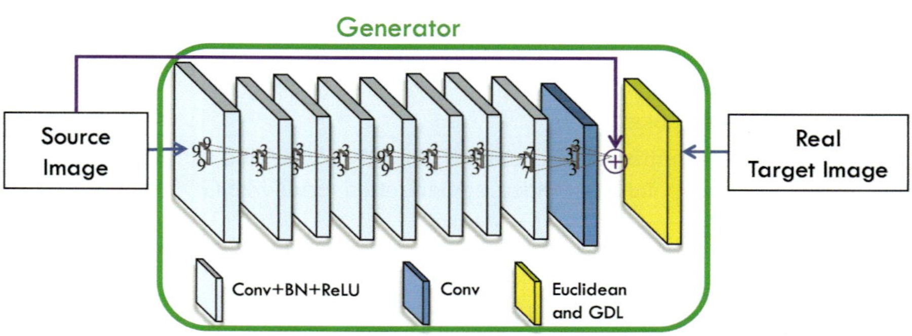

FIGURE 1.5 Generator architecture used in the GAN setting for estimation of synthetic target image. Note the solid-purple-line arrow from source image to the "plus" sign, which expresses the long-term residual connection.

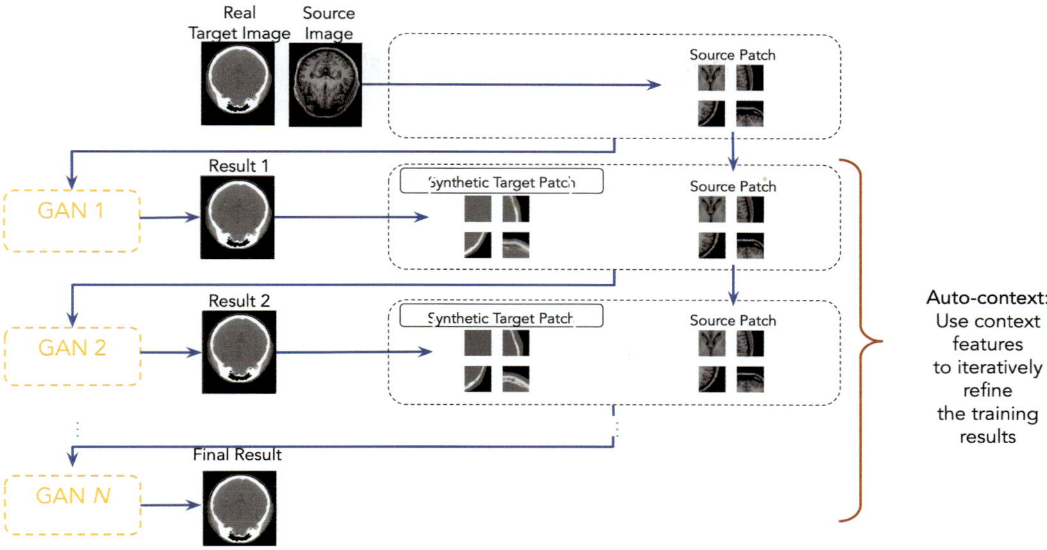

FIGURE 1.6 Illustration of ACM refinement with GAN.

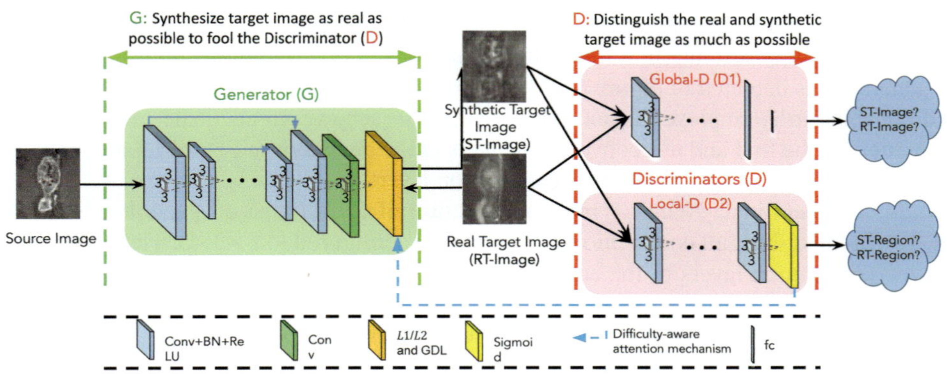

FIGURE 1.7 Architecture used in the deep supervised generative adversarial setting to synthesize target image. This framework contains one generator and two discriminators. A difficult-region aware attention mechanism is also included in the framework.

1. Global Discriminator (D1): This is typically a standard CNN that assesses the overall realism of the entire generated image. It provides a holistic judgment on whether the synthetic image looks plausible as a whole. WGAN-GP loss is often used for D1 for better training stability.
2. Local Discriminator (D2): This is often an FCN-based discriminator designed to evaluate the realism of local regions or patches within the image, producing a dense output map. Each element in this map can indicate the quality or "realness" of a specific part of the synthetic image. The output can be used to derive a confidence map. Using dual discriminators can help alleviate issues like adversarial gradient vanishing and ensures that the generator is scrutinized at both global and local levels. This architecture is depicted in Figure 1.7.

1.3.4.5 Difficult-Region-Aware Attention Mechanisms

Medical images often contain small but clinically critical regions (e.g., tumors, lesions) that are hard to synthesize accurately because they might be underrepresented or have complex appearances.

Difficult-region-aware attention mechanisms [5] aim to address this. These mechanisms typically leverage the output from a local discriminator (D2), which can identify poorly synthesized regions (low confidence). This information is then used to modulate the generator's training loss, for instance, by up-weighting the loss contribution from these difficult regions.

A common approach is to apply voxel-level attention weights F to the reconstruction loss:

$$L_{\text{AttG}}(X,Y) = F \odot \| Y - G(X) \|^{p} \tag{1.15}$$

where $\odot$ is the element-wise multiplication and $F = (1 - M)^{\beta}$, and β is the voxel-level attention parameter. Note, F here works as a scaling factor, which is used to largely suppress the contribution of easy-to-synthesize regions to the training loss and emphasize the hard-to-synthesize regions.

1.3.4.6 Details of Layer in the Generator

Details of Layers in FCN: A typical architecture of an FCN-based generator network G is illustrated in Figure 1.3, where the numbers denote the filter sizes. This network processes a source image as input and attempts to generate the corresponding target image. Specifically, it comprises nine layers that include convolution, BN, and ReLU operations. The kernel sizes for these layers are 9^3, 3^3, 3^3, 3^3, 9^3, 3^3, 3^3, 7^3, and 3^3, respectively. The number of filters for each layer is 32, 32, 32, 64, 64, 64, 32, 32, and 1, respectively. The final layer contains a single convolutional filter, and its output is regarded as the estimated target image. Notably, pooling operations are omitted in this architecture to preserve the spatial resolution of the feature maps. Given that traditional convolution operations in the generator, as depicted in Figure 1.3, may not ensure a sufficiently effective receptive field [6], dilated convolution is employed as an alternative [7] to achieve an adequate receptive field. The dilation rates for the first and last convolution layers of the generator in Figure 1.3 are set to 1, while a dilation rate of 2 is applied to all other convolution layers.

Details of Layers in U-Net: A typical architecture of a U-Net-based generator is depicted in Figure 1.4. In the U-Net, all convolution filter sizes are configured to $3 \times 3 \times 3$. The number of channels in the convolution layers of the encoder is set to 32, 64, 64, 128, 128, 256, and 512, with the decoder convolution layers symmetrically configured. It is important to note that the number of channels in the final layer is 1. The encoder phase includes three pooling layers, while the decoder phase incorporates three strided convolutions. For each convolution layer, except the last one, a combination of Conv+BN+ReLU is utilized as the basic neuron, whereas only Conv is used for the final layer.

1.4 DIFFUSION MODELS FOR MEDICAL IMAGE SYNTHESIS

In recent years, diffusion probabilistic models [8–10] have emerged as a powerful class of generative models, demonstrating remarkable success in synthesizing high-fidelity and diverse images, often outperforming established techniques like GANs. Initially popularized in the nonmedical domain by models generating realistic images from text (e.g., DALL-E2 [11], Imagen [12], Stable Diffusion [8,9]), their application to the complexities of 3D medical image generation is an active and promising area of research.

The application of diffusion models, especially latent diffusion models (LDMs), to 3D medical image synthesis has shown promising results [10]:

- High-Quality 3D Data Generation: Studies have successfully demonstrated the generation of realistic 3D volumes for various modalities and anatomical regions, including brain MRI (e.g., ADNI dataset), chest CT (e.g., LIDC-IDRI dataset), breast MRI (e.g., DUKE dataset), and knee MRI (e.g., MRNet dataset).

- Adaptability to Various Resolutions: These models have shown the ability to handle different image resolutions inherent in medical datasets, such as 64×64×64 for brain MRI, 128×128×128 for chest CT, and anisotropic resolutions like 256×256×32 for breast and knee MRI.
- Perceptual Realism: A crucial aspect is the realism of generated images to medical experts. Synthetic images generated by diffusion models have been rated favorably by radiologists in terms of "realistic image appearance," "anatomical correctness," and "consistency between slices." This qualitative validation by domain experts is vital, as standard quantitative metrics may not fully capture clinical acceptability.
- Downstream Task Enhancement: Synthetic data generated by diffusion models can be valuable for improving the performance of other AI models, particularly in low data regimes common in medical imaging. For example, pretraining a segmentation model (like Swin UNETR) in a self-supervised fashion using synthetic breast MR images has been shown to substantially improve breast segmentation performance when only limited labeled data from a target institution is available for fine-tuning. This highlights the potential for using synthetic data to bridge data scarcity gaps and improve model generalization across different institutions or datasets.
- The robust training, ability to generate diverse and high-quality 3D medical data, and potential for enhancing downstream applications make diffusion models a highly promising avenue for future advancements in medical image synthesis, particularly within the demanding context of precision radiation therapy.

1.5 AI IN TREATMENT PREPARATION: ADVANCED IMAGING AND AUTOMATED CONTOURING

The initial stages of radiotherapy planning are foundational for successful treatment, involving precise medical imaging and the accurate delineation of target volumes and critical normal tissues. AI is making substantial contributions to these preparatory phases by enhancing imaging capabilities and automating the traditionally laborious contouring process. This section will delve into AI-driven techniques for advanced image acquisition and synthesis, such as the generation of sCT data from MRI to support MR-only workflows and improve visualization. Furthermore, it will explore intelligent automated contouring methods, including the use of sophisticated CNN architectures for segmenting tumors and OARs, and innovative approaches to address and learn from the inherent uncertainties in medical image segmentation, thereby improving the robustness and reliability of treatment planning inputs.

1.5.1 AI-Enhanced Image Acquisition and Synthesis

MRI offers superior soft-tissue contrast compared to CT, making it invaluable for delineating tumors and OARs in radiation therapy, especially in anatomical sites like the brain and abdomen [13]. For treatments such as prostate SBRT, the enhanced visualization of structures like the urethra on MRI is critical. Despite these advantages, conventional radiotherapy workflows necessitate CT scans for their electron density information, which is essential for accurate dose calculation. While registering MR images to planning CTs is standard practice, this step can introduce geometric uncertainties of 2–3 mm and requires patients to undergo additional imaging procedures [13].

To address these limitations, the concept of an MR-only radiotherapy workflow has gained considerable interest. This approach aims to streamline the treatment process, reduce the imaging burden on patients, and minimize errors associated with multimodal image registration. A pivotal technology enabling MR-only workflows is the generation of sCT images directly from the acquired MR data. AI, particularly deep learning methodologies, has shown significant promise in this domain by learning the complex, nonlinear mapping from MR image intensities to CT HU.

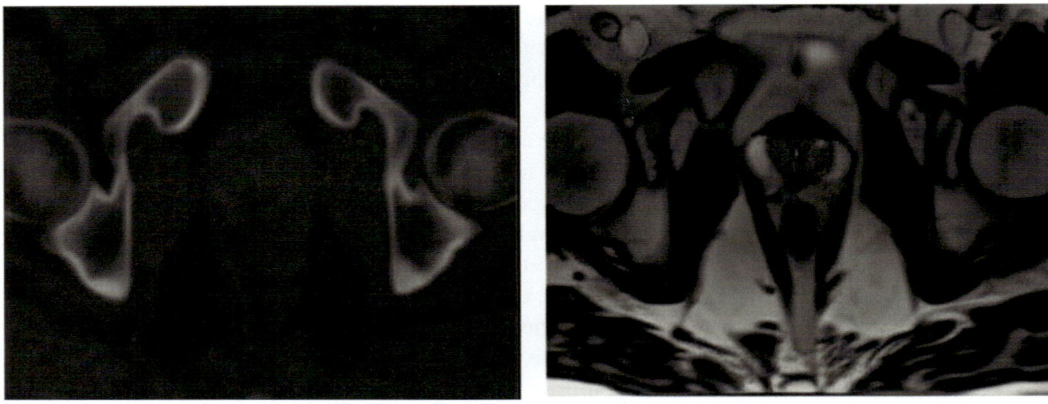

(a) CT (b) Generated MRI

FIGURE 1.8 A side-by-side comparison of a planning CT showing a fiducial and a preprocessed MR image simulating fiducial enhancement.

A notable application of AI in this area is the work by Szalkowski et al. [13], who developed a machine learning model to create sCTs from pelvic MR images for prostate cancer treatments. Their approach utilized a deep convolutional adversarial network, a type of GAN, which was previously demonstrated by their group to produce CTs with accuracy comparable to or exceeding that of methods like atlas-based registration. A key focus of their 2021 study was to ensure that these sCTs, and subsequently the synthetic digitally reconstructed radiographs (sDRRs) generated from them, could accurately visualize implanted fiducial markers. This is crucial for image-guided robotic radiosurgery systems, such as the CyberKnife, which rely on fiducial tracking for precise treatment delivery. As a proof of concept, since fiducial-enhancing MR sequences were not routinely acquired, Szalkowski et al. [13] preprocessed existing clinical T2 MR images to mimic the appearance of fiducial-enhancing MRIs (fe-MRI), as depicted in Figure 1.8.

The AI model structure employed by Szalkowski et al. [13] comprised a 3D FCN as the generator to synthesize the CT images from MR patches, and a CNN as the discriminator. The discriminator's role is to differentiate between the generated sCT patches and real CT patches, thereby guiding the generator to produce more realistic sCTs. This network architecture is illustrated in Figure 1.9. The training of such models involves careful selection of parameters; for instance, Szalkowski et al. [13] found a patch size of 128 × 128 pixels and a training set of nine patient image pairs to be optimal for their pelvic MR-to-CT synthesis task.

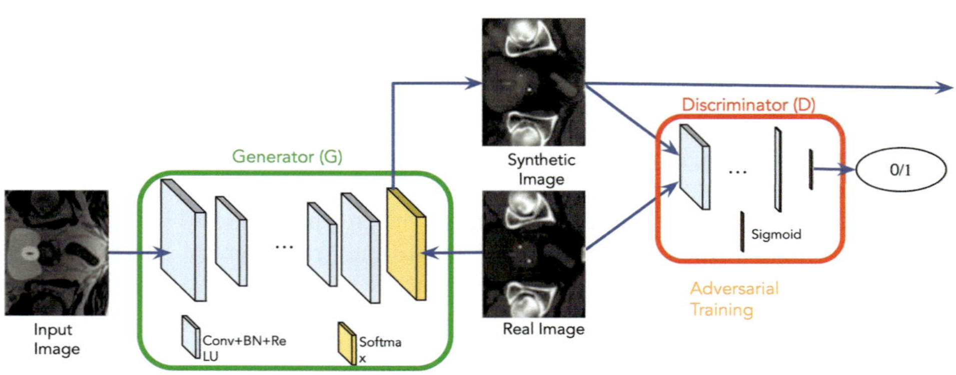

FIGURE 1.9 A diagram illustrating the generative adversarial network architecture, showing the generator and discriminator components.

FIGURE 1.10 Comparative images of DRRs generated from real CTs versus synthetic CTs, showing fiducial markers.

The performance of this AI-driven synthesis was rigorously evaluated. The sCTs generated for prostate cases demonstrated a mean absolute error (MAE) of 72.9±88.1 HU and a mean peak signal-to-noise ratio (PSNR) of 31.23±2.16dB relative to the ground-truth CT images. More importantly for image guidance, the sDRRs created from these sCTs also showed high fidelity, with a mean MSE of 0.66±0.42 and a mean PSNR of 22.88±3.74dB when compared to digitally reconstructed radiographs (DRRs) from actual CTs. Figure 1.10 illustrates the visual similarity between real and synthetic DRRs, highlighting fiducial visibility.

Crucially, the study confirmed that the visualization and localization of fiducial markers were not compromised. Human observer studies found no statistically significant difference in the number of fiducials identified or their centroid locations between the real and synthetic images, with mean localization differences of 0.5±0.4mm for CTs and 1.4±0.96mm for DRRs [13]. Furthermore, the dosimetric accuracy of the sCTs was validated, with 3D gamma analysis of treatment plans calculated on sCTs showing a 97.7±0.7 agreement (3%/2mm criteria) with plans on real CTs. This indicates that the sCTs are suitable for accurate dose calculations.

In conclusion, AI-powered image synthesis, particularly the generation of sCT and sDRR from MRI, is a promising avenue for enhancing image acquisition strategies in radiotherapy. These techniques facilitate MR-only workflows, offering the potential to improve treatment accuracy by leveraging MRI's superior soft-tissue contrast while providing the necessary data for dose calculation and image guidance, including critical fiducial visualization for systems like robotic radiosurgery [13]. This reduces the reliance on multimodal registration and can lead to a more efficient and patient-friendly radiotherapy process.

1.5.2 Intelligent Contouring of PTVs and OARs

Accurate delineation of the planning target volume (PTV) and surrounding OARs is a cornerstone of precision radiation therapy. Manual contouring, however, is a time-consuming, labor-intensive process prone to inter- and intra-observer variability [14]. AI, particularly deep learning, has emerged as a powerful tool to automate and standardize this critical step.

CNNs, with architectures like U-Net [2] and its numerous variants, have become the de facto standard for medical image segmentation tasks, including those in radiotherapy [14]. These networks learn hierarchical features from images to perform pixel-wise or voxel-wise classification, thereby identifying the boundaries of anatomical structures.

A significant challenge in medical image segmentation is the inherent uncertainty, which can arise from ambiguous boundaries, image noise, or variations in anatomy. Traditional deep learning models output a probability map, and a fixed threshold is often used to derive the final segmentation. However, as Tang et al. [14] point out, the confidence of the network in this probability map is often unclear, and segmentation results can be unreliable even with high probabilities if the underlying uncertainty is also high. This is particularly problematic for defining precise boundaries, which is crucial in radiotherapy. Figure 1.11 illustrates how uncertain regions, often found at the target boundaries, can be visualized.

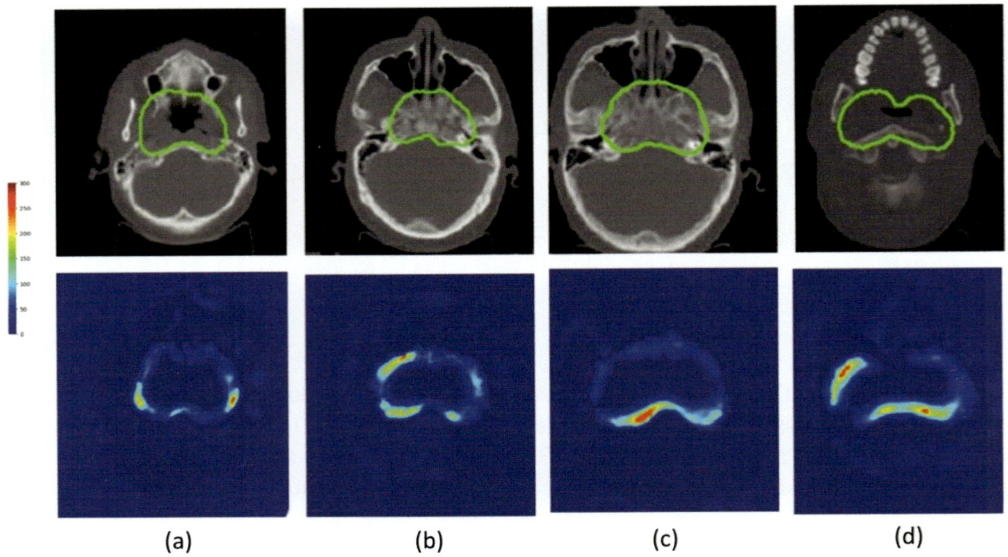

FIGURE 1.11 Examples of uncertainty maps in medical image segmentation, showing higher uncertainty (e.g., deeper color) at the boundaries of structures.

To address this, Tang et al. [14] proposed the uncertainty guided network (UG-Net), an end-to-end framework designed to learn from and contend with segmentation uncertainty. UG-Net consists of a coarse segmentation module (CSM) that generates an initial segmentation and an associated uncertainty map (e.g., using Monte Carlo dropout sampling). This uncertainty map is then fed into an uncertainty guided module (UGM) to extract discriminative features from unreliable regions. A feature refinement module (FRM), embedded with dual attention (DAT) blocks, subsequently refines the features from the CSM's decoder, incorporating the uncertainty-related features to produce a final, more robust segmentation. The overall architecture of UG-Net is depicted in Figure 1.12. This approach allows the network to actively learn to handle difficult cases rather than simply thresholding or ignoring uncertain predictions.

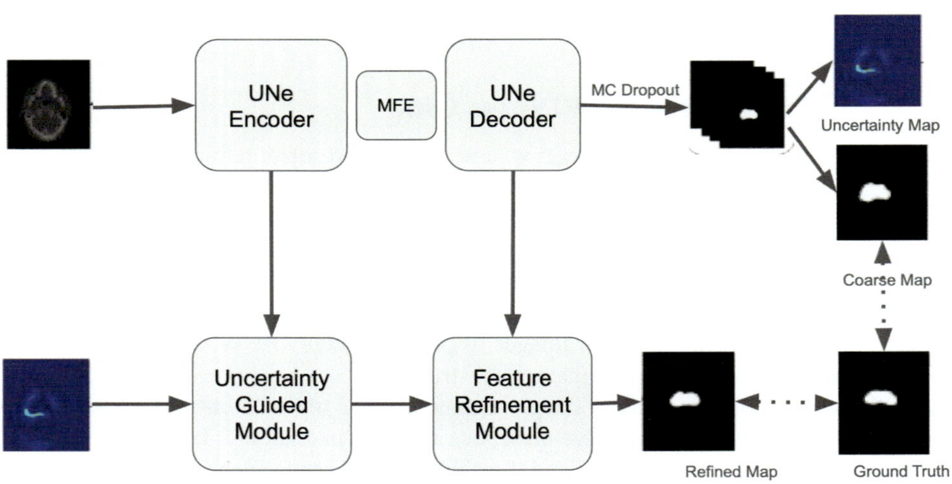

FIGURE 1.12 A schematic diagram of the UG-Net architecture, highlighting the coarse segmentation module (CSM) with MC dropout sampling, the uncertainty guided module (UGM), and the feature refinement module (FRM).

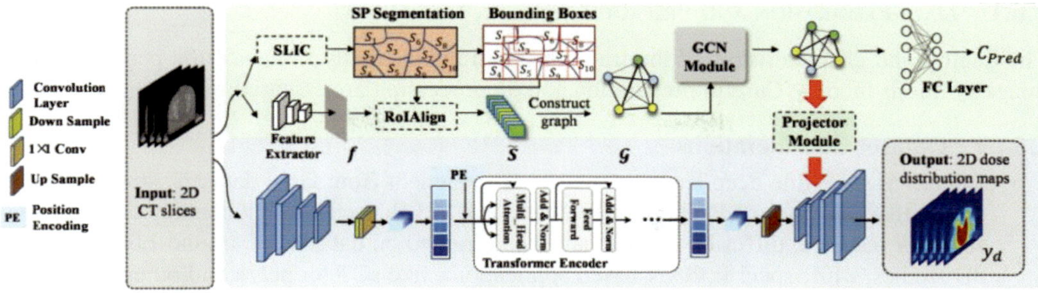

FIGURE 1.13 An illustration of a GCN-based auxiliary branch for extracting anatomical information via super-pixel classification, as part of a larger dose prediction network.

The importance of precise boundary information is paramount. CNN architectures often employ pooling layers or strided convolutions that can lead to the loss of fine spatial details, potentially blurring segmentation boundaries [14]. To counteract this, techniques like skip connections (as in U-Net) are used to combine low-level detail with high-level semantic information. Furthermore, modules like the multi-scale feature extractor (MFE) in UG-Net [14] help capture context at various resolutions, which can be beneficial for objects of different sizes and for refining boundaries. The FRM in UG-Net also plays a role in highlighting valuable features related to the segmentation task and suppressing irrelevant information, which is crucial for accurate boundary definition.

Beyond dedicated segmentation models, AI-driven segmentation capabilities are also being integrated as auxiliary components within larger radiotherapy planning frameworks. For instance, Li et al. [15] proposed a multitask attention adversarial network (MtAANET) for 3D radiotherapy dose distribution prediction that uses only CT images as input. Their framework includes an auxiliary segmentation task for PTV and OARs, implemented with a shared encoder and a dedicated segmentation decoder. The anatomical information derived from this auxiliary segmentation task is then fused with features for the primary dose prediction task, demonstrating that segmentation can provide essential anatomical context even when explicit masks are not the final output.

Similarly, Jiao et al. [16], in their TransDose model for dose prediction from CT images, utilize a super-pixel-based graph convolutional network (GCN) classification as an auxiliary branch. This branch excavates category-specific anatomical features by classifying super-pixels into PTV, OARs, or background. While not producing fine-grained segmentation masks in the traditional sense, this super-pixel classification provides crucial anatomical knowledge to the main dose prediction network, compensating for the absence of explicit input segmentation masks, as shown in Figure 1.13. This highlights a trend where AI models internally derive or utilize segmentation-like anatomical understanding to inform complex downstream tasks in the radiotherapy workflow.

In summary, AI, predominantly through CNN-based architectures, is revolutionizing the delineation of tumors and OARs. Advanced methods not only automate the process but also explicitly address challenges like segmentation uncertainty and boundary precision. Moreover, the anatomical insights gleaned from AI-driven segmentation prove valuable as integral components in more comprehensive AI systems for tasks such as automated dose prediction, even when explicit segmentation masks are not the primary input to these systems.

1.6 TRAINING AND EVALUATION OF IMAGE SYNTHESIS MODELS

The development of robust and clinically relevant AI-based image synthesis models relies not only on sophisticated architectures but also on meticulous data preparation, effective training strategies, and comprehensive evaluation methodologies. This section details these critical aspects, drawing from practices reported in the literature.

1.6.1 Data Preparation and Preprocessing

The quality and characteristics of the training data fundamentally influence the performance of image synthesis models. Careful preparation and preprocessing are essential steps.

1.6.1.1 Dataset Considerations

- Dataset Size: While deep learning models often benefit from large datasets, studies have shown that effective medical image synthesis can be achieved with moderately sized datasets. For instance, diffusion models have been trained on datasets of around 1,000–1,844 3D studies, while specific GAN-based applications, like sCT for pelvic radiotherapy, have utilized smaller, highly curated datasets of as few as 11 subjects for development and testing, with training sets sometimes as small as 9 patient image pairs. The required dataset size often depends on the complexity of the synthesis task and the diversity of the patient population.
- Paired vs. Unpaired Data: Many supervised synthesis methods, particularly those aiming for direct source-to-target modality translation (e.g., MRI to CT), require accurately co-registered paired image datasets. Unpaired image synthesis (e.g., using CycleGAN-like architectures) is also an area of research but may present additional challenges in ensuring anatomical and content fidelity for clinical applications.
- Data Source and Diversity: Using multi-institutional data can improve model generalization, though it may also introduce variability due to different scanners and protocols.

1.6.1.2 Common Preprocessing Steps

Standard preprocessing steps are crucial for normalizing data and preparing it for model training:

- Image Registration: For paired training, accurate spatial alignment between source and target images is paramount. This typically involves (1) rigid registration (e.g., using tools like FLIRT) to correct for global differences in patient positioning and (2) deformable or nonrigid registration (e.g. using ANTs–SyN or Diffeomorphic Demons) to account for local anatomical variations and ensure voxel-wise correspondence.
- Intensity Normalization: Image intensities are scaled to a consistent range to aid model convergence. Common methods include min–max normalization (e.g., to a range of –1 to 1) or *Z*-score normalization (subtracting the mean and dividing by the standard deviation across the training data).
- Resampling and Resizing: Images are often resampled to a uniform voxel spacing (e.g., $1 \times 1 \times 1\,\text{mm}^3$) and resized to consistent matrix dimensions suitable for the network architecture.
- Cropping: Regions of interest may be cropped to reduce computational load or focus the model on relevant anatomy.
- Anatomical Standardization: For specific applications like brain imaging, skull stripping or removal of non-brain areas is a common step.
- Data Augmentation: To increase the effective size of the training set and improve model robustness, data augmentation techniques like random flipping (e.g., vertical flipping) or affine transformations may be applied during training.
- Application-Specific Processing: In some cases, further processing is needed. For example, in a study aiming to synthesize CTs with visible fiducials from MRI, clinical T2 MRIs were processed to simulate the appearance of fiducial-enhancing sequences as a proof of principle. Images may also be padded to meet specific input size requirements of clinical software like treatment planning systems.

1.6.2 Training Strategies

Effective training involves careful selection of methods, optimizers, and parameters.

1.6.2.1 Input Strategy: Patch-Based vs. Full Image

1. Patch-Based Training: This approach involves dividing the input images into smaller 2D or 3D patches, which are then fed into the network. The synthesized patches are subsequently stitched back together to form the complete output image, often by averaging intensities in overlapping regions. This method is memory-efficient, allowing for the use of deeper networks or higher resolution processing on limited hardware. The size of the patch is an important hyperparameter; for instance, a patch size of 128×128 pixels was found to provide a good balance of fiducial contrast and overall image quality in one sCT synthesis study.
2. Full Image Training: Alternatively, entire images (or volumes) can be processed at once, which is common for FCNs, U-Nets, and diffusion models, provided that sufficient GPU memory is available. This approach can better preserve global context but may be computationally more demanding.

1.6.2.2 Model-Specific Training Procedures

- GANs: Training GANs involves an alternating optimization procedure where the generator and discriminator are updated iteratively. The balance between generator and discriminator updates, and the weighting of different loss components (e.g., adversarial, reconstruction, GDL), are crucial for stable training.
- Diffusion Models: These are typically trained by optimizing the U-Net to predict the noise added during the forward diffusion process over many time steps. LDMs involve a two-stage approach: first, training an autoencoder (e.g., VQ-GAN), and then training the diffusion model in the learned latent space.
- Iterative Refinement: Techniques like the ACM involve training multiple models (e.g., GANs) sequentially, where the output of one model provides additional contextual input to the next, leading to iterative refinement of the synthesis.

1.6.3 Quantitative Evaluation Metrics

Objective, quantitative metrics are essential for comparing different synthesis methods and optimizing model parameters.

In medical image synthesis tasks, MAE, PSNR, and structural similarity (SSIM) index [17] are commonly used evaluation metrics for quantitatively assessing performance. Let I be the ground-truth image with dimensions $m \times n$, and U be the synthesized image:

$$\text{MAE} = \frac{1}{mn} \sum_{i=0}^{m-1} \sum_{j=0}^{n-1} \left| I(i,j) - U(i,j) \right| \tag{1.16}$$

$$\text{PSNR} = 10 \cdot \log_{10} \left(\frac{\text{MAX}_I^2}{\text{MSE}} \right) \tag{1.17}$$

where MAX_I represents the maximum possible pixel value of the image, and MSE denotes the mean squared error:

$$\text{MSE} = \frac{1}{mn} \sum_{i=0}^{m-1} \sum_{j=0}^{n-1} \left[I(i,j) - U(i,j) \right]^2 \tag{1.18}$$

$$\mathrm{SSIM}(x,y)=\frac{\left(2\mu_x u_y+C_1\right)\left(2\sigma_{xy}+C_2\right)}{\left(\mu_x^2+\mu_y^2+C_1\right)\left(\sigma_x^2+\sigma_y^2+C_2\right)} \tag{1.19}$$

where μ_x and μ_y are the means of images x and y, respectively. σ_x and σ_y are the variances of x and y, respectively, while σ_{xy} is the covariance between x and y. C_1 and C_2 are constants used to stabilize the division when the denominator is weak, with $C_1=(k_1L)^2$ and $C_2=(k_2L)^2$, where L is the dynamic range of the pixel values (typically 2^n-1, where n is the number of bits per pixel), $k1=0.01$, and $k2=0.03$. Note that Equation 1.19 yields a local SSIM map, and an additional averaging step is required to obtain a global SSIM (scalar).

While quantitative metrics provide objective measures, they may not fully capture the perceptual quality or clinical utility of synthetic images. Therefore, qualitative and task-based evaluations are indispensable.

1.7 FUTURE DIRECTIONS

AI-driven medical image synthesis has made substantial strides, yet the field is continuously evolving, with numerous exciting avenues for future research and development. These advancements promise to further enhance the capabilities and clinical impact of synthetic imaging, particularly in precision radiation therapy.

1.7.1 Enhanced Model Architectures and Hybrid Approaches

The quest for higher fidelity, diversity, and stability in image synthesis will continue to drive innovation in model architectures. Future work will likely focus on developing more sophisticated neural networks. A promising direction is the exploration of hybrid models that synergistically combine the strengths of different generative paradigms. For instance, integrating the sharp image generation capabilities of GANs with the stable training and high sample diversity of diffusion models could lead to superior synthesis outcomes. Transformer-based architectures, which have shown success in other vision tasks, may also find broader application in medical image synthesis.

1.7.2 Advanced Conditional and Controllable Synthesis

Current synthesis often focuses on translating one modality to another. The future will likely see a shift toward more controllable and conditional synthesis. This includes generating images conditioned not just on another image but also on a richer set of inputs such as detailed clinical parameters, genomic data, textual reports (a capability already demonstrated by some diffusion models in other domains), or user-defined sketches and annotations. Furthermore, enhancing the ability to predict future anatomical changes or image appearances, such as disease progression, remains a key area of interest.

1.7.3 Improving Data Handling and Computational Efficiency

The processing of large, high-resolution 3D medical images remains computationally demanding. Future research will need to address methods for reducing the computational burden associated with training complex models and processing extensive datasets. This includes algorithmic optimizations, leveraging more powerful hardware, and developing techniques to effectively train with and process larger image volumes to capture complete patient anatomy for applications like comprehensive treatment planning. Scaling models to higher image resolutions, reflective of state-of-the-art clinical acquisitions, is also an important goal.

1.7.4 Federated Learning and Privacy Preservation

To address challenges related to data privacy and limited dataset sizes at individual institutions, federated learning presents a promising approach. This would allow models to be trained on decentralized datasets from multiple institutions without the need to share raw patient data, thereby fostering collaboration and enabling the development of more generalizable synthesis models.

1.8 CONCLUSION

This chapter has navigated the rapidly evolving landscape of AI-driven medical image synthesis, elucidating its fundamental principles, core techniques, and significant applications, particularly within the domain of precision radiation therapy. We have explored how foundational deep learning architectures like CNNs, FCNs, and U-Nets have paved the way for sophisticated image-to-image translation tasks. Building upon these, advanced generative frameworks, most notably GANs and denoising diffusion probabilistic models (DDPMs), have demonstrated remarkable capabilities in producing high-fidelity, realistic synthetic medical images. For GANs, we detailed the adversarial training process, common architectural choices for generators and discriminators, the critical role of combined loss functions (including reconstruction and GDLs), and innovative enhancements such as residual learning, ACMs, dual-discriminator systems, and attention mechanisms designed to tackle challenging synthesis scenarios like pathological regions. Similarly, for diffusion models, we outlined the elegant noising and denoising paradigm, the adaptation of U-Net architectures for 3D data, and the advent of LDMs that offer computational efficiency by operating in a compressed latent space.

In conclusion, AI-driven medical image synthesis represents a transformative technology with the potential to significantly enhance various facets of precision radiation therapy. By enabling the generation of desired imaging information that might otherwise be unavailable, these techniques are helping to optimize treatment planning, improve therapeutic accuracy, and ultimately, contribute to better patient outcomes. Continued research, interdisciplinary collaboration, and careful clinical translation will be key to realizing the full potential of these powerful tools in the ongoing evolution of cancer care.

REFERENCES

1. D. Nie, X. Cao, Y. Gao, L. Wang, D. Shen, Estimating CT image from MRI data using 3D fully convolutional networks, in: *1st International Workshop on Large-Scale Annotation of Biomedical Data and Expert Label Synthesis, LABELS 2016 and 2nd International Workshop on Deep Learning in Medical Image Analysis*, DLMIA 2016 held in conjunction with 19th International Conference on Medical Image Computing and Computer Assisted Intervention, MICCAI 2016 - Athens, Greece, Springer, 2016, pp. 170–178.
2. O. Ronneberger, P. Fischer, T. Brox, U-net: Convolutional networks for biomedical image segmentation, in: *International Conference on Medical Image Computing and Computer-Assisted Intervention*, Springer, 18th International Conference, Munich, Germany, October 5-9, 2015, pp. 234–241.
3. I. Goodfellow, J. Pouget-Abadie, M. Mirza, B. Xu, D. Warde-Farley, S. Ozair, A. Courville, Y. Bengio, Generative adversarial nets, in: Z. Ghahramani and M. Welling and C. Cortes and N. Lawrence and K.Q. Weinberger (eds), *Advances in Neural Information Processing Systems*, Curran Associates, Inc., 2014, pp. 2672–2680. https://proceedings.neurips.cc/paper_files/paper/2014/file/f033ed80deb0234979a61f95710dbe25-Paper.pdf}
4. D. Nie, R. Trullo, J. Lian, C. Petitjean, S. Ruan, Q. Wang, D. Shen, Medical image synthesis with context-aware generative adversarial networks, in: *20th International Conference on Medical Image Computing and Computer-Assisted Intervention, MICCAI 2017,* Quebec City, Canada, Springer, 2017, pp. 417–425.
5. Q. Xiao, D. Nie, Fine-grained medical image synthesis with dual-attention adversarial learning, in: *Annual Conference on Medical Image Understanding and Analysis*, Medical Image Understanding and Analysis, 28th Annual Conference, MIUA 2024, Manchester, UK, Springer, July 24–26, 2024, pp. 298–306.

6. W. Luo, Y. Li, R. Urtasun, R. Zemel, Understanding the effective receptive field in deep convolutional neural networks, in: D. Lee and M. Sugiyama and U. Luxburg and I. Guyon and R. Garnett (eds), *Advances in Neural Information Processing Systems*, Curran Associates, Inc., 2016, pp. 4898–4906. https://proceedings.neurips.cc/paper_files/paper/2016/file/c8067ad1937f728f51288b3eb986afaa-Paper.pdf
7. F. Yu, V. Koltun, Multi-scale context aggregation by dilated convolutions, arXiv preprint arXiv:1511.07122.
8. J. Ho, A. Jain, P. Abbeel, Denoising diffusion probabilistic models, in: H. Larochelle and M. Ranzato and R. Hadsell and M.F. Balcan and H. Lin (eds), *Advances in Neural Information Processing Systems*, vol. 33, Curran Associates, Inc., 2020, pp. 6840–6851. https://proceedings.neurips.cc/paper_files/paper/2020/file/4c5bcfec8584af0d967f1ab10179ca4b-Paper.pdf
9. R. Rombach, A. Blattmann, D. Lorenz, P. Esser, B. Ommer, High-resolution image synthesis with latent diffusion models, in: *Proceedings of the IEEE/CVF Conference on Computer Vision and Pattern Recognition*, 2022 IEEE/CVF Conference on Computer Vision and Pattern Recognition (CVPR), New Orleans, LA, USA, 18-24 June 2022. In: 2022 IEEE/CVF Conference on Computer Vision and Pattern Recognition (CVPR), New York: IEEE, 2022, pp. 10684–10695.
10. F. Khader, G. Müller-Franzes, S. TayebiArasteh, T. Han, C. Haarburger, M. SchulzeHagen, P. Schad, S. Engelhardt, B. Baeßler, S. Foersch, et al., Denoising diffusion probabilistic models for 3D medical image generation, *Scientific Reports* 13 (1) (2023) 7303.
11. A. Ramesh, P. Dhariwal, A. Nichol, C. Chu, M. Chen, Hierarchical text-conditional image generation with clip latents, arXiv preprint arXiv:2204.06125 1 (2) (2022) 3.
12. C. Saharia, W. Chan, S. Saxena, L. Li, J. Whang, E. L. Denton, K. Ghasemipour, R. Gontijo Lopes, B. Karagol Ayan, T. Salimans, et al., Photorealistic text-to-image diffusionmodelswithdeeplangua-geunderstanding, in: S. Koyejo and S. Mohamed and A. Agarwal and D. Belgrave and K. Cho and A. Oh (eds), *Advances in Neural Information Processing Systems*, Curran Associates, Inc., vol. 35, 2022, pp. 36479–36494. https://proceedings.neurips.cc/paper_files/paper/2022/file/ec795aeadae0b7d230fa35cbaf04c041-Paper-Conference.pdf
13. G. Szalkowski, D. Nie, T. Zhu, P.-T. Yap, J. Lian, Synthetic digital reconstructed radiographs for MR-only robotic stereotactic radiation therapy: A proof of concept, *Computers in Biology and Medicine* 138 (2021) 104917.
14. P. Tang, P. Yang, D. Nie, X. Wu, J. Zhou, Y. Wang, Unified medical image segmentation by learning from uncertainty in an end-to-end manner, *Knowledge-Based Systems* 241 (2022) 108215.
15. H. Li, X. Peng, J. Zeng, J. Xiao, D. Nie, C. Zu, X. Wu, J. Zhou, Y. Wang, Explainable attention guided adversarial deep network for 3D radiotherapy dose distribution prediction, *Knowledge-Based Systems* 241 (2022) 108324.
16. Z. Jiao, X. Peng, Y. Wang, J. Xiao, D. Nie, X. Wu, X. Wang, J. Zhou, D. Shen, Transdose: Transformer-based radiotherapy dose prediction from CT images guided by super-pixel-level gcn classification, *Medical Image Analysis* 89 (2023) 102902.
17. Z. Wang, A. C. Bovik, H. R. Sheikh, E. P. Simoncelli, Image quality assessment: From error visibility to structural similarity, *IEEE Transactions on Image Processing* 13 (4) (2004) 600–612.

2 Medical Image Segmentation

Jue Jiang

2.1 INTRODUCTION

Precision radiation therapy relies on accurate medical image analysis to identify tumors and critical organs for treatment planning. Traditionally, this process of contouring anatomical structures on computed tomography (CT), magnetic resonance imaging (MRI), or positron emission tomography (PET) scans has been manual, time-consuming, and subject to inter-observer variability. In recent years, artificial intelligence (AI) and deep learning have shown tremendous potential to automate and enhance medical image segmentation, leading to greater consistency and efficiency in radiotherapy workflows. Deep learning models have already surpassed conventional methods in general imaging tasks such as object detection and segmentation, and these advances have quickly translated to medical imaging applications. For example, convolutional neural networks (CNNs) like the U-Net [1] introduced a powerful encoder–decoder architecture that enabled highly accurate segmentation of biomedical images, fueling a wave of research into AI-driven contouring tools. Such methods have been leveraged for tasks ranging from detection of lesions to fully automated delineation of tumors and organs at risk, increasing the degree of automation in radiation treatment planning for various cancers (e.g., pancreatic tumor segmentation on CT scans [2]).

Despite these successes, applying deep learning in the medical domain faces several key challenges. First, training effective models usually requires large amounts of expert annotated data, yet obtaining sufficiently large and well curated labeled datasets in medicine is difficult and labor-intensive. Domain experts (radiologists, radiation oncologists) must carefully segment images, and this is especially burdensome when volumes of 3D scans are involved. Second, medical imaging encompasses a wide variety of modalities and acquisition protocols. Images from different scanners, hospitals, or modalities (CT, MRI, X-ray, etc.) often have substantial differences in appearance and resolution. Models trained on one dataset or modality can suffer a drop in performance when applied to another due to this domain shift. These issues of data scarcity and domain variability motivate the development of advanced techniques that can learn effectively from limited labels and generalize across domains. In this chapter, we present an overview of AI-driven medical image segmentation approaches in the context of precision radiation therapy, with an emphasis on how they address the challenges above. We begin with fully supervised deep learning models that have become the foundation for segmentation tasks (Section 1.2), including the U-shape Net and a number of its high-performing variants. We then describe semi-supervised segmentation methods (Section 1.3) that leverage unlabeled images to improve performance when annotations are sparse; these include pseudo-labeling strategies, consistency regularization techniques, adversarial (GAN-based) approaches, and contrastive learning. Next, we examine unsupervised domain adaptation (UDA) methods (Section 1.4) which enable models trained in a source domain to adapt to a different target domain without target labels. We cover approaches based on image and feature distribution alignment, teacher–student frameworks with pseudo-labeling, and uncertainty-aware alignment to handle unreliably labeled regions. Finally, we explore the emergence of large foundation models for medical image segmentation (Section 1.5). These are models trained on massive datasets (often with self-supervision or weak labels) that aim to provide general segmentation capabilities transferable to many tasks. Throughout the chapter, we highlight how these AI techniques contribute to more precise and automated image analysis in radiotherapy, and we consider remaining challenges and future directions in this rapidly evolving field.

DOI: 10.1201/9781003480365-3

2.2 SUPERVISED SEGMENTATION WITH DEEP NEURAL NETWORKS

Fully supervised deep learning models have achieved state-of-the-art accuracy in medical image segmentation when provided with sufficient annotated training data. In this section, we review several influential neural network architectures for supervised segmentation, which have become widely adopted for delineating tumors and organs in radiotherapy planning. These models typically learn a direct mapping from input medical images to pixel-wise segmentation masks, and they are trained end-to-end using large sets of images with expert-drawn contours as ground truth.

2.2.1 U-Net

The U-Net [1] is a CNN architecture introduced by Ronneberger et al. in 2015 that is specifically designed for biomedical image segmentation. It has a characteristic U-shaped structure that consists of a contracting encoder path for feature extraction and an expansive decoder path for precise localization. This symmetric encoder–decoder design, coupled with skip connections that transfer feature maps from encoder layers to corresponding decoder layers, allows U-Net to capture both high-level semantic information and fine-grained spatial details. In the encoder (downsampling) path, successive convolutional layers and pooling operations reduce the spatial resolution of feature maps while increasing their depth, enabling the network to learn abstract representations of the image content. In the decoder (upsampling) path, transposed convolutions (up-convolutions) progressively restore the spatial resolution. U-Net introduces skip connections that concatenate feature maps from an encoder layer to a decoder layer at the same level. These skip connections provide the decoder with high-resolution contextual features from earlier in the network, helping it recover detailed structures that might otherwise be lost during encoding. Since its introduction, U-Net has become a de facto standard for medical image segmentation and has been widely applied to problems in radiology, pathology, and beyond. It provides a powerful balance between localization accuracy and use of global context, making it well-suited for segmenting anatomical structures in radiotherapy planning (e.g., delineating gross tumor volume and organs at risk on CT scans).

2.2.2 nnU-Net

While models like U-Net require manual expert tuning for each new task, the nnU-Net ("no new U-Net") framework introduced by Isensee et al. [3] represents a paradigm shift by automating the design and configuration of segmentation pipelines. nnU-Net builds upon the U-Net architecture but eliminates the need for task-specific tailoring: it dynamically adapts its architecture, hyperparameters, and preprocessing steps to any new dataset in a standardized way. This automated approach allows nnU-Net to achieve top performance across diverse tasks without manual intervention, effectively becoming a robust baseline for medical image segmentation. At its core, nnU-Net provides three architecture configurations out-of-the-box: a 2D U-Net, a 3D U-Net, and a cascaded 2-stage 3D U-Net. The choice of configuration is determined by the dataset properties (such as image dimensions and spacing). By selecting an appropriate model configuration, nnU-Net balances segmentation accuracy with computational efficiency for each task. Beyond architecture selection, nnU-Net's most innovative aspect is its automated, data-driven hyperparameter optimization and processing. When applied to a new dataset, nnU-Net analyzes the data (intensity distributions, image sizes, class balance, etc.) and then automatically configures crucial settings such as image normalization, resampling resolution, patch size, batch size, learning rate schedule, and even network depth and number of convolutional features.

The result is that nnU-Net often achieves state-of-the-art segmentation performance out-of-the-box on a wide range of benchmarks and challenges, from multi-organ CT segmentation to brain tumor MRI segmentation. Indeed, it won multiple competitions (such as the Medical Segmentation Decathlon and BraTS brain tumor challenge) with minimal or no manual tuning, demonstrating the generality of its approach.

2.2.3 Multi-Resolution Residual Network (MRRN)

Segmenting medical images often requires capturing both fine details and broader contextual information. The multi-resolution residual network (MRRN) [4] was developed as an advanced architecture to address this need by combining multi-scale processing with residual learning. MRRN extends traditional CNNs with parallel pathways at multiple resolutions and weaves in residual connections (skip connections within the network layers) to ease the flow of gradients. This design is particularly advantageous for medical image segmentation, where anatomical structures can vary greatly in size, shape, and location. By simultaneously analyzing images at different scales, MRRN can identify small, subtle structures (e.g., thin anatomical boundaries) while also maintaining awareness of larger contextual features. To be specific, in an MRRN, input images are processed through multiple resolution streams. For instance, one stream operates on the full-resolution image, while another operates on a downsampled version. Each stream has a series of convolutional layers, and crucially, residual blocks are used so that each layer also receives a shortcut connection from earlier layers, alleviating vanishing gradient issues and encouraging feature reuse. The multi-resolution outputs are then fused by concatenation so that the final segmentation prediction is informed by features at all considered scales. The residual connections across layers within each resolution help the network learn complex representations without losing low-level information, as they effectively "add" learned refinements to features rather than completely transforming them.

2.2.4 TransUNet

TransUNet [5] is a hybrid architecture that integrates CNNs with Transformer modules to leverage the strengths of both in medical image segmentation. Proposed by Chen et al. in 2021, TransUNet was among the first to introduce Transformers (which had revolutionized natural language processing and later computer vision) into a U-Net-like segmentation framework. The motivation is to allow the model not only to extract local features via CNNs, but also to capture long-range dependencies and global context through the self-attention mechanism of Transformers. This is particularly useful in biomedical images, where important contextual relationships (e.g., between distant regions of an organ) may not be captured by the localized receptive fields of CNNs alone.

The TransUNet architecture typically consists of a CNN-based encoder followed by a Transformer that serves as a bottleneck layer, and then a CNN-based decoder resembling the U-Net decoder. The encoder first produces a set of feature maps from the input image. These feature maps are then flattened and fed into a Transformer encoder which applies self-attention to model interactions between all patch embeddings of the image. Essentially, each patch of the image (or each spatial location in the feature map) can attend to every other patch, allowing the network to learn global feature dependencies (e.g., the relationship between a tumor and distant anatomical structures). After the Transformer module, the enriched feature representations are reshaped back and passed into the decoder network which uses upsampling and skip connections (from the CNN encoder) to produce the final segmentation.

2.2.5 Swin-UNet

Swin-UNet [6] is another hybrid architecture for medical image segmentation that fuses the U-Net paradigm with the Swin Transformer [7]. The Swin Transformer is a vision Transformer that introduces the concept of shifted windows for efficient self-attention, limiting attention computation to local windows while still allowing cross-window information flow. Swin-UNet uses the Swin Transformer as its encoder and a U-Net-style CNN decoder, effectively combining a purely Transformer-based encoding of the image with a convolutional decoding path for segmentation. In Swin-UNet, the input image is partitioned into nonoverlapping patches which are treated similar to tokens in a Transformer. These patches pass through multiple Swin Transformer layers in the encoder.

Each Swin Transformer layer performs self-attention in localized windows of the image, capturing local patterns, and then shifts the window positions in the next layer so that information is also shared across neighboring windows. This approach greatly reduces the computational cost compared to global attention, yet can approximate global context by stacking layers with window shifts. The encoder produces a multi-scale representation of the image akin to feature maps at different resolutions. The decoder of Swin-UNet typically mirrors the multi-resolution structure, using upsampling and skip connections to recombine the Transformer features into a full-resolution segmentation map. Skip connections can be taken either directly from intermediate stages of the Swin Transformer encoder (projected to appropriate dimensions for the decoder) or from convolutional projections of the encoder features, ensuring that fine detail information is fed into the decoder. The decoder might be composed of convolutional blocks or even inverse Transformer blocks to progressively increase resolution, but in practice convolutional upsampling blocks work well.

2.3 SEMI-SUPERVISED SEGMENTATION

In medical imaging, labeled data can be limited due to the time and expertise required for annotation. Semi-supervised segmentation methods aim to improve model performance by leveraging both labeled and unlabeled data during training. These approaches use the information contained in unlabeled images—often far more abundant than labeled ones—to regularize or augment the learning process, thus compensating for scarce annotations. In the context of radiotherapy, semi-supervised methods are valuable because they can produce accurate segmentations without the need for exhaustively labeling every imaging slice, which is especially useful for delineating tumors or organs in large 3D scans.

Several families of techniques exist for semi-supervised segmentation. We cover four prominent categories here: (1) Pseudo-labeling-based methods, where the model's own predictions on unlabeled data are treated as proxy labels for further training; (2) Consistency regularization methods, which impose that the model's output remain stable under input perturbations or model perturbations; (3) GAN-based methods, which use generative adversarial networks (GANs) to utilize unlabeled data by enforcing that predicted segmentations look realistic; and (4) Contrastive learning methods, which learn robust feature representations from unlabeled images by comparing augmented views of the data. These methods are often complementary and can be combined in practice.

2.3.1 Pseudo-Labeling Approaches

Pseudo-labeling is a straightforward yet powerful semi-supervised technique [8].

The idea is to use a model trained on the labeled data to predict labels for the unlabeled data, and then include those confident predictions as additional "pseudo" ground truth to further train the model. Two common variations of pseudo-labeling in segmentation are self-training (using a single model's predictions) and co-training (using multiple models or multiple views of the data to generate and cross-update pseudo-labels).

2.3.1.1 Self-Training

Self-training starts by training an initial segmentation model on the small labeled dataset. Once this model has reasonably learned the task, it was then applied to the unlabeled images to predict segmentation masks. Rather than trust all predictions, a confidence threshold is applied to only regions of the unlabeled images for which the model is highly confident in its prediction are kept as pseudo-labels. For example, if the model outputs a probability map, one might take only pixels where some class probability exceeds, say, 0.9 as "pseudo-annotated." These confident pseudo-labeled images are then added to the training set (with their newly assigned labels), and the model is retrained or fine-tuned on the combination of original labeled data and pseudo-labeled data [8].

2.3.1.2 Co-Training

Co-training goes one step further by involving two or more models (or one model applied to two different "views" of the data) that teach each other. In a co-training setup [9], one could train two segmentation models on the labeled data, perhaps with different architectures or initialized differently. Each model then generates pseudo-labels for the unlabeled set. However, instead of each model just training on its own pseudo-labels, the models exchange information: model A is retrained using the pseudo-labeled outputs provided by model B, and vice versa. Since the two models may make different errors, this cross-training can correct some mistakes—each model benefits from the other's "second opinion." Co-training implicitly assumes that the two models (or views) are at least somewhat independent in their errors, so that one model's confident predictions are reliable for the other.

In medical images field, one can implement the idea of "multiple views" by, for example, providing different input channels or augmentation to two models. For instance, in a multimodal case (CT and MRI available for the same anatomy), one model could focus on CT and the other on MRI; each one labels unlabeled cases and helps train the other with its modality's perspective. Even if only one modality is present, one could use different data augmentations or patches vs. whole images as two views. The general outcome is that co-training can result in more robust learning from unlabeled data than self-training, as it mitigates some risk of reinforcing a single model's blind spots.

2.3.2 Consistency Regularization Approaches

Another major class of semi-supervised techniques is consistency regularization, which rests on the principle that a good model should produce stable, consistent outputs even when its inputs (or its internal parameters) undergo small permutation changes in the context of noise. In the context of segmentation, consistency regularization enforces that the segmentation result for an unlabeled image remains the same under various transformations or perturbations. This idea is grounded in the smoothness assumption: data points (in our case, medical images) that are close to each other in the input space are likely to have the same label. By making the model's predictions insensitive to minor perturbations, we effectively encourage the decision boundary to lie in regions of low data density, which is desirable for generalization [10]. We summarize the commonly used consistency regularization from three perspectives: enforcing consistency with respect to (1) input data perturbations, (2) model perturbations, and (3) task perturbations.

Many semi-supervised segmentation methods incorporate one or more of these consistency types.

2.3.2.1 Data Consistency

Data consistency means that if we apply augmentations or noise to an input image, the segmentation output should remain unchanged (after undoing the transformation on the output if needed). For example, if we take an unlabeled MRI and slightly rotate it or adjust its brightness, a well-trained model's segmentation of a tumor in that MRI should still segment the same region. In practice, to implement data consistency, we can feed an unlabeled image I through the model to get a prediction, then feed a transformed version T(I) through the model to get another prediction. We then constrain these two predictions to be the same once we account for the known effect of T (for instance, if T was a rotation, we would inverse-rotate one of the predictions before comparing). A consistency loss (often L2 or a cross-entropy between the two outputs) is added to the training objective, penalizing differences. Common perturbations T include random geometric transformations (flip, rotation, scale), elastic deformations, adding Gaussian noise, or even using different patch crops of a larger image. By training with this loss on unlabeled data, the model learns more invariant and smoother mappings.

2.3.2.2 Model Consistency

Model consistency (sometimes called temporal consistency or self-ensembling) involves perturbing the model itself and requiring consistent predictions. One approach is to maintain two versions of the model: a student and a teacher. The teacher could be an exponential moving average (EMA) of the student's weights (as in the "Mean Teacher" model). At each training step, the student learns to match the teacher's predictions for unlabeled inputs [11]. Because the teacher's parameters change slowly (averaging the student over time) or because we add noise/dropout to the student, the teacher–student discrepancy acts as a model perturbation. The student is penalized if its output deviates from the teacher's output on the same image.

2.3.2.3 Task Consistency

Task consistency refers to consistency across different but related prediction tasks. In a multitask learning scenario, one can train an auxiliary task on unlabeled data and ensure that the primary segmentation task is consistent with it. For instance, one might train a model to perform both segmentation and another task like edge detection, or reconstruction of the input image, or classification of a property, using the unlabeled data. Consistency between tasks might mean that the segmentation output, when processed appropriately, aligns with the output of the auxiliary task. A concrete example is ensuring that if a model segments an organ and also predicts a bounding box for that organ as an auxiliary task, the segmentation mask's bounding box matches the predicted bounding box.

2.3.3 GAN-Based Methods

GANs [12] have also been employed to tackles semi-supervised segmentation by taking advantage of unlabeled data in a unique way. In a typical GAN, a generator creates synthetic data and a discriminator (or critic) tries to distinguish between real and generated data. For semi-supervised learning, one can use a variant where the discriminator is trained not only to differentiate real vs. fake, but also to classify real data into the correct classes. In segmentation, this idea can be applied by having a discriminator network that looks at the predicted segmentation masks (or some combination of image and mask) and judges whether they look like plausible segmentations.

In a semi-supervised setting, GANs can utilize unlabeled images by feeding them to the segmentation network and then into the discriminator. Even though no ground truth mask exists for these images, the discriminator will treat the segmentation output as a "fake" it should critique, unless the segmentation happens to look like ones from the labeled set. The segmentation network is trained to fool the discriminator on these unlabeled cases, effectively learning from the discriminator's feedback what constitutes a plausible segmentation shape or structure. For example, the discriminator might learn the typical shape of a liver in CT from the labeled examples; when an unlabeled CT is given, if the segmentation network's output liver mask has an odd shape or unrealistic boundary, the discriminator will likely flag it as fake, and the segmentation network will adjust to make it more realistic. One of the earliest examples of using GANs for semi-supervised segmentation is Souly et al. [13], which used adversarial training to improve segmentation of images with few labels. In medical imaging, adversarial losses have been used to enforce that segmented structures look like real anatomies, adding a sort of shape prior learned implicitly from data. This is especially useful in radiotherapy segmentation where one might want to ensure, say, that a segmented organ contour is anatomically plausible even if the model is uncertain (unlabeled data can help in that regard by enforcing the anatomy prior through the GAN).

2.3.4 Contrastive Learning for Segmentation

Contrastive learning has emerged as a powerful form of self-supervised learning, and it has been adapted to semi-supervised segmentation to learn robust visual representations from unlabeled images [14]. The core idea of contrastive learning is to encourage representations of similar data points (e.g., two different augmentations of the same image) to be close in feature space, and representations of dissimilar points (e.g., different images) to be far apart. By doing soon a large amount of unlabeled data, the model can learn informative features that make downstream tasks (like segmentation) easier to train with few labels.

In segmentation, there are typically two levels at which contrastive learning can be applied: the image level and the region/patch level.

Image-Level Contrastive Learning: In image-level contrastive learning, each entire image is treated as an instance for contrast. For example, given an unlabeled medical image, one can create two different augmented versions of it (through random rotations, scaling, intensity jitter, etc.). These two augmented images are fed through the encoder network (which could be the encoder part of a U-Net, for instance) to produce two feature vectors (perhaps by global average pooling the encoder's feature map). The model is then trained to maximize the agreement (e.g., via cosine similarity) between these two feature vectors, while simultaneously pushing them apart from feature vectors of other images in the batch [15]. This way, the encoder learns to extract features that are invariant to the chosen augmentations but distinctive for each image. Over many images, the encoder's feature space becomes organized such that images with similar content end up closer together.

Patch-Level Contrastive Learning: Patch-level (or region-level) contrastive learning goes one step finer. Instead of treating a whole image as one entity, this approach divides images into patches or regions and learns representations for these smaller parts [16]. For instance, one might take an image and sample a pair of patches from it that overlap significantly (so they depict mostly the same content).

These two patches, after augmentation, are fed through the network to produce feature vectors (maybe using a patch-based encoder or a spatial pooling around the patch region in a feature map). The objective is to make the features of these two patches similar, while differentiating them from patches sampled from different parts of the image or from different images. Patch-level contrastive learning forces the model to pay attention to local details and ensures that corresponding regions of an image (e.g., two different crops that both contain the same tumor) map to a similar representation. This is particularly beneficial for medical segmentation because the task is inherently local deciding the label of a pixel involves looking at its local neighborhood. By using patch-level contrast, the model learns a feature space where local regions are distinguished by their anatomical or pathological content. For example, patches that contain tumor tissue might end up clustered in feature space distinct from patches of normal tissue, even without labels saying "tumor" or "normal." When a small number of labeled examples are introduced, the model can quickly learn the mapping from these learned features to actual segmentation labels.

In radiotherapy, where one might have many unsegmented scans and only a handful with painstaking contours, contrastive learning can allow those unsegmented scans to contribute to the model training. Ultimately, contrastive methods and adversarial or consistency methods are not mutually exclusive some of the best semi-supervised frameworks might integrate contrastive learning for representation learning with consistency training or pseudo-labeling for directly improving the segmentation outputs, exploiting unlabeled data in complementary ways.

2.4 UNSUPERVISED DOMAIN ADAPTATION FOR SEGMENTATION

Supervised deep learning models often assume that training (source) data and test (target) data come from the same distribution. In medical imaging, this assumption frequently breaks down: a model trained on CT scans from one hospital might underperform on CT scans from a different hospital due to differences in scanners or protocols; likewise, a model trained on one modality (say CT) cannot directly segment another modality (like MRI) because of the domain gap. UDA aims to adapt a model trained on a labeled source domain to perform well on an unlabeled target domain. In the context of segmentation, UDA methods allow us to leverage existing annotated datasets (which might be in a different imaging modality or acquired with different settings) to segment new kinds of images for which we have little or no annotations.

The goal of UDA for segmentation is to minimize the reduction in accuracy that occurs when applying a model to a target domain with different characteristics. This is achieved by finding domain-invariant features or by otherwise aligning the source and target data distributions so that the segmentation network generalizes across them [15,17]. A variety of approaches exist, which we can group into three broad categories: (1) Image-level and feature-level alignment methods, which attempt to make the source domain images or features look like those from the target domain (or vice versa); (2) Teacher–student self-training methods, which involve generating pseudo-labels on target data and refining them (many of these were discussed in the semi-supervised context but are equally applicable for domain adaptation by treating target domain as unlabeled); and (3) Uncertainty-aware and other advanced domain adaptation techniques, which explicitly model the uncertainty or structure of domain shifts to better transfer knowledge.

In recent years, numerous UDA methods have been proposed in the medical imaging community, given the prevalence of cross-institutional and cross-modality problems. Below, we outline some key approaches within these categories.

2.4.1 Image and Feature Alignment-Based Methods

A common strategy for domain adaptation is to directly align either the input images or the learned feature representations between source and target domains. If successful, this makes the domain of origin irrelevant to the segmentation network—that is, the network sees inputs or features that are "normalized" across domains.

Image Alignment via Style Transfer: Image alignment techniques operate in the pixel space: The idea is to transform images from one domain to resemble those of another. This is often done using GAN-based style transfer. For example, one could train a CycleGAN to translate CT scans into MRI-like scans (if adapting from CT to MRI) without needing paired images [18]. By creating such "pseudo-target" images from the source labeled images, one can then apply the segmentation model on images that look as if they came from the target domain. The model can be trained either on these transformed source images with known labels, or one can transform target images into source style and then apply a source-trained model. In practice, if one has labeled CT and wants to adapt to unlabeled MRI, a CycleGAN can yield synthetic MRI (with CT structures) and synthetic CT (from real MRI). The segmentation model can then be trained on synthetic MRI with labels (the labels from the original CT). This reduces appearance differences: the segmentation network doesn't have to account for CT vs MRI contrast, since it only sees one style. Still, image alignment is a powerful tool, effectively augmenting or converting data across domains so that a standard segmentation pipeline can be applied.

Feature Alignment via Distribution Matching: Feature alignment focuses on the latent representation (feature space) of the network. The objective here is to train the segmentation model such that the feature distributions of source and target domains are made similar. One influential approach is using an adversarial loss at the feature level [19]. For instance, one can attach a domain discriminator network to the output of the encoder of a U-Net. This discriminator tries to distinguish whether a given feature map comes from a source or target image. Meanwhile, the encoder is trained to fool this discriminator (in adversarial training fashion), making its output features domain indistinguishable. As a result, the encoder learns domain-invariant features. In practice, this might mean the encoder focuses on structures common to both CT and MRI (like edges or shapes of organs) and ignores modality-specific cues (like absolute intensity differences). DANN (domain-adversarial neural network) is a well-known framework that implements this via a gradient reversal layer [20]. In segmentation, we apply this concept such that after a certain layer (often the final encoder layer), the features cannot tell the domain apart.

The segmentation head then uses these aligned features to make predictions. If alignment is successful, a model trained on source labels can directly apply to target features since they live in the same distribution. Another popular feature alignment technique is maximum mean discrepancy (MMD) minimization [21] or correlation alignment (CORAL) [22]. These are statistical measures of distribution difference. MMD, for instance, computes a distance between feature distributions of source and target by comparing moments (like means in a high-dimensional kernel space). By adding an MMD loss between source and target feature representations, one can encourage their distributions to overlap. CORAL aligns the covariance of source and target feature distributions by a simpler loss on covariance matrices [22]. These methods do not use a discriminator and are often easier to train, though possibly less flexible in capturing complex distribution differences compared to adversarial training.

Often, feature alignment and image alignment are combined for best effect. For example, a pipeline might use CycleGAN to bring images closer and then still use a feature-level adversarial alignment. The combination addresses both low-level (appearance) and mid-level (feature) disparities. The primary assumption of alignment methods is that there exists a common feature space where both domains can be represented such that the task remains feasible. If the domains differ in content (not just style), alignment might not suffice. In medical imaging, however, many domain shifts are indeed largely "stylistic" (different scanners, protocols, or modalities imaging the same anatomy). Alignment has been effectively applied to problems like cross-modality organ segmentation (CT to MRI, etc.), where even though MRI intensity is not directly comparable to CT Hounsfield units, the underlying organ shapes and relative positions are consistent and can serve as domain-invariant cues.

2.4.2 Teacher–Student Self-Training Methods

Another major category for domain adaptation builds on the pseudo-labeling and self-training ideas we discussed in the semi-supervised section, but now explicitly for transferring knowledge to the target domain. The common work flow is: train an initial segmentation model on the labeled source data, then use that model to predict labels for the target domain images (which are unlabeled), and finally refine the model using those target predictions as pseudo-labels. This procedure effectively iteratively adapts the model to the target domain data. A simple version is often called "Direct Self-Training" or just pseudo-label refinement. The initial source-trained model likely produces imperfect masks on target images, but some regions might be segmented correctly or with high confidence. By applying a confidence threshold and taking the confident regions of the target predictions as pseudo-ground truth, one can retrain or fine-tune the model. For example, if the model is quite sure about the center of an organ but unsure about edges, one might add a loss to make sure it at least gets the center right (where it's confident). Over a few iterations, the area of confident predictions may expand. This is analogous to semi-supervised self-training [23], except that initially the model only saw source domain data. In practice, this technique can incrementally adapt a model from one modality to another by "bootstrapping" on its own predictions. An enhanced approach is the noisy student training (NST) and mean teacher models which we described earlier, but applied to domain adaptation [11,24]. In NST, for instance, the source-trained model plays the role of the teacher that labels target data; then a student model is trained on those noisy labels while noise (augmentations) is added to the student during training to improve robustness. In mean teacher adaptation, one could maintain a teacher (EMA of the student) continuously while training on both source (labeled) and target (unlabeled with consistency loss). The teacher generates pseudo-labels for target images and the student is trained to predict similarly. Over time the student adapts to target data and the teacher (being EMA) always lags somewhat behind, providing a stable target. One example is adversarial dropout regularization [25], where dropout in the model is used to create a form of teacher–student: two different dropout masks on the same target image yield two predictions, and the model is trained to make them consistent (a form of self-ensemble on target). This was specifically proposed for domain adaptation and relates to the model consistency idea we discussed.

A variant of this idea is mutual learning or co-training for adaptation [26], where instead of one model, two models adapt together (similar to co-training earlier). Each model might generate pseudo-labels for target and teach the other, helping to reduce bias. For example, two different architectures could segment a target MRI; where they agree, it's likely correct, where they disagree, one or both are wrong. You could focus training on agreed regions.

A more recent focus in domain adaptation is being uncertainty-aware, which means explicitly modeling what the network is unsure about on target data and using that information to guide adaptation [27,28]. The rationale is that domain shift often causes increased uncertainty in the model's predictions (e.g., lower prediction probabilities, or variability in predictions under augmentations). By quantifying this, one can, for instance, choose where to trust pseudo-labels or enforce consistency.

In conclusion, UDA techniques enable models to transfer segmentation capability from one setting to another without target labels. Image and feature alignment approaches (e.g., GAN-based style transfer, MMD, adversarial feature alignment) make the source and target data more similar in appearance or representation [18,19,22,29]. Teacher–student and self-training approaches leverage the source-trained model to generate proxy labels and refine the model on the target domain, often enhanced by consistency and ensemble strategies [23,24,26]. Uncertainty-aware methods add a refinement by guiding the adaptation based on model confidence, preventing the model from learning from or being misled by highly uncertain predictions [25,30]. In practice, the best performing adaptation frameworks in medical imaging tend to integrate multiple components: for instance, adversarial feature alignment combined with self-training and entropy minimization has shown very strong results in cross-modality organ segmentation benchmarks. As a result, we now see models that can train on one modality (e.g., CT with labels) and successfully segment another modality (e.g., MRI) nearly as well as if we had a moderate amount of supervised data for that modality, thus greatly expanding the utility of AI models across different clinical scenarios and imaging technologies.

2.5 FOUNDATION MODELS FOR MEDICAL IMAGE SEGMENTATION

In the realm of AI, a foundation model refers to a large model (often with hundreds of millions or even billions of parameters) trained on a broad dataset at scale, such that it can serve as a general-purpose model for a variety of downstream tasks. In natural language processing, models like GPT-3 or BERT are foundation models, and in computer vision, models like Vision Transformers or CLIP trained on massive image datasets fulfill a similar role. Recently, there has been a push to develop foundation models specifically for medical imaging and segmentation. The idea is to train a very large model on diverse medical images (possibly across institutions, anatomies, and tasks) in a mostly self-supervised or weakly supervised manner, so that the model learns a rich representation of medical images. This model can then be fine-tuned or prompted to perform specific segmentation tasks with minimal additional training effect in context of training example or training time. In precision radiation therapy, foundation models hold the promise of providing out-of-the-box segmentation solutions that are robust across different image modalities and patient populations, thereby reducing the need for extensive training data for each new segmentation task. In this section, we discuss some emerging examples of foundation models applied to medical image segmentation and their key components: extremely large training datasets, transformer-based architectures, and sometimes federated or distributed training schemes to gather diversity.

2.5.1 SMIT: Self-Distilled Masked Image Transformer

One example of a foundation model concept is SMIT (Self-distilled Masked Image Transformer) [31], which has been explored for medical image segmentation as a self-supervised pretraining approach. The SMIT model has been pretrained with 10k CT scans (unlabeled) by randomly masking patches of the images and training a transformer to reconstruct them in a self-distillation manner. Through this process, the transformer structure (the foundation model) learns strong low-level and mid-level representations of medical images (edges, textures, typical anatomical patterns), without needing any manual labels. Once trained, the model can then be fine-tuned for segmentation with fewer labeled examples with accelerated training convergence [32].

2.5.2 MedSAM: Segment Anything Model for Medical Image

The segment anything model (SAM) from Meta AI is a foundation model for general image segmentation that can produce a segmentation mask for any prompt (like a point or bounding box) on any image. SAM was originally trained on over 1 billion masks from natural images (SA-1B dataset). It uses a promptable design: it has an image encoder (a Vision Transformer) that computes image embeddings, a prompt encoder (for points, boxes, text queries, etc.), and a mask decoder that combines image and prompt information to output a segmentation mask. MedSAM [28] takes the architecture of SAM and adapts it to the medical domain by training it on a large collection of medical images and segmentation masks. In one approach, the SAM model was fine-tuned using over 1.5 million image-mask pairs across 10 modalities and 30+ anatomical classes [28]. These data were pulled from public medical segmentation datasets (like those from the medical segmentation decathlon, etc.), covering CT, MRI, ultrasound, X-ray, pathology images, etc. The result is a single model that can perform interactive segmentation on a wide range of medical imaging modalities and segmentation targets after being given a simple prompt. Recent research about medical image foundation based on SAM include SegVol [33] and Vista [34]. One disadvantage of SAM related method is the manual input prompt which might prevent SAM for clinical workflow use.

2.5.3 FedFMS: Federated Foundation Models for Segmentation

Federated learning is a technique to train models on data from multiple institutions without the data leaving its source, thus preserving privacy. FedFMS [35] stands for federated foundation models for medical image segmentation. The motivation is to build a foundation model collaboratively across institutions/hospitals, which each might have a lot of images but cannot share them directly due to patient privacy.

In a federated setup, each hospital (client) trains the model on its local data and shares only the model weights (or weight updates) with a central server. The server aggregates the updates (e.g., by averaging) to form a global model, which is then sent back to clients for another round of local training. Over many such federated rounds, the global model learns from data at all sites, yet no raw image ever leaves a hospital's firewall.

FedFMS specifically is a framework where two types of models were explored: FedSAM: Federated training of the full segment anything model (where each client fine-tunes SAM and gradients are aggregated). However, transmitting the full SAM model (which is very large) and aggregating it might be bandwidth and memory intensive. FedMSA: A more communication-efficient approach introduced by Liu et al., where instead of fine-tuning all of SAM's parameters, they freeze the large backbone and fine-tune only small adapter modules (MSA: medical SAM adapter) at each client. These adapters (like small additional layers inserted in SAM's architecture) have far fewer parameters, so sending them around in federated learning is much easier. FedMSA involves averaging those adapter weights across sites. Essentially, each site slightly adapts SAM to its local data (like adding a slight local bias), and these small changes are combined to make a globally effective model.

This approach allowed training a federated segmentation model on multiple institutions' datasets (including different modalities and anatomies). The results showed that the federated models (especially FedMSA) achieved performance close to a model trained on the pooled data (which is the ideal but not possible due to privacy) and better than a model trained only on each single-institution data. That demonstrates the benefit of the collaborative learning. For radiation therapy, where data is often private in each hospital or cancer center, federated foundation models mean we can leverage knowledge from many centers without violating privacy. For example, one hospital might have more head-and-neck cancer cases and another more lung cancer cases; a foundation model trained via FedFMS could learn from both and be capable of segmenting anatomy or tumors in both contexts.

2.6 CONCLUSION

AI has made significant strides in automating and improving medical image segmentation, a critical component of precision radiation therapy. In this chapter, we explored a series of AI-driven approaches, from supervised deep neural networks to semi-supervised learning techniques, UDA strategies, and large-scale foundation models. Each of these developments addresses specific challenges: supervised architectures have greatly improved segmentation accuracy given sufficient training data; semi- and unsupervised methods alleviate the dependence on large labeled datasets and enable models to generalize across different imaging domains; and foundation models promise a new level of generality and robustness by leveraging large amounts of data and compute. A common theme throughout these approaches is the focus on generalization, whether across data-limited scenarios, across domain shifts, or across diverse tasks. Techniques like pseudo-label self-training and consistency regularization allow models to effectively use unlabeled images, which is particularly valuable in medicine where annotations are expensive and sometimes subjective. Domain adaptation methods ensure that a model trained in one setting (e.g., one hospital's scanner or one modality) remains effective in another, which is essential for real-world deployment. Foundation models, trained on millions of images, encapsulate a prior knowledge that can be adapted to many specific segmentation problems with relatively little additional input, representing the culmination of these generalization efforts. For precision radiation therapy, these advancements translate into practical benefits: improved efficiency: automated and semiautomated segmentation tools can significantly reduce the time clinicians spend on manual contouring of tumors and organs, thereby accelerating the treatment planning process. As models become more accurate and reliable, the need for manual corrections diminishes.

Consistency and Quality: AI-driven segmentation provides consistent results that are less prone to inter-observer variation. This consistency can lead to more standardized treatment plans. Moreover, complex structures or subtle tumor boundaries that might be missed by the human could be detected by an AI that has learned from large datasets of similar cases.

Adaptability: With domain adaptation, a model trained on one institution's data can be ported to another's with minimal loss of performance, facilitating wider adoption. While the technology is advancing rapidly, clinical integration requires careful validation. Models should be extensively tested against expert benchmarks and in prospective settings to ensure safety and efficacy. Interpretability and user control are also key: clinicians need to understand when to trust the model and when to be cautious. Features such as uncertainty estimates can be instrumental in this regard by highlighting which parts of an AI-generated contour are less certain and might need review.

The convergence of large foundation models with federated learning opens the door for continuously improving AI systems that learn from the collective experience of many centers without compromising patient privacy. Such systems could be updated regularly as new data becomes available, constantly refining their knowledge. In radiation oncology, this means the AI assisting treatment planning could keep getting better with time, potentially learning from outcomes and adapting accordingly. AI-driven medical image analysis has evolved from research to approaches that are on the concept of practical, widespread use. By maintaining the technical content and rigor in developing these models while also framing them in an intuitive, clinically relevant manner, we underscore their value: enabling more precise, efficient, and individualized radiation therapy. As these technologies mature, the collaboration between clinicians and AI will likely become a cornerstone of the workflow, ultimately aiming for improved patient outcomes and advancing the quality of cancer treatment.

REFERENCES

1. O. Ronneberger, P. Fischer, and T. Brox, "U-net: Convolutional networks for biomedical image segmentation," in *Medical Image Computing and Computer-Assisted Intervention–MICCAI 2015: 18th International Conference*, Munich, Germany, October 5–9, 2015, proceedings, part III 18, Springer International Publishing, 2015, pp. 234–241.
2. V. Asadpour, R. A. Parker, P. R. Mayock, S. E. Sampson, W. Chen, and B. Wu, "Pancreatic cancer tumor analysis in CT images using patch-based multi-resolution convolutional neural network," *Biomedical Signal Processing and Control*, vol. 68, p. 102652, 2021.
3. F. Isensee, P. F. Jaeger, S. A. Kohl, J. Petersen, and K. H. Maier-Hein, "nnU-Net: A self-configuring method for deep learning-based biomedical image segmentation," *Nature Methods*, vol. 18, no. 2, pp. 203–211, 2021.
4. J. Jiang, Y.-C. Hu, C.-J. Liu, D. Halpenny, M. D. Hell-mann, J. O. Deasy, G. Mageras, and H. Veeraraghavan, "Multiple resolution residually connected feature streams for automatic lung tumor segmentation from CT images," *IEEE Transactions on Medical Imaging*, vol. 38, no. 1, pp. 134–144, 2018.
5. J. Chen, Y. Lu, Q. Yu, X. Luo, E. Adeli, Y. Wang, et al., "Transunet: Transformers make strong encoders for medical image segmentation," arXiv preprint arXiv:2102.04306, 2021.
6. H. Cao, Y. Wang, J. Chen, D. Jiang, X. Zhang, Q. Tian, and M. Wang, "Swin-unet: Unet-like pure transformer for medical image segmentation," in *European Conference on Computer Vision*, Computer Vision – ECCV 2022 Workshops, Tel Aviv, Israel, October 23–27, 2022, Cham: Springer Nature Switzerland, 2022, pp. 205–218.
7. Z. Liu, Y. Lin, Y. Cao, H. Hu, Y. Wei, Z. Zhang, S. Lin, and B. Guo, "Swin transformer: Hierarchical vision transformer using shifted windows," In *Proceedings of the IEEE/CVF International Conference on Computer Vision*, 2021 IEEE/CVF International Conference on Computer Vision (ICCV), Montreal, QC, Canada, 2021, pp. 10012–10022.
8. D. H. Lee, "Pseudo-label: The simple and efficient semi-supervised learning method for deep neural networks," in *Workshop on Challenges in Representation Learning*, Atlanta, ICML, vol. 3, no. 2, Jun. 2013, p. 896.
9. Z. Shen, P. Cao, H. Yang, X. Liu, J. Yang, and O. R. Zaiane, "Co-training with high-confidence pseudo labels for semi-supervised medical image segmentation," arXiv preprint arXiv:2301.04465, 2023.
10. X. Yang, Z. Song, I. King, and Z. Xu, "A survey on deep semi-supervised learning," *IEEE Transactions on Knowledge and Data Engineering*, vol. 35, no. 9, pp. 8934–8954, 2022.
11. Y. Ge, D. Chen, and H. Li, "Mutual mean-teaching: Pseudo label refinery for unsupervised domain adaptation on person re-identification," arXiv preprint arXiv:2001.01526, 2020.
12. I. J. Goodfellow, J. Pouget-Abadie, M. Mirza, B. Xu, D. Warde-Farley, S. Ozair, A. Courville, and Y. Bengio, "Generative adversarial nets," In Z. Ghahramani and M. Welling and C. Cortes and N. Lawrence and K.Q. Weinberger (eds), *Advances in Neural Information Processing Systems*, Curran Associates, Inc., 2014, p. 27. https://proceedings.neurips.cc/paper_files/paper/2014/file/f033ed80deb0234979a61f95710dbe25-Paper.pdf
13. N. Souly, C. Spampinato, and M. Shah, "Semi supervised semantic segmen-tation using generative adversarial network," in *Proceedings of the IEEE International Conference on Computer Vision*, 2017 IEEE International Conference on Computer Vision (ICCV), Venice, Italy, 2017, pp. 5688–5696.
14. X. Hu, D. Zeng, X. Xu, and Y. Shi, "Semi-supervised contrastive learning for label-efficient medical image segmentation," in *Medical Image Comput-ing and Computer Assisted Intervention–MICCAI 2021: 24th International Conference*, Strasbourg, France, September 27–October 1, 2021, Proceedings, Part II 24, Springer International Publishing, 2021, pp. 481–490.

15. J. Jiang, Y.-C. Hu, N. Tyagi, P. Zhang, A. Rimner, G. S. Mageras, J. O. Deasy, and H. Veeraraghavan, "Tumor-aware, adversarial domain adaptation from CT to MRI for lung cancer segmentation," in *Medical Image Computing and Computer Assisted Intervention–MICCAI 2018: 21st International Conference*, Granada, Spain, September 16–20, 2018, Proceedings, Part II 11, pages 777–785. Springer, 2018.
16. H. Wu, Z. Wang, Y. Song, L. Yang, and J. Qin, "Cross-patch dense contrastive learning for semi-supervised segmentation of cellular nuclei in histopathologic images," in *Proceedings of the IEEE/CVF Conference on Computer Vision and Pattern Recognition*, 2022 IEEE/CVF Conference on Computer Vision and Pattern Recognition (CVPR), New Orleans, LA, USA, 2022, pp. 11666–11675.
17. M. Toldo, A. Maracani, U. Michieli, and P. Zanuttigh, "Unsupervised domain adaptation in semantic segmentation: A review," *Technologies*, vol. 8, no. 2, p. 35, 2020.
18. J. Y. Zhu, T. Park, P. Isola, and A. A. Efros, "Unpaired image-to-image translation using cycle-consistent adversarial networks," in *Proceedings of the IEEE International Conference on Computer Vision*, 2017 IEEE International Conference on Computer Vision (ICCV), Venice, Italy, 2017, pp. 2223–2232.
19. Q. Tian, J. Zhou, and Y. Chu, "Joint biadversarial learning for unsupervised domain adaptation," *Knowledge-Based Systems*, vol. 248, p. 108903, 2022.
20. Y. Ganin and V. Lempitsky, "Unsupervised domain adaptation by back propagation," in Bach, Francis and Blei, David (eds), *Proceedings of the 32nd International Conference on Machine Learning,*{Proceedings of Machine Learning Research PMLR Lille, France, 2015, pp. 1180–1189.
21. A. Kumagai and T. Iwata, "Unsupervised domain adaptation by matching distributions based on the maximum mean discrepancy via unilateral transformations," in *Proceedings of the Thirty-Third AAAI Conference on Artificial Intelligence and Thirty-First Innovative Applications of Artificial Intelligence Conference and Ninth AAAI Symposium on Educational Advances in Artificial Intelligence,,* AAAI Press, Honolulu, Hawaii, USA, vol. 33, no. 01, 2019, pp. 4106–4113.
22. B. Sun, J. Feng, and K. Saenko, "Correlation alignment for unsupervised domain adaptation," in Csurka, G. (ed.), *Domain Adaptation in Computer Vision Applications. Advances in Computer Vision and Pattern Recognition*. Springer, Cham, 2017, pp. 153–171.
23. P. Zhang, B. Zhang, T. Zhang, D. Chen, Y. Wang, and F. Wen, "Prototypical pseudo label denoising and target structure learning for domain adaptive semantic segmentation," in *Proceedings of the IEEE/CVF Conference on Computer Vision and Pattern Recognition*, 2021 IEEE/CVF Conference on Computer Vision and Pattern Recognition (CVPR), Nashville, TN, USA, 2021, pp. 12414–12424.
24. V. Manohar, P. Ghahremani, D. Povey, and S. Khudanpur, "A teacher–student learning approach for unsupervised domain adaptation of sequence trained ASR models," in *2018 IEEE Spoken Language Technology Workshop (SLT)*, Athens, Greece, 2018, pp. 250–257.
25. K. Saito, Y. Ushiku, T. Harada, and K. Saenko, "Adversarial dropout regularization," arXiv preprint arXiv:1711.01575, 2017.
26. J. L. G´omez, G. Villalonga, and A. M. L´opez, "Co-training for unsupervised domain adaptation of semantic segmentation models," *Sensors*, vol. 23, no. 2, p. 621, 2023.
27. X. Wu, S. Zhang, Q. Zhou, Z. Yang, C. Zhao, and L. J. Latecki, "Entropy minimization versus diversity maximization for domain adaptation," *IEEE Transactions on Neural Networks and Learning Systems*, vol. 34, no. 6, pp. 2896–2907, 2021.
28. J. Ma, Y. He, F. Li, L. Han, C. You, and B. Wang, "Segment anything in medical images," *Nature Communications*, vol. 15, no. 1, p. 654, 2024.
29. T. Chen, S. H. Wang, Q. Wang, Z. Zhang, G. S. Xie, and Z. Tang, "Enhanced feature alignment for unsupervised domain adaptation of semantic segmentation," *IEEE Transactions on Multimedia*, vol. 24, pp. 1042–1054, 2021.
30. D. Guan, J. Huang, A. Xiao, S. Lu, and Y. Cao, "Uncertainty-aware unsupervised domain adaptation in object detection," *IEEE Transactions on Multimedia*, vol. 24, pp. 2502–2514, 2021.
31. J. Jiang, N. Tyagi, K. Tringale, C. Crane, and H. Veeraraghavan, "Self-supervised 3D anatomy segmentation using self distilled masked image transformer (smit)," In *Medical Image Computing and Computer Assisted Intervention – MICCAI 2022: 25th International Conference, Singapore, September 18–22, 2022, Proceedings, Part IV*, Singapore. Springer, Berlin, Heidelberg, 2022, pp. 556–566. doi: 10.1007/978-3-031-16440-8_53
32. J. Jiang and H. Veeraraghavan, "Self-supervised pretraining in the wild imparts image acquisition robustness to medical image transformers: An application to lung cancer segmentation," *Proceedings of Machine Learning Research*, vol. 250, p. 708, 2024.
33. Y. Du, F. Bai, T. Huang, and B. Zhao, "Segvol: Universal and interactive volumetric medical image segmentation," *Advances in Neural Information Processing Systems*, vol. 37, pp. 110746–110783, 2024.

34. Y. He, P. Guo, Y. Tang, A. Myronenko, V. Nath, Z. Xu, D. Yang, C. Zhao, B. Simon, M. Belue, et al., "Vista3d: Versatile imaging segmentation and annotation model for 3D computed tomography," arXiv preprint arXiv:2406.05285, 2024.
35. Y. Liu, G. Luo, and Y. Zhu, "Fedfms: Exploring federated foundation models for medical image segmentation," in *Medical Image Computing and Computer Assisted Intervention – MICCAI 2024: 27th International Conference, Marrakesh, Morocco, October 6–10, 2024, Proceedings, Part VIII*, Marrakesh, Morocco, Cham: Springer Nature Switzerland, Berlin, Heidelberg, 2024, pp. 283–293.

3 Medical Image Registration

Xinrui Song and Pingkun Yan

Section 1: An Overview of Medical Image Registration

3.1.1 DEFINITION

While imaging modalities and patient-specific characteristics impact the intensity, resolution, and morphology of the resulting medical image, the anatomical structures and regions of interest (ROIs) stay consistent across images. The art of registering one image to another via identifying the correspondence between similar anatomical structures is called **medical image registration**.

Medical image registration is also referred to as image fusion or image alignment. As the task is usually performed on images pairs, one image is considered the moving image, and the other is the reference image, or the fixed image. Image registration then is defined as transforming the moving image into the space of the reference image. Note that the key outcome of image registration is mainly the transformation itself. The transformation can be used to warp the moving image into the reference space. The warped image can be used in various applications, including quantifying movement, quantifying growth, aligning the atlas, and segmenting images. More example applications will be introduced in the following section.

3.1.2 CLINICAL APPLICATIONS OF MEDICAL IMAGE REGISTRATION

The need for registering images arises from multiple clinical settings. Registration can be performed between images from the same patient but different modalities, or from the same modality but at different time points (longitudinal tracking).

3.1.2.1 Longitudinal Tracking

Longitudinal tracking can serve multiple purposes, such as monitoring tumor growth. Benign tumors, which do not grow or invade surrounding tissues, may not require immediate treatment but should always be monitored closely. The same applies to treatment monitoring. During radiotherapy, tumors can change in response to treatment, necessitating registration for adaptive planning to adjust radiation dose and delivery. By registering follow-up images with the original treatment planning images, clinicians can quantify the tumor's response and update treatment plans accordingly. In these cases, image registration serves as a tool to quantify both growth and movement of cancerous tissue over time. Unlike segmentation, which only quantifies volume, deformable registration allows for tracking nonuniform growth or shrinkage, as well as changes in the tumor's shape and position relative to surrounding anatomy. Growth or shrinkage is visible and quantifiable as inflation or deflation in the displacement field—an output of deformable registration algorithms. Additionally, patient-related factors, such as weight loss, can result in shrinkage of soft tissue while bony tissue remains relatively unchanged, further highlighting the need for precise registration to account for these anatomical variations.

DOI: 10.1201/9781003480365-4

3.1.2.2 Treatment Planning

Surgery or treatment planning also benefits from image registration. For radiotherapy planning, MR could provide much better soft-tissue detail than CT, while CT is the gold standard for providing spatial accuracy, bony anatomy definition, and electron density information for dose calculations. Therefore, the alignment between MR and CT, and possibly subsequent CTs are very helpful. Another use case is the validation of surgical success. In procedures like tumor ablation, the goal is to remove the entire tumor while preserving as much healthy tissue as possible. Achieving this balance can be challenging, and postoperative imaging is often necessary to confirm the complete removal of cancerous tissue. By registering post-surgery images with presurgery scans, we can visualize whether the ablated region aligns with the original surgical plan.

Registration across different modalities, however, is innately more challenging due to intensity and contrast differences, field of view (FOV) differences, and disparate anatomical depiction, as structures that are visible in one modality may be concealed in another.

3.1.2.3 Real-time Guidance

The need for real-time imaging guidance results from the trade-off between spatial resolution and temporal resolution. While imaging modalities such as ultrasound excel in capturing real-time images, the signal-to-noise ratio is usually low, and the resolution also isn't satisfactory. Differentiating target lesions from imaging artifacts could be challenging even for experienced surgeons. Therefore, the registration between such real-time imaging methods and a preoperative high-resolution image, such as CT or MR, would largely enhance the accuracy of such operations. One clinical example would be a prostate cancer biopsy. Traditionally, the procedure is only guided with ultrasound. The ultrasound image shows a noisy representation of the prostate region, where only very limited anatomical structures would be visible. The urologists take 12 samples uniformly distributed throughout the prostate, and the procedure is named a random biopsy. When preoperative MR images are available, the urologists would perform what they call a *cognitive registration* between the two images, thereby providing an educated guess of whether the current ultrasound footage is showing the biopsy target they saw in the MR. This practice signals progress from random biopsy to targeted biopsy. Later, many image fusion platforms came to the market, using different tracking systems to assist the fusion between ultrasound and MRI.

3.1.2.4 Template Registration

Template registration refers to the process of aligning an input image (or a series of images) to a predefined reference image or a standardized anatomical "template." The template typically represents a normative or average anatomy (e.g., an average brain MRI), and individual subject images are registered to this template for comparison, analysis, or image segmentation.

One of the most common applications of template registration is brain imaging. Templates such as the *MNI*-152 *brain* template are used to align individual MRI or functional MRI (fMRI) scans for group studies. This allows for comparison of anatomical or functional data across individuals or populations. The go-to image processing pipeline for brain MRI analysis is FreeSurfer [1], a tool built for studying the cortical and subcortical anatomy. The whole pipeline starts with the registration of the processing image and an atlas template. Similarly, Klein et al. [2] used atlas registration for the segmentation of prostate in MR images.

3.1.2.5 Image Recon Patient Motion

Medical image registration is crucial in image reconstruction, particularly for managing patient motion. Movements, whether voluntary like breathing or involuntary like small shifts, can blur images and hinder accurate interpretation. Registration techniques align images taken at different times or from various angles, correcting for these shifts and enabling clearer, more cohesive images. In MRI, for example, registration helps correct head motion artifacts in fMRI or diffusion MRI scans, while in CT, respiratory gating uses registration to align images across different breathing phases. By addressing motion, registration ensures higher quality images for precise diagnosis, treatment planning, and monitoring.

3.1.3 GEOMETRICAL FLEXIBILITY OF DIFFERENT TYPES OF REGISTRATION

In medical image registration, the choice of registration type plays a crucial role in determining how images from different sources (or at different time points) are aligned. Each registration type offers different levels of geometrical flexibility, allowing for varying degrees of movement and deformation between the source and target images. Different types of registration have different applications, and higher flexibility does not always lead to a better result (Figure 3.1).

3.1.3.1 Rigid and Affine Registration

Rigid Registration limits the degree of freedom to translation, rotation, and uniform scaling. Originally, scaling was not classified as a part of rigid registration. The move to include scaling happened around the 2000s and 2010s, when more studies on deformable registration emerged, and rigid registration was commonly used as a preprocessing step. Image registration, especially for 3D images, is a very challenging task for humans; rigid registration is the highest flexibility that human annotators can handle.

Suppose the original coordinate of a voxel is represented as

$$\mathbf{v} = \begin{pmatrix} v_x \\ v_y \\ v_z \\ 1 \end{pmatrix}$$

The 3D scaling transformation can be represented as

$$S = \begin{pmatrix} s_x & 0 & 0 & 0 \\ 0 & s_y & 0 & 0 \\ 0 & 0 & s_z & 0 \\ 0 & 0 & 0 & 1 \end{pmatrix}$$

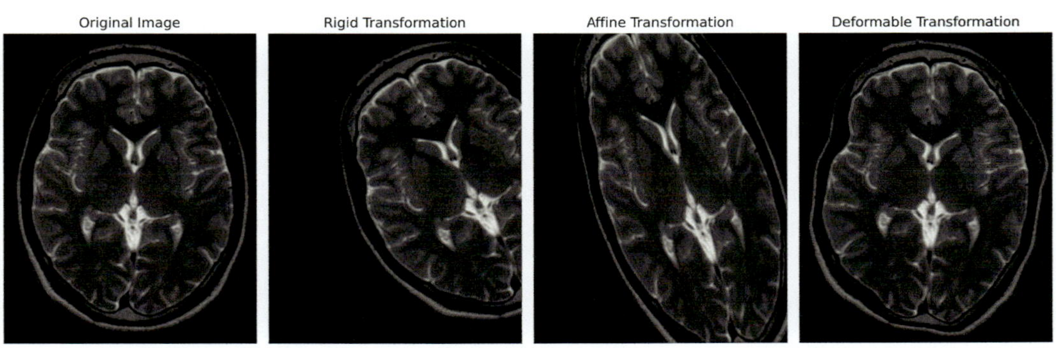

FIGURE 3.1 Visualization of different types of registration.

where s_x, s_y, s_z are the scaling factors along the *x*, *y*, and *z* axes, respectively.

The 3D translation can be represented as

$$T = \begin{pmatrix} 1 & 0 & 0 & t_x \\ 0 & 1 & 0 & t_y \\ 0 & 0 & 1 & t_z \\ 0 & 0 & 0 & 1 \end{pmatrix}$$

where t_x, t_y, t_z are the translations along the *x*, *y*, and *z* axes, respectively.

Rotation in 3D space is a more complicated issue. The most commonly used and basic description of 3D rotation is the Euler rotation angles. The Euler system consists of three rotations around the *x*, *y*, and *z* axes, respectively. Note that the combination of these three rotations is not commutative, meaning that a rotation defined as *x-y-z* (the convention) cannot be interpreted and implemented in the *x-z-y* order.

The rotation matrix about the *x*-axis by an angle θ_x

$$R_x(\theta_x) = \begin{pmatrix} 1 & 0 & 0 & 0 \\ 0 & \cos\theta_x & -\sin\theta_x & 0 \\ 0 & \sin\theta_x & \cos\theta_x & 0 \\ 0 & 0 & 0 & 1 \end{pmatrix}$$

The rotation matrix about the *y*-axis by an angle θ_y

$$R_y(\theta_y) = \begin{pmatrix} \cos\theta_y & 0 & \sin\theta_y & 0 \\ 0 & 1 & 0 & 0 \\ -\sin\theta_y & 0 & \cos\theta_y & 0 \\ 0 & 0 & 0 & 1 \end{pmatrix}$$

The rotation matrix about the *z*-axis by an angle θ_z

$$\mathrm{R}_z(\theta_z) = \begin{pmatrix} \cos\theta_z & -\sin\theta_z & 0 & 0 \\ \sin\theta_z & \cos\theta_z & 0 & 0 \\ 0 & 0 & 1 & 0 \\ 0 & 0 & 0 & 1 \end{pmatrix}$$

For a rotation applied in the *x-y-z* order, the combined rotation matrix is obtained by multiplying the subsequent rotation matrix on the right side:

$$R(\theta_x, \theta_y, \theta_z) = R_z(\theta_z) R_y(\theta_y) R_x(\theta_x)$$

The matrix expands into

$$R = \begin{pmatrix} \cos\theta_y \cos\theta_z & -\cos\theta_y \sin\theta_z & \sin\theta_y & 0 \\ \sin\theta_x \sin\theta_y \cos\theta_z + \cos\theta_x \sin\theta_z & -\sin\theta_x \sin\theta_y \sin\theta_z + \cos\theta_x \cos\theta_z & -\sin\theta_x \cos\theta_y & 0 \\ -\cos\theta_x \sin\theta_y \cos\theta_z + \sin\theta_x \sin\theta_z & \cos\theta_x \sin\theta_y \sin\theta_z + \sin\theta_x \cos\theta_z & \cos\theta_x \cos\theta_y & 0 \\ 0 & 0 & 0 & 1 \end{pmatrix}$$

Note that when applying a rigid transformation, the convention is to start with scaling, followed by rotation, and then translation. This process is also noncommutative.

Other representations of 3D rotations used in registration include Lie algebra [3], quaternion [4], etc.; some proven numerically more stable for optimization. Refer to external sources for more information.

Affine registration extends the rigid transformation matrix with nonuniform scaling and shearing. However, since neither of these is physically plausible, their application in medical image registration is limited.

3.1.3.2 Deformable Registration

Early deformable registration methods were inspired by physical models, such as elastic body models, which treat the image as an elastic material that deforms under forces. This approach, first proposed in the 1980s, allows for smooth, continuous deformations that preserve the overall structure of anatomical regions. Another foundational technique was derived from interpolation theory, such as thin-plate splines (TPS), which used a sparse set of landmarks to interpolate smooth deformations across the image. These early methods enabled local deformations but were computationally expensive and limited in their ability to handle large, complex changes.

As the field progressed, more sophisticated methods were developed. Fluid models, for instance, treated the deforming image like a viscous fluid, capable of capturing large, nonlinear deformations. These models are based on the Navier–Stokes equations, which allow for a more flexible representation of changes across time and space. Later, large deformation diffeomorphic metric mapping (LDDMM) frameworks were introduced, providing a mathematically rigorous approach that ensures smooth and invertible transformations, making them ideal for capturing large deformations while preserving topology. Finally, statistical models were developed to account for anatomical variability across populations, using learned patterns of deformation to guide the registration process. For a detailed explanation of each method, refer to the review article by Sotiras et al. [5].

Many of the previously introduced methods are results of compromises made to the computation capacity at the time of invention. With the introduction of power GPUs in the 2010s, the field has started to shift toward dense displacement fields (DDFs). DDFs emerged from the need to accurately map every voxel from a source image to a target image, providing a dense vector field that captures fine-scale deformations. Unlike early parametric models, which used a limited set of control points, DDFs estimate displacements for each voxel, allowing for highly flexible, nonparametric transformations. For 3D images, the displacement fields take the dimension of $[X,Y,Z,3]$, also written as $[X,Y,Z,[x,y,z]]$. The first three dimensions represent the original coordinate of a voxel, and the last channel encodes the displacement of that voxel in all three directions. For identity transformation, the entire field would be zero. Displacement fields are calculated either through optimization or deep learning-based neural network inference. Further details are provided in Section 3.2.

3.1.4 EVALUATION METRICS FOR MEDICAL IMAGE REGISTRATION

3.1.4.1 Accuracy Metrics

Quantitative evaluation of medical image registration quality reflects how accurate each anatomical structures from the image pair are aligned. Similar to segmentation tasks where the Dice coefficient is used to quantify the overlap between predicted and ground truth segmentation masks, in the registration task, Dice is also used to evaluate the overlap between the two corresponding organs in the image pair. The Dice coefficient is defined as

$$D(A,B) = \frac{2|A \cap B|}{|A| + |B|}$$

where A and B are the segmentation of the same organ from the image pair. However, while the Dice coefficient effectively measures the overall alignment between organs, it does not capture the internal structure of these organs. A good example is lung imaging. Aligning the five lobes of the lung is relatively straightforward, but the more critical task is registering the vascular structures within the lungs. For this reason, we also need metrics that assess registration quality at a finer level of detail. The target registration error (TRE) measures the millimeter distance between corresponding target points in an image pair, providing a reflection of registration quality at the finest level. However, the limitation of TRE lies in the difficulty of accurately defining these target points. If annotators lack experience, the TRE may be unreliable, or even misleading.

3.1.4.2 Smoothness Metrics

Another important metric for assessing the quality of image registration is smoothness, which can be evaluated using the standard deviation of the Jacobian determinant. This metric quantifies how smoothly the transformation field behaves across the image. Mathematically, the Jacobian determinant $J_T(x)$ at each point x measures how much the local volume is distorted by the transformation T. A rigid transformation would have a constant Jacobian determinant of 1, meaning that the local volumes do not change across the image. However, large deviations in the Jacobian determinant indicate areas where the transformation is irregular, which may result in unrealistic or biologically implausible deformations. A negative local Jacobian determinant indicates folding in the displacement field, representing a physically implausible deformation that should be avoided. The number of negative Jacobian determinants could be used as an indicator of smoothness.

The standard deviation of the Jacobian determinant provides a single value summarizing the variability in local volume changes throughout the image. A lower standard deviation reflects a smoother transformation, while a higher value indicates more irregularities in the registration. This is particularly useful for ensuring that the transformation does not introduce artifacts, such as folding or extreme stretching, which could distort anatomical structures. The mathematical formula for the standard deviation of the Jacobian determinant is as follows:

$$\sigma(J_T) = \sqrt{\frac{1}{N}\sum_x \left(J_T(x) - \overline{J_T}\right)^2}$$

where $J_T(x)$ is the Jacobian determinant at point x. Deformable image registration is often described as an ill-posed task, which is an accurate description. The objective is to generate a displacement field that perfectly warps the moving image to match the fixed image. However, the smoothness constraint, which ensures the transformation remains biologically plausible, can interfere with accuracy. The challenge lies in finding a balance between smoothness and accuracy, so the resulting transformation is both physically realistic and aligns images as closely as possible.

Section 2: Methods for Medical Image Registration

3.2.1 CONVENTIONAL OPTIMIZATION-BASED METHODS

Algorithmic design often roots in how humans carry out the same task. For an experienced annotator, image registration is performed iteratively. The annotator would overlap the image pair on top of each other, compare if all the structures and contours match, and then adjust the alignment and compare again. Conventional optimization-based registration methods are designed with the same spirit. A similarity metric is chosen to evaluate the alignment, and an optimizer is used to update the alignment. The conventional methods with handcrafted similarity metrics are known for their stability, explainability, and generalizability (Figure 3.2).

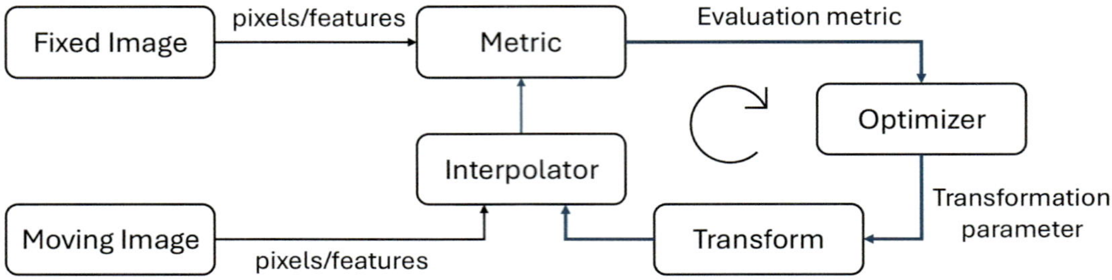

FIGURE 3.2 Optimization-based registration framework.

3.2.1.1 Similarity Metric

The simplest and most efficient metric is mean squared error (MSE), which compares the differences between corresponding voxel intensities. When both images are of the same modality, MSE would often. However, since MSE is very sensitive to noise and intensity variations, this metric is not recommended for multimodal registration or noisy images (e.g., MRI with bias field). MSE is defined as

$$\mathrm{MSE} = \frac{1}{N}\sum_{i=1}^{N}\left(I_1(i) - I_2(i)\right)^2$$

where N is the number of pixels and $I_1(i)$ stands for the intensity of a pixel i from image I_1. Note that the sum of squared distance (SSD) represents the same concept and is equivalent to MSE N.

Normalized cross-correlation (NCC) is another intensity-based similarity metric. As opposed to directly computing the difference in intensity, NCC compares how well the trend of intensity value correlates with the trend in another image. This metric is therefore more robust to noise and intensity scaling than MSE. The intensity still has to follow a similar overall trend for this metric to be effective:

$$\mathrm{NCC} = \frac{\sum_{i=1}^{N}\left(I_1(i) - \overline{I_1}\right)\left(I_2(i) - \overline{I_2}\right)}{\sqrt{\sum_{i=1}^{N}\left(I_1(i) - \overline{I_1}\right)^2}\sqrt{\sum_{i=1}^{N}\left(I_2(i) - \overline{I_2}\right)^2}}$$

Mutual information (MI) measures the mutual dependence between two variables. In the definition below, $p_{I_1 I_2}(i,j)$ is the joint probability distribution of intensities i in image I_1 and j in image I_2; $p_{I_1}(i)$ and $p_{I_2}(j)$ are the marginal probability distributions of intensities in each image. As opposed to matching intensity values or trends, MI quantifies the correspondence in intensity values. For example, if the same structure in both images has similar spatial alignment and intensity patterns, even if the images are from different modalities, the MI would be very high. The main drawback of this metric is speed:

$$\mathrm{MI}(I_1, I_2) = \sum_{i,j} p_{I_1 I_2}(i,j)\log\left(\frac{p_{I_1 I_2}(i,j)}{p_{I_1}(i)\, p_{I_2}(j)}\right)$$

In image registration algorithms, MI is typically computed using the joint histogram of the two images, where the two axes represent the intensity values of the two images. Each bin in the joint histogram counts how often a specific pair of intensity values from the two images occurs at corresponding locations. For 3D images with a large range of intensity, the computation could be very slow. To mitigate this, the images are often downsampled, or intensities are quantized to reduce the number of bins.

3.2.1.2 Optimization Techniques

Optimization techniques iteratively update transformation parameters to maximize or minimize a similarity metric (such as MI or MSE). A commonly used technique is gradient descent, which adjusts parameters in the direction of the steepest descent in the similarity metric. This method works well when the metric is smooth and differentiable, gradually improving alignment by updating the parameters according to the negative gradient of the cost function. However, it can be slow and prone to getting stuck in local minima. Another approach, Powell's method, is a derivative-free optimization technique that minimizes the similarity metric along one direction at a time. This method is useful when gradient information is unavailable or noisy, but it can be inefficient in high-dimensional spaces as it does not leverage gradient information.

More advanced methods, like Quasi-Newton methods such as the Broyden–Fletcher–Goldfarb–Shanno (BFGS) algorithm, offer faster convergence by approximating the second derivatives (the Hessian matrix) without the computational cost of calculating the full matrix. This allows for more efficient optimization compared to standard gradient descent, especially in nonlinear and large-scale problems. Finally, evolutionary algorithms (e.g., genetic algorithms) take a probabilistic approach, inspired by natural selection, to explore the solution space. They rely on operations like mutation, crossover, and selection to iteratively improve the registration. These algorithms are less likely to get trapped in local minima and can handle highly complex or noisy optimization landscapes, but they are computationally expensive and slower than traditional methods. Evolutionary algorithms are especially useful when the optimization problem is non-convex or when gradient-based methods struggle.

3.2.2 DEEP LEARNING-BASED PREDICTION MODELS

Deep learning-based prediction models have revolutionized the field of image registration, allowing for more accurate and efficient estimation of similarity, rigid registration, and deformable registration. These models leverage the powerful representation learning capabilities of deep neural networks, bypassing the need for manual feature engineering. With the increasing availability of medical imaging data and advancements in computational power, deep learning approaches have shown tremendous potential in both rigid and deformable registration tasks.

3.2.2.1 Estimating Similarity

The estimation of similarity between images is conventionally performed with metrics such as MSE and MI, as introduced in Section 3.2.1. Deep learning models, particularly convolutional neural networks (CNNs), have been employed to learn similarity metrics [6–9]. By training CNNs on paired images with known transformations, the network learns to predict a similarity score that can guide the registration process. Reinforcement learning (RL) has also been explored in estimating similarity, where the network acts as an agent that iteratively adjusts the transformation parameters to maximize a reward function based on the alignment of the images [10–12]. The RL is akin to similarity estimation since the algorithm relies on a reward/Q-value to correctly reflect the quality of image registration. Based on the reward, the trained "agent" predicts the next action to better align the images.

3.2.2.2 Estimating Rigid/Affine Registration

Rigid registration involves aligning two images using transformations such as rotation and translation, without allowing any local deformation. The output of such networks is typically a set of transformation parameters:

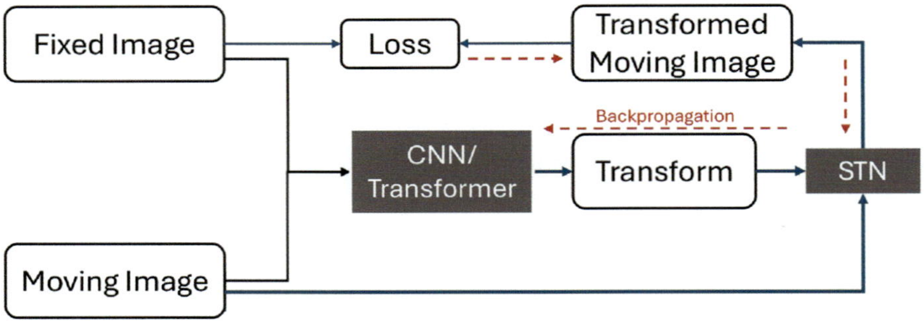

FIGURE 3.3 Deep learning-based predictive registration framework.

$$T = \left[t_x, t_y, t_z, \alpha_x, \alpha_y, \alpha_z\right]$$

where t stands for translation along a particular axis, and α stands for rotation. Counterintuitively, training a neural network to predict the rigid transformation parameters is much harder than training the network for deformable registration. This is because the transformation parameters, unlike a displacement field which has the same shape as the original image, are very abstract compared to the input image. Many efforts are put in this direction to ensure that a robust prediction can be made. One of the key components is to have a training set that is representative of the inference time challenges, as neural networks tend to pick up bias quickly. For example, Hoffmann et al. [13] proposed to use synthetic images to train a predictor that covers all possible misalignment and misorientation. Using a more complex neural network, for example incorporating a self-attention mechanism [14] and transformers [15], could also help the performance.

Rigid/affine registration is not always inferior to deformable registration. In some applications, only rigid registration is applicable. For example, when performing out-of-plane registration of 2D images [16–20], rigid registration retrieves the orientation of the 2D image in 3D space.

3.2.2.3 Estimating Deformable Registration

Deformable registration is a more complex problem, as it requires the model to account for local deformations and nonlinear transformations to align images. The cornerstone of deep learning-based deformable registration is Voxelmorph [21]. In Voxelmorph, a U-Net is trained to predict displacement fields that can warp the moving image to align with the fixed image. The network is supervised either with conventional similarity metrics such as MSE and NCC, or with the Dice coefficient computed from segmentation labels when available. This approach allows the model to learn to predict complex, spatially varying deformations instantly during inference time. The method was later adapted to different applications with different neural network architectures [22–25], but the overall framework stays unchanged (Figure 3.3).

3.2.3 FEATURE-BASED REGISTRATION

Iterative registration could be performed with similarity metrics calculated from not only voxel intensities, but higher dimensional features, too. Handcrafted features were the dominant approach before the rise of deep learning; although more research has been focusing on deep learning prediction models, many challenges [26] show that well-designed handcrafted features are still achieving state-of-the-art performance.

3.2.3.1 Handcrafted Features

In image processing, various handcrafted features like SIFT (scale-invariant feature transform), Gabor filters, and edge detection are widely used for tasks such as feature extraction, registration, and object recognition. SIFT [27] detects and describes key points in an image that are invariant to scale, rotation, and illumination, making it highly effective for matching objects across different views. The method is later generalized to 3D medical image registration [28–30]. Gabor filters, on the other hand, capture frequency and orientation information, mimicking the human visual system to analyze textures and patterns in images. Edge detection techniques, such as Canny or Sobel operators, focus on identifying the boundaries of objects by detecting sharp intensity changes, helping in object localization and segmentation tasks. Lastly, modality-independent neighborhood descriptor (MIND) [31] is specifically designed for multimodal image registration, generating descriptors that capture the local image structure independently of intensity variations, making it particularly robust for aligning images from different modalities like CT and MRI. Together, these techniques offer powerful, complementary ways to extract and analyze important features in images.

3.2.3.2 Learning-Based Features

With the development of deep learning, researchers realized that neural networks can also be used to extract/encode features that assist registration. Yan et al. [32] used contrastive learning to train a feature encoder optimized to capture global and local features. The work was later adapted for optimization-based image registration [33] and generalized to multimodal registration tasks [34,35], too. Siebert et al. [36] proposed that when sufficient label is present, training an nnUNet [37] for segmentation, then use the network's feature for image registration yields the best result. Though achieving the highest Dice on most datasets, the nnUNet features are homogenous within organs, omitting details such as vasculatures. Song et al. [38,39] proposed to use the feature from DINOv2 [40] for medical image registration. The DINOv2 image encoder is trained on 2D natural images but shows shocking generalizability to 3D medical images with no tuning, also hitting state-of-the-art performance on multiple challenges.

Section 3: Resources to Get Started

You have read a lot about medical image registration, but nothing compares to the hands-on experience of applying these techniques yourself. In this section, we offer practical guidance and resources to help you dive into image registration tasks and experiment with various algorithms. Whether you're a beginner seeking foundational exercises or an advanced user looking to explore specialized methods, these resources are designed to support your journey from theory to application, providing the tools and examples you need to truly understand medical image registration.

3.3.1 COMMON DATASETS

The dataset defines the task. There are abundant public medical image datasets, but obtaining images from the same patient with segmentation or target landmark labels is not easy. The Learn2Reg challenge [26] provides the most comprehensive collection of datasets for benchmarking different image registration methods on different tasks/data points. Here you can find well-curated and pre-processed datasets with expert annotated labels; each of these steps could take you days or weeks if starting from scratch.

If you are looking for a larger dataset and would not mind processing it yourself, the TCIA (the cancer image archive) website contains millions of raw data. Whatever anatomies, diseases, or imaging modalities you are interested in, you can find them there. When seeking for scans from the same patient, pay attention to how each dataset is organized, as there is no unified standard; but most of the times scans from the same patient would be stored in the same folder. Always refer to the readme file.

3.3.2 COMMON TOOLKITS

Several open-source toolkits offer robust tools for implementing and experimenting with image registration algorithms. Here, we introduce some of the most commonly used toolkits in the field, highlighting each toolkit's strengths for various registration tasks and providing sample code to help you get started.

3.3.2.1 ITK (Insight Segmentation and Registration Toolkit)

The insight segmentation and registration toolkit (ITK) is one of the most established toolkits for medical image registration and segmentation, offering a broad range of registration algorithms from rigid and affine transformations to complex deformable models. ITK is written in C++ but also provides Python bindings through SimpleITK, making it accessible to researchers and developers working in both languages. With strong support for multimodal registration, ITK enables users to apply robust techniques on various imaging modalities. Below is an example using SimpleITK to perform rigid registration between two images:

```
import SimpleITK as sitk

# Load images
fixed_image=sitk.ReadImage("fixed_image.nii")
moving_image=sitk.ReadImage("moving_image.nii")

# Set up the registration method
registration=sitk.ImageRegistrationMethod()
registration.SetMetricAsMeanSquares()
registration.SetOptimizerAsRegularStepGradientDescent(learningR
ate=2.0, minStep=1e-4, numberOfIterations=500)
registration.SetInterpolator(sitk.sitkLinear)

# Set the transformation type
transform=sitk.CenteredTransformInitializer(fixed_image, moving_
image, sitk.Euler3DTransform())
registration.SetInitialTransform(transform, inPlace=False)

# Execute the registration
final_transform=registration.Execute(fixed_image, moving_image)
print("Final metric value:", registration.GetMetricValue())
```

3.3.2.2 Elastix

Elastix is a specialized registration toolkit particularly known for its flexibility and strong support for deformable registration. It builds on ITK and provides additional registration methods and metrics tailored for medical images, making it a popular choice in clinical research. Users define parameter files to specify the registration configuration, which enables a high degree of customization without requiring code changes. Elastix is available as a command-line tool, and it can also be accessed through Python using PyElastix.

In typical use, Elastix is employed for nonrigid (deformable) registration tasks, such as aligning brain MRI scans, lung CT images, or other medical images where anatomical structures may vary in shape or size. The deformable registration approach in Elastix can be controlled with a B-spline transformation, which enables smooth, local deformations across the image based on a grid of control points. This approach provides significant flexibility to adapt to local anatomical differences while maintaining a coherent global structure. The example provided in Python shows a basic setup using PyElastix:

```
import elastix

# Define file paths
fixed_image = "fixed_image.nii"
moving_image = "moving_image.nii"
output_dir = "output"

# Set up and run Elastix registration

elastix = elastix.ElastixInterface()
elastix.register(fixed_image=fixed_image, moving_image=moving_image,
output_dir=output_dir, parameters=["parameters.txt"])

# Read and display the results

result_image = elastix.get_transformix_output_image()
```

REFERENCES

1. FreeSurfer, Fischl B. *NeuroImage* 62.2 (2012):774–781.
2. Klein, Stefan, et al. "Automatic segmentation of the prostate in 3D MR images by atlas matching using localized mutual information." *Medical Physics* 35.4 (2008): 1407–1417.
3. Liu, Li, Haocheng Sun, and Fanzhang Li. "A Lie group kernel learning method for medical image classification." *Pattern Recognition* 142 (2023): 109735.
4. Song, Xinrui, et al. "Transformed grid distance loss for supervised image registration." In Alessa Hering, Julia Schnabel, Miaomiao Zhang, Enzo Ferrante, Mattias Heinrich, Daniel Rueckert (eds), *Biomedical Image Registration*. Cham: Springer International Publishing, 2022.177–181.
5. Sotiras, Aristeidis, Christos Davatzikos, and Nikos Paragios. "Deformable medical image registration: A survey." *IEEE Transactions on Medical Imaging* 32.7 (2013): 1153–1190.
6. Cheng, Xi, Li Zhang, and Yefeng Zheng. "Deep similarity learning for multi-modal medical images." *Computer Methods in Biomechanics and Biomedical Engineering: Imaging & Visualization* 6 (2016): 1–5.
7. Simonovsky, Martin, Benjamín Gutirrez-Becker, Diana Mateus, Nassir Navab, and Nikos Komodakis. "A deep metric for multimodal registration." *Medical Image Computing and Computer-Assisted Intervention—MICCAI: 19th International Conference,* Athens, Greece, October 17–21, 2016, Proceedings, Part III, pp. 10–18.
8. Zagoruyko, Sergey, and Nikos Komodakis. "Learning to compare image patches via convolutional neural networks." *IEEE Conference on Computer Vision and Pattern Recognition (CVPR)*, Boston, MA, June 7–12, 2015, pp. 4353–4361.
9. Haskins, Grant, et al. "Learning deep similarity metric for 3D MR–TRUS image registration." *International Journal of Computer Assisted Radiology and Surgery* 14 (2019): 417–425.
10. Liao, Rui, Shun Miao, Pierre de Tournemire, Sasa Grbic, Ali Kamen, Tommaso Mansi, and Dorin Comaniciu. "An artificial agent for robust image registration." *AAAI'17: Proceedings of the Thirty-First AAAI Conference on Artificial Intelligence*, San Francisco, CA, February 4, 2017, pp. 4168–4175.
11. Ma, Kai, Jiangping Wang, Vivek Singh, Birgi Tamersoy, Yao-Jen Chang, Andreas Wimmer, and Terrence Chen. "Multimodal image registration with deep context reinforcement learning." *International Conference on Medical Image Computing and Computer-Assisted Intervention—MICCAI 2017: 20th International Conference*, Quebec City, QC, Canada,, September 11–13, 2017, pp. 240–248. Springer.
12. Wang, Ziyu, Tom Schaul, Matteo Hessel, Hado Van Hasselt, Marc Lanctot, and Nando De Freitas. "Dueling network architectures for deep reinforcement learning." arXiv preprint arXiv:1511.06581, 2015.

13. Hoffmann, Malte, et al. "Anatomy-aware and acquisition-agnostic joint registration with synthmorph." *Imaging Neuroscience* 2 (2024), 2 imag–2–00197.
14. Song, Xinrui, et al. "Cross-modal attention for multi-modal image registration." *Medical Image Analysis* 82 (2022): 102612.
15. Mok, Tony C. W., and Albert Chung. "Affine medical image registration with coarse-to-fine vision transformer." *2022 IEEE/CVF Conference on Computer Vision and Pattern Recognition (CVPR)*, New Orleans, LA, USA, 2022, pp. 20803-20812.
16. Guo, Hengtao, et al. "Sensorless freehand 3D ultrasound reconstruction via deep contextual learning." *Medical Image Computing and Computer Assisted Intervention–MICCAI 2020: 23rd International Conference*, Lima, Peru, October 4–8, 2020, Proceedings, Part III 23. Springer International Publishing, 2020.
17. Guo, Hengtao, et al. "End-to-end ultrasound frame to volume registration." *Medical Image Computing and Computer Assisted Intervention–MICCAI 2021: 24th International Conference,* Strasbourg, France, September 27–October 1, 2021, Proceedings, Part IV 24. Springer International Publishing, 2021.
18. Guo, Hengtao, et al. "Ultrasound frame-to-volume registration via deep learning for interventional guidance." *IEEE Transactions on Ultrasonics, Ferroelectrics, and Frequency Control* 70.9 (2022): 1016–1025.
19. Luo, Mingyuan, et al. "Deep motion network for freehand 3D ultrasound reconstruction." In *Medical Image Computing and Computer Assisted Intervention – MICCAI 2022: 25th International Conference*, Singapore, September 18–22, 2022, Proceedings, Part IV, Singapore, Cham: Springer Nature Switzerland, 2022.https://doi.org/10.1007/978-3-031-16440-8_28
20. Prevost, Raphael, et al. "3D freehand ultrasound without external tracking using deep learning." *Medical Image Analysis* 48 (2018): 187–202.
21. Balakrishnan, Guha, et al. "Voxelmorph: A learning framework for deformable medical image registration." *IEEE Transactions on Medical Imaging* 38.8 (2019): 1788–1800.
22. Chen, Junyu, et al. "Transmorph: Transformer for unsupervised medical image registration." *Medical Image Analysis* 82 (2022): 102615.
23. Shi, Jiacheng, et al. "Xmorpher: Full transformer for deformable medical image registration via cross attention." *Medical Image Computing and Computer Assisted Intervention – MICCAI 2022: 25th International Conference, Singapore, September 18–22, 2022, Proceedings, Part VI*, Singapore, Cham: Springer Nature Switzerland, 2022. https://doi.org/10.1007/978-3-031-16446-0_21
24. Jia, Xi, et al. "U-net vs transformer: Is u-net outdated in medical image registration?" *Machine Learning in Medical Imaging: 13th International Workshop, MLMI 2022, Held in Conjunction with MICCAI 2022*, Singapore, September 18, 2022, Proceedings, Singapore, 2022, Cham: Springer Nature Switzerland,. https://doi.org/10.1007/978-3-031-21014-3_16
25. Hu, Yipeng, et al. "Weakly-supervised convolutional neural networks for multimodal image registration." *Medical Image Analysis* 49 (2018): 1–13.
26. Hering, Alessa, et al. "Learn2Reg: Comprehensive multi-task medical image registration challenge, dataset and evaluation in the era of deep learning." *IEEE Transactions on Medical Imaging* 42.3 (2022): 697–712.
27. Lowe, David G. "Distinctive image features from scale-invariant keypoints." *International Journal of Computer Vision* 60 (2004): 91–110.
28. Rister, Blaine, Mark A. Horowitz, and Daniel L. Rubin. "Volumetric image registration from invariant keypoints." *IEEE Transactions on Image Processing* 26.10 (2017): 4900–4910.
29. Allaire, Stephane, John J. Kim, Stephen L. Breen, David A. Jaffray, and Vladimir Pekar. "Full orientation invariance and improved feature selectivity of 3D SIFT with application to medical image analysis," *2008 IEEE Computer Society Conference on Computer Vision and Pattern Recognition Workshops*, Anchorage, AK, June 23–28, 2008, pp. 1–8.
30. Ni, Dong, et al. "Volumetric ultrasound panorama based on 3D SIFT." *Medical Image Computing and Computer Assisted Intervention* 11 (2008): 52–60.
31. Heinrich, Mattias P., et al. "MIND: Modality independent neighbourhood descriptor for multi-modal deformable registration." *Medical Image Analysis* 16.7 (2012): 1423–1435.
32. Yan, Ke, et al. "SAM: Self-supervised learning of pixel-wise anatomical embeddings in radiological images." *IEEE Transactions on Medical Imaging* 41.10 (2022): 2658–2669.
33. Li, Zi, et al. "Samconvex: Fast discrete optimization for ct registration using self-supervised anatomical embedding and correlation pyramid." *Medical Image Computing and Computer Assisted Intervention – MICCAI 2023: 26th International Conference*, Vancouver, BC, Canada, October 8–12, 2023, Proceedings, Part X, Vancouver, BC, Canada,. Cham: Springer Nature Switzerland, 2023.

34. Mok, Tony C. W., et al. "Modality-agnostic structural image representation learning for deformable multi-modality medical image registration." *Proceedings of the IEEE/CVF Conference on Computer Vision and Pattern Recognition*. Seattle, WA, USA, 2024, pp. 11215–11225.
35. Bai, Xiaoyu, Fan Bai, Xiaofei Huo, Jia Ge, Jingjing Lu, Xianghua Ye, Ke Yan, and Yong Xia. "UAE: Universal anatomical embedding on multi-modality medical images." 2023.
36. Siebert, Hanna, et al. "ConvexAdam: Self-configuring dual-optimisation-based 3D multitask medical image registration." *IEEE Transactions on Medical Imaging* 44.2 (2024): 738–748.
37. Isensee, Fabian, et al. "nnU-Net: A self-configuring method for deep learning-based biomedical image segmentation." *Nature Methods* 18.2 (2021): 203–211.
38. Song, Xinrui, Xuanang Xu, and Pingkun Yan. "General purpose image encoder DINOv2 for medical image registration." arXiv preprint arXiv:2402.15687 (2024).
39. Song, Xinrui, Xuanang Xu, and Pingkun Yan. "DINO-Reg: General purpose image encoder for training-free multi-modal deformable medical image registration." *Medical Image Computing and Computer Assisted Intervention – MICCAI 2024: 27th International Conference*, Marrakesh, Morocco, October 6–10, 2024, Proceedings, Part II, Marrakesh, Morocco. Cham: Springer Nature Switzerland, 2024, pp. 608–617. https://doi.org/10.1007/978-3-031-72069-7_57
40. Oquab, Maxime, et al. "Dinov2: Learning robust visual features without supervision." arXiv preprint arXiv:2304.07193 (2023).

4 Empowering Innovation in Medical Imaging with AI-Based Radiomics

Amgad Muneer, Joe Y. Chang, and Jia Wu

4.1 INTRODUCTION

Radiomics, a transformative field in medical imaging, marks a shift toward extracting and analyzing quantitative data from medical images [1], especially in oncology applications [2–4]. It converts standard imaging modalities—such as computed tomography (CT), magnetic resonance imaging (MRI), and positron emission tomography (PET)—into high-dimensional data that captures detailed tissue and lesion characteristics. These quantitative imaging features, often imperceptible to the human eye, capture vital information about shape, texture, intensity, and spatial relationships within the image [5,6]. By doing so, radiomics transitions imaging from a primarily qualitative field into a data-driven, quantifiable one, offering deeper insights into disease biology [5,7,8].

Traditionally, the analysis of medical images has been subjective, relying on the visual interpretation of radiologists or oncologists, who assess features such as tumor size, shape, and density [9]. While this form of visual assessment has been integral to diagnostic and therapeutic decision-making for decades, it is inherently limited by interobserver variability and the qualitative nature of image interpretation [10]. Radiomics offers an objective alternative by converting these visual assessments into a comprehensive set of quantitative features [11]. For example, rather than describing a tumor as simply "round" or "irregular," radiomics provides detailed shape metrics, such as surface area and volume, or mathematical descriptions of texture variations. This wealth of data can then be incorporated into predictive models, offering clinicians a robust tool for risk stratification [12], treatment response prediction [13], and long-term prognosis [10].

One of the core strengths of radiomics lies in its ability to capture subtle imaging patterns and heterogeneity within tumors [10]. Tumor heterogeneity (variations in cellular composition, microenvironment, and genetic mutations) plays a critical role in disease progression and therapeutic response [14,15]. Radiomics enables the quantitative characterization of this heterogeneity, allowing for the identification of imaging biomarkers that may correlate with the underlying pathophysiology [16–18].

Artificial intelligence (AI) refers to computational techniques that enable machines to perform tasks typically done by humans [19]. AI is increasingly used in cancer research for diagnosing cancer [20], predicting outcomes [21], optimizing treatments, and improving clinical trial designs by analyzing large datasets like medical images and genomic information [1,22]. Deep learning (DL) algorithms are divided into supervised, unsupervised, and reinforcement learning (Figure 4.1).

Supervised learning is the most widely used, where models are trained on labeled datasets [23]. For each input (e.g., a medical image), a corresponding label is provided (e.g., tumor vs. non-tumor). The model learns to make predictions by identifying patterns between the input and its label. This approach is often used in cancer imaging to classify tumor types or predict treatment outcomes using well-labeled datasets of medical scans. Unsupervised learning does not require labeled data. The model detects patterns or structures within the data without explicit guidance [24]. It is useful for tasks like clustering tumors with similar characteristics, identifying anomalies, or discovering

DOI: 10.1201/9781003480365-5

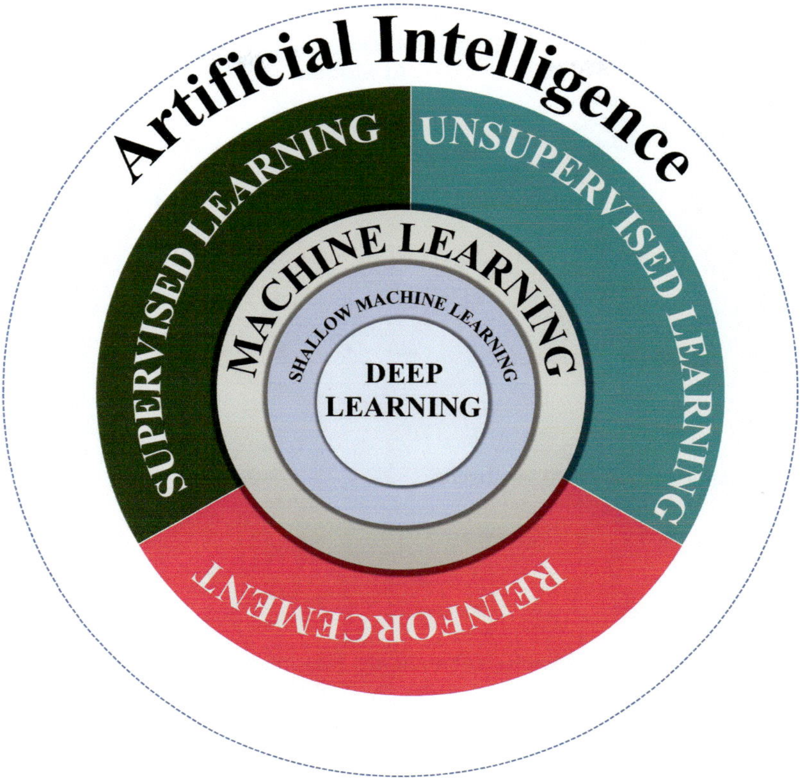

FIGURE 4.1 Hierarchical structure of artificial intelligence and its subfields.

hidden subtypes of cancer based on imaging or genomic data [25,26]. Self-supervised learning (SSL) [27], a subset of unsupervised learning, involves the model generating its own labels through tasks like reconstructing incomplete medical images [28] or predicting missing genetic sequences [29]. This technique is often used for pretraining models before fine-tuning them with supervised methods for cancer detection or prognosis [27]. Reinforcement learning (RL) involves an agent interacting with its environment, learning from feedback in the form of rewards and penalties. The goal is to optimize decisions over time [30]. In cancer research, RL is applied to personalize treatment regimens, where the agent learns to adjust treatment strategies (like chemotherapy or radiotherapy dosing) to maximize patient outcomes based on individual responses, or to optimize clinical trial designs for better treatment efficacy [31,32].

The integration of AI with radiomics has advanced the field, allowing for the analysis of large-scale imaging datasets and the development of predictive models, as shown in Figure 4.2. Machine learning (ML) and DL techniques have proven highly effective in automating feature extraction, identifying complex nonlinear relationships between radiomic features and clinical outcomes [33,34]. AI-based radiomics surpasses traditional methods by enabling models to learn directly from data, reducing the need for manual feature selection [35]. The synergy between AI and radiomics enhances prediction accuracy and helps discover novel imaging biomarkers often missed with traditional techniques.

In precision radiation therapy (RT), AI-driven radiomics offers the potential to personalize treatment plans [33]. By analyzing pre- and intra-treatment imaging, radiomics provides insights into tumor biology, guiding decisions on radiation dose, fractionation, and adaptive therapy. It also aids

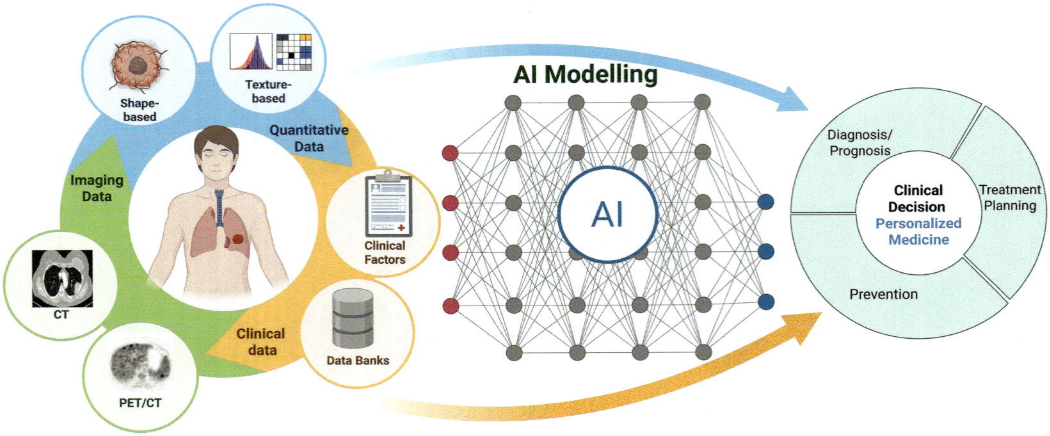

FIGURE 4.2 Radiomics and artificial intelligence.

in predicting radiation-induced toxicities, balancing treatment efficacy, and minimizing adverse effects [8]. Additionally, early radiomic changes can indicate treatment response, allowing timely adjustments to radiation plans. Therefore, combining radiomic, clinical, and genomic data, AI models can improve patient stratification, predict outcomes, and tailor treatments to individual tumor characteristics, aligning with precision medicine principles.

This chapter presents a comprehensive exploration of AI-based radiomics in RT. It begins with an overview of the fundamental concepts and principles of radiomics analysis, including image acquisition, segmentation, feature extraction, and modeling. Following this, the methods of radiomics analysis are examined, highlighting both hand-crafted radiomics and DL techniques. The chapter then explores AI's role in radiomics applications for detection, tumor characterization, and treatment response in RT. Key factors influencing radiomic features and strategies for harmonizing these features, including feature selection and correction methods, are also discussed.

4.2 CONCEPT AND PRINCIPLES OF RADIOMICS ANALYSIS

Based on the guidelines set by the National Cancer Institute's (NCI) Quantitative Imaging Network (QIN), radiomics workflow typically involves four steps, as presented in Figure 4.3, image acquisition, imaging segmentation, feature extraction, radiomics analysis, and modeling. These steps of radiomics workflow are discussed in technical depth in the following subsection.

4.2.1 Image Acquisition and Imaging Modalities in Radiotherapy

Medical imaging is fundamental to the success of modern radiotherapy, serving as a cornerstone for precise treatment planning, accurate delivery, and thorough posttreatment monitoring [10]. The primary imaging modalities used in radiotherapy are CT, PET with fluorodeoxyglucose (FDG), and MRI, which offer unique insights into tumor anatomy, metabolism, and functional characteristics (Figure 4.4). These imaging techniques complement each other, providing crucial data that guide clinicians in designing personalized radiation treatment plans that maximize tumor control while minimizing damage to surrounding healthy tissues.

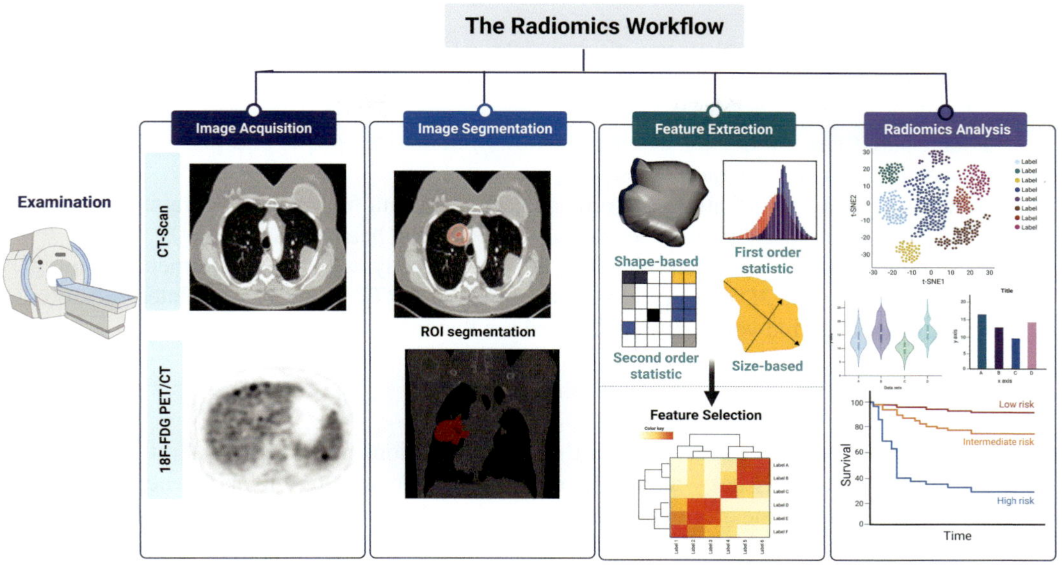

FIGURE 4.3 The radiomics workflow. First, high-quality medical images like CT or PET/CT scans are acquired. These images are then processed to segment the region of interest (ROI), such as tumors or specific subregions (i.e., habitats). Following segmentation, various quantitative features, including shape, texture, and intensity, are extracted. Finally, these features are analyzed, often combined with clinical and genomic data, to develop diagnostic, predictive, or prognostic models, enabling prediction of key outcomes.

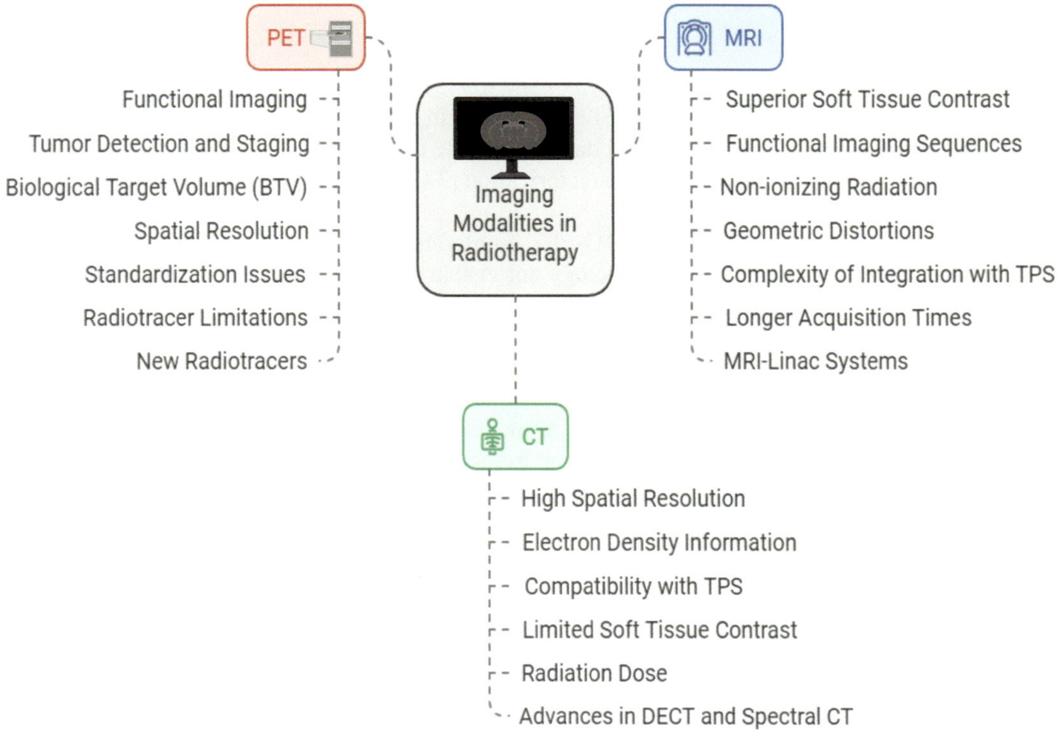

FIGURE 4.4 Significant and limitations of imaging modalities.

4.2.1.1 CT

CT is crucial for radiotherapy planning, offering detailed anatomical images to define tumor boundaries and nearby critical organs (OARs) [36]. Its key benefits include:

- High Spatial Resolution: CT accurately shows tumor size, shape, and position, enabling precise targeting during radiotherapy [37].
- Electron Density Information: CT provides essential data for dose calculations, ensuring precise radiation distribution to the tumor while sparing healthy tissues.
- Treatment Planning Compatibility: CT integrates easily with most treatment planning systems (TPS), like 3D conformal radiotherapy (3D-CRT), intensity-modulated radiation therapy (IMRT), and volumetric modulated arc therapy (VMAT).

On the other hand, CT has some limitations in RT:

- Limited Soft Tissue Contrast: One of the main limitations of CT is its inability to distinguish between soft tissues with similar densities. This can be problematic when targeting tumors located in or near critical structures such as the brain or pelvic organs, where high soft tissue contrast is essential.
- Radiation Dose: CT exposes patients to additional ionizing radiation. While the doses are relatively low compared to therapeutic radiation doses, repeated scans or CT simulations may contribute to cumulative radiation exposure.

To this end, advances in dual-energy CT (DECT) and spectral CT hold promise for improving the tissue characterization capabilities of CT in radiotherapy. These emerging technologies offer enhanced tissue contrast and improved material differentiation, which could be valuable for delineating tumors and OARs with greater accuracy.

4.2.1.2 PET in Radiotherapy with FDG (FDG-PET)

PET in radiotherapy with FDG (FDG-PET) is essential in radiotherapy, particularly for metabolically active tumors. It provides functional data on glucose metabolism, complementing anatomical imaging (CT or MRI) for better tumor characterization [37]. Key advantages include:

- Functional Imaging: Unlike CT, FDG-PET highlights areas of increased glucose metabolism, offering insights into tumor biology not visible on anatomical scans. This is particularly useful in identifying active tumor regions that may not be apparent on anatomical imaging alone.
- Tumor Detection and Staging: FDG-PET is highly sensitive for detecting metastases and staging cancers, such as in lung, lymphoma, and head and neck cancers.
- Biological Target Volume (BTV): PET helps define metabolically active tumor regions, enabling more precise radiation targeting, especially in advanced techniques like stereotactic body radiation therapy (SBRT) and IMRT.

On the side, FDG-PET imaging has some limitations in RT:

- Spatial Resolution: PET has lower spatial resolution than CT or MRI, leading to blurred images and potential inaccuracies in delineating tumor boundaries.
- Standardization Issues: Variability in FDG uptake can complicate consistency across institutions, affecting treatment planning.
- Radiotracer Limitations: FDG's non-specificity can cause false positives in inflammatory or infectious tissues, complicating scan interpretation.

To address this, newer radiotracers, such as F-MISO for hypoxia imaging and FLT for cellular proliferation, are being developed to overcome FDG's limitations. These tracers could provide more specific information about tumor biology, including hypoxic regions that may require dose escalation or areas of rapid proliferation that could influence treatment strategies.

4.2.1.3 MRI in RT

MRI is highly valuable in radiotherapy due to its excellent soft tissue contrast, which enables precise tumor delineation, especially in complex areas like the brain, prostate, and pelvis. MRI also offers various imaging sequences for anatomical, functional, and metabolic information without ionizing radiation [37]. Key advantages include:

- Superior Soft Tissue Contrast: MRI excels at differentiating soft tissues, crucial for accurate tumor localization in areas like the brain, where CT may struggle.
- Functional Imaging Sequences: Techniques like DWI and DCE-MRI provide insights into tumor cellularity and vascularity, enhancing RT planning.
- Nonionizing Radiation: MRI allows for repeated imaging without radiation exposure, supporting real-time monitoring and adaptive radiotherapy (MRIgRT) in response to anatomical changes during treatment.

On the other hand, MRI imaging has some limitations, such as:

- Geometric Distortions: MRI can produce geometric distortions, particularly near air-tissue interfaces or metallic implants, which may affect accuracy in treatment planning.
- Complex Integration with Treatment Planning Systems (TPS): MRI lacks electron density data, requiring multi-modality image registration with CT, which can introduce uncertainties.
- Longer Acquisition Times: MRI scans are slower than CT or PET, potentially leading to patient discomfort and motion artifacts.

To this end, MRI-Linac systems, which combine an MRI scanner with a linear accelerator (LINAC), represent a cutting-edge advancement in RT. These systems allow for real-time MRI imaging during radiation delivery, enabling adaptive RT that responds to changes in tumor position, size, and shape during treatment. Finally, variations in acquisition parameters, such as slice thickness, contrast administration, and timing, can significantly affect the accuracy of tumor delineation and the reproducibility of radiomic features. Standardizing these protocols across different imaging modalities is essential to ensure that RT treatments are based on consistent, high-quality imaging data.

4.2.2 Segmentation

Segmentation is a crucial step in the radiomics workflow, where the region of interest (ROI) or the volume of interest (VOI), often a tumor, is delineated from surrounding tissues on medical images, as well as the organs at risk (OAR). The ROI typically refers to a 2D area, such as a specific slice of an X-ray or MRI, while the VOI applies to 3D volumetric acquisitions (e.g., CT or MRI scans), allowing for the entire tumor to be analyzed in three dimensions. The accuracy of this segmentation process directly influences the quality of the extracted radiomic features [38,39], which are used for downstream analysis, including treatment planning and outcome prediction. Whether the segmentation is performed on 2D images or 3D volumes, the reliability of this process determines the precision of the radiomics map generated for the tumor [38,39]. Errors in segmentation, whether due to variability between algorithms or differences in operator input, can introduce significant variability in the extracted radiomic features, ultimately affecting the robustness and reproducibility of

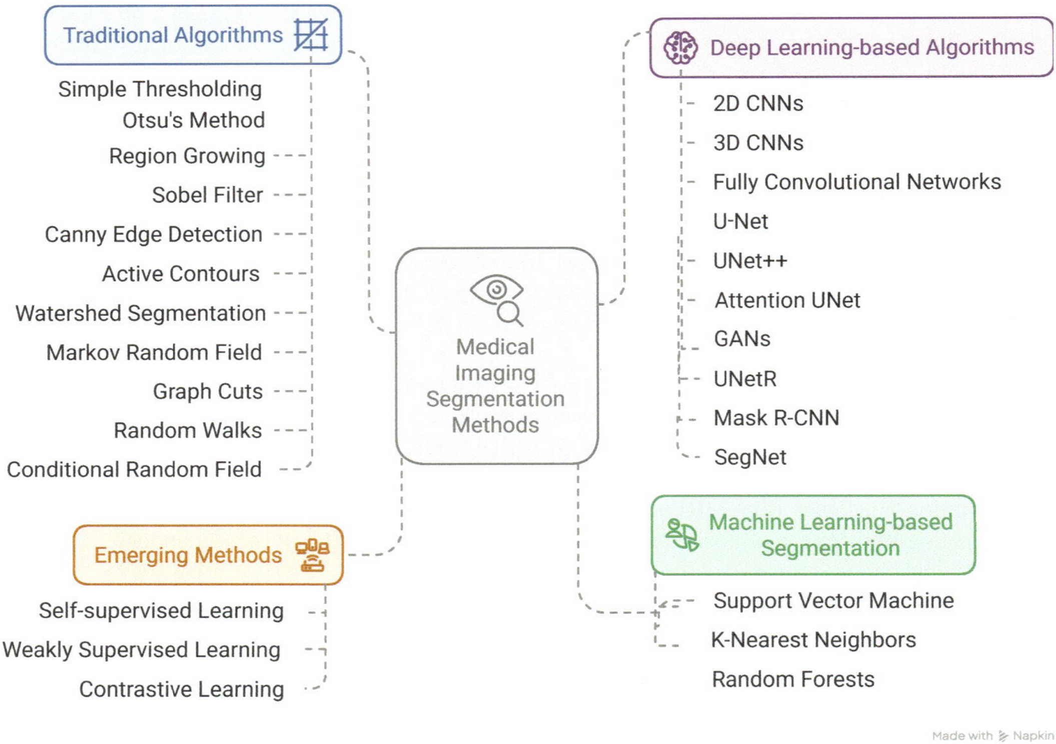

FIGURE 4.5 Overview of medical imaging segmentation methods.

radiomics-based models [37]. Tumor segmentation is particularly challenging because of indistinct or complex borders, and debates continue about how to establish a reliable and reproducible ground truth. Many segmentation methods have been proposed and studied in the last 20 years; such algorithms are summarized in Figure 4.5.

4.2.2.1 Traditional Algorithms

Traditional medical imaging segmentation methods, while effective in specific cases, often face limitations when dealing with complex or high-dimensional images [37]. As a result, they have been increasingly supplemented by advanced techniques like ML and DL. One of the most fundamental methods is simple thresholding, which converts an image into a binary format based on a predefined intensity threshold. Pixels with intensities above the threshold are classified as the foreground (object of interest), while those below are designated as the background [40]. Though simple thresholding is fast and computationally efficient, it tends to perform poorly in images with uneven lighting or when clear intensity distinctions between regions are lacking. Otsu's method improves upon simple thresholding by automatically determining the optimal threshold value [41]. It calculates this threshold by minimizing the intraclass variance, which ensures that the differences within the segmented regions are minimal. Otsu's method is highly effective for images with a bimodal intensity distribution but can produce suboptimal results for images with a unimodal or multimodal intensity histogram.

Region growing begins from a seed point and expands the segmented area by incorporating neighboring pixels with similar properties, like intensity or texture [42]. This method is beneficial for segmenting connected regions but is sensitive to noise and depends on the accurate selection of the initial seed. Poor seed placement or noise can lead to incorrect region expansion. The Sobel filter is a gradient-based technique used for detecting edges in an image by highlighting regions of high spatial frequency [43]. It works by calculating the gradient magnitude of the image, emphasizing boundaries between different regions. While Sobel is simple and effective for detecting edges, it may amplify noise, particularly in areas where the gradient is not well-defined. Canny edge detection is an algorithm with multiple stages: noise reduction, gradient calculation, non-maximum suppression, and edge tracking by hysteresis. It excels at detecting strong edges while minimizing the effects of noise, making it a robust option for boundary detection, though it requires more computational resources than simpler edge detection techniques.

Active contours, also known as snakes, use an iterative approach to evolve an initial contour around the tumor based on image gradient and boundary information. While effective for well-defined lesions, active contour models struggle with tumors that have complex or poorly defined margins [44]. The evolution is guided by image forces (such as gradient) and internal forces (to maintain smoothness). This method is particularly effective for capturing object shapes, but its success is highly dependent on the initialization and may get stuck in local minima if not properly tuned. Watershed segmentation treats the image's pixel intensities as a topographic surface, where high intensity corresponds to peaks and low intensity to valleys [45]. The algorithm "floods" the image from local minima, segmenting it into distinct regions at watershed lines. While this approach is useful for separating overlapping objects, it is prone to over-segmentation [46], particularly in noisy images. Markov random field (MRF) models the relationships between neighboring pixels, treating them as dependent random variables [47]. This method is useful for segmentation tasks that require spatial context, as it encourages smoothness within regions. MRFs can be powerful, but their computational complexity increases significantly with larger images or more complex spatial relationships. Graph cuts reformulate image segmentation as a graph partitioning problem, where each pixel is treated as a node in the graph, and edges represent the similarity between neighboring pixels [48]. The algorithm segments the image by cutting the graph in a way that separates foreground from background. This method is robust and produces high-quality results, though it can be computationally demanding [49].

Random walks are a probabilistic method in which a random walker starts from predefined seed points and traverses the image [50]. The probability of a walker reaching a certain pixel determines its classification as either foreground or background. Random walks are effective in handling noisy images and uncertain regions but can require significant computational resources depending on the image size. Conditional random fields (CRF) extend Markov random fields by incorporating additional observation-based features, making them more flexible and capable of capturing complex contextual relationships in images [51]. CRFs are widely used for labeling tasks and offer superior performance in applications where contextual dependencies between pixels are important. However, their flexibility comes at the cost of increased computational complexity, particularly during training and inference [52].

4.2.2.2 Machine Learning-Based Algorithms

ML-based algorithms have been widely applied in medical imaging for tumor segmentation and cancer detection [53,54]. These methods rely on predefined features extracted from images and use statistical models to classify regions of interest, helping differentiate between tumor and healthy tissues based on learned patterns. Support vector machine (SVM) is a supervised algorithm that distinguishes tumor regions by identifying the optimal boundary (hyperplane) separating different tissue types. It is particularly effective in binary classification tasks but may struggle with highly imbalanced datasets [54]. Ayachi and Amor [55] used SVM as a segmentation method for brain tumor segmentation, demonstrating its application in distinguishing tumor tissue from normal brain tissue. Similarly, Amin et al. [56] developed an automated method to classify brain tumors as malignant or benign using MRI images, where an SVM classifier, combined with cross-validation, yielded high-performance metrics: 97.1% accuracy, 91.9% sensitivity, and 98.0% specificity.

Additionally, Padlia et al. [43] applied SVM for brain tumor detection using T1-weighted and FLAIR images, utilizing feature extraction techniques to enhance segmentation accuracy. K-nearest neighbors (K-NN) classifies pixels based on the labels of their "k" closest neighbors in the feature space [57]. In tumor segmentation, K-NN assigns a label (tumor or non-tumor) based on a majority vote from nearby pixels. It is simple but computationally expensive for large datasets and sensitive to noisy data. Khalid et al. [58] proposed K-NN for segmenting abnormalities in MRI brain images. The method analyses characteristics like minimum, maximum, and mean gray-level pixel values for different brain components. The K-NN segmentation involves determining the k value, calculating Euclidean distances, sorting minimum distances, and assigning the majority class. Purwono et al. [59] used K-NN for segmenting cervical cancer in CT-scan images. Two feature extraction methods were applied, and experiments were conducted with different K values (K=3, 5, and 9). Results indicated that accuracy was around 59.4%, with larger K values slightly reducing accuracy. Random forests (RFs) use an ensemble of decision trees to segment tumor regions. Each tree in the forest provides a classification, and the final segmentation is determined by majority voting [60]. RFs are robust and can handle high-dimensional, complex medical data, making them effective for segmenting tumors with varying features. However, they can be computationally intensive with large datasets. Hartmann et al. [61] used RF for medical image segmentation, and they compared its performance with deep convolutional neural networks (DCNN). Cao et al. [62] demonstrated the effectiveness of RF for automated segmentation of the glomerular basement membrane in transmission electron microscopy images. These algorithms offer efficient segmentation, though they are often surpassed by DL methods in handling large and complex medical imaging datasets.

4.2.2.3 Deep Learning-Based Segmentation Methods

DL-based segmentation methods have revolutionized medical imaging by enabling automatic feature extraction and end-to-end learning, which significantly improves the accuracy and robustness of tumor and cancer segmentation [63]. These methods leverage large datasets and advanced architectures to learn complex patterns directly from imaging, offering superior performance in challenging segmentation tasks [64]. 2D and 3D convolutional neural networks (CNNs) are foundational DL architectures for medical image segmentation [64–66]. In cancer segmentation, 2D CNNs process individual image slices, while 3D CNNs can analyze volumetric data, making them more effective for segmenting tumors with intricate spatial structures. CNNs automatically learn hierarchical features from the images, improving segmentation accuracy, especially in high-resolution datasets. Fully convolutional networks (FCNs) extend CNNs by replacing the fully connected layers with convolutional layers, allowing the network to produce pixel-wise segmentation maps. FCNs are widely used in medical image segmentation, particularly for delineating tumor boundaries, as they enable the entire image to be processed in one forward pass, improving both speed and accuracy. Gan et al. [66] implemented a hybrid 2D and 3D convolutional neural network for automated delineation of lung tumors from CT images. 3D CNN, designed based on V-Net, extracted tumor context information from the sequences of CT images, and a 2D CNN with an encoder–decoder structure and dense connections enhanced feature propagation. The hybrid module was used to fuse 2D and 3D features. The hybrid CNN was comparatively studied with individual 2D and 3D CNNs, and in addition, the relation that existed between the segmentation performance of the proposed hybrid CNN models and the GTV volume size is analyzed. Hassanzadeh et al. [64] further explore the development of 3D networks from 2D images and Neuro-evolutionary 2D networks for 3D volume segmentation. They advocate the creation of evolutional deep 2D networks on medical image segmentation, then the conversion to 3D networks. This approach significantly reduces computational time while maintaining high accuracy for 3D medical image segmentation across nine datasets.

U-net and U-net++ are popular DL architectures specifically designed for biomedical image segmentation [63,65,67]. U-net uses an encoder–decoder structure with skip connections to capture both low-level and high-level features, making it highly effective for precise tumor segmentation [67]. U-Net++ builds on this by introducing denser skip connections, further improving segmentation performance, especially in complex tumor shapes and structures [68]. Attention U-net enhances the traditional U-net by integrating attention mechanisms that allow the network to focus on the most relevant regions in the image, such as tumors [69,70]. This attention-guided approach helps in identifying subtle details in medical images, making it particularly useful for segmenting small or poorly defined tumors [68]. Generative adversarial networks (GANs) are used to improve segmentation by generating synthetic data that enhances the model's robustness [71]. Salehjahromi et al. [72] have introduced a conditional generative adversarial network (cGAN) pipeline capable of generating FDG-PET images from diagnostic CT scans, specifically designed for multicenter. In tumor segmentation, GANs can refine segmentation outputs by learning from real and generated examples, leading to more accurate predictions, particularly in cases with limited labeled data. UNetR [73] and Mask R-CNN [74] are advanced models that incorporate transformer-based architectures and region-based segmentation, respectively. UNetR leverages vision transformers for better context understanding, making it suitable for large tumor regions or cases with substantial anatomical variability [73]. Mask R-CNN, on the other hand, extends traditional object detection methods by adding a mask prediction branch [74], making it effective for precise tumor segmentation and localization. SegNet is another encoder–decoder architecture that focuses on efficient pixel-wise segmentation [75], and it performs well in terms of computational efficiency and memory usage, making it suitable for segmenting large 3D datasets [76].

4.2.2.4 Emerging Segmentation Methods

Emerging segmentation methods like self-supervised, weakly supervised, and contrastive learning are gaining significant attention and driving innovation in medical imaging. These methods integrate advanced learning techniques to overcome the limitations of traditional, ML and DL approaches [77]. They offer novel solutions for handling complex medical images, such as tumor or cancer segmentation, where labeled data may be scarce, or tumors exhibit significant variability in appearance [78,79]. SSL is a cutting-edge approach where the model learns representations from unlabeled data by solving auxiliary tasks, such as predicting missing parts of an image or reconstructing images [78]. In tumor segmentation, SSL allows models to pretrain on vast amounts of unlabeled medical images, enhancing their ability to generalize and segment tumors accurately even with limited labeled data [80]. Dhere and Sivaswamy [77] applied SSL for kidney cancer segmentation using CT images, introducing a novel proxy task to enhance the segmentation process. Bai et al. [79] present an SSL approach for training a cardiac MR image segmentation network where features are learned by predicting anatomical positions. These positions act as supervisory signals without the need for additional manual annotations. The SSL method outperforms or matches a U-net trained from scratch in small data settings. Compared to the baseline U-net, the SSL [79] method improves the average Dice metric for short-axis image segmentation from 0.811 to 0.852 using only five annotated subjects. Ouyang et al. [78] proposed a novel self-supervised few-shot semantic segmentation for medical images called SSLALPNet that does away with the need for annotations during its training process. The method uses superpixel-based pseudo-labels as supervision signals and introduces an adaptive local prototype pooling module to enhance segmentation accuracy. The approach was validated across three tasks: organ segmentation in abdominal CT and MRI images, and cardiac segmentation in MRI images.

Weakly supervised learning addresses the challenge of acquiring precise pixel-wise annotations for medical images, which can be time-consuming and costly. This method uses weak labels, such as image-level or region-level annotations, to guide the segmentation process. In tumor segmentation, weakly supervised models can learn to segment tumors from coarse or partial labels, reducing the need for extensive manual annotation while maintaining accuracy [81]. Feng et al. [82] propose a two-stage, weakly supervised framework for medical image segmentation. The first stage performs coarse segmentation using class activation maps (CAM) generated by an image classification model to detect the presence or absence of a nodule in each slice. In the second stage, fine-grained instance-level segmentation is achieved by selecting the ROI around each localized instance in the

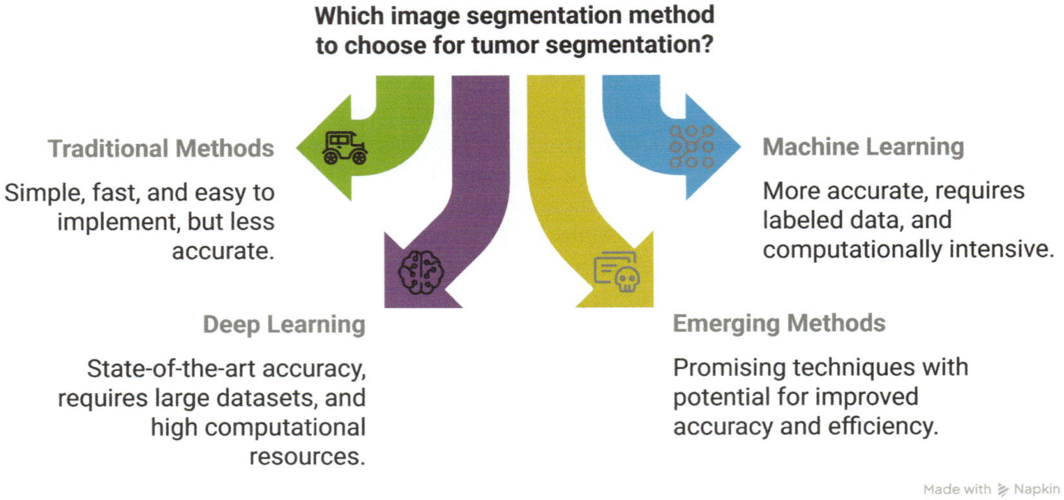

FIGURE 4.6 Comparison of image segmentation methods for tumor segmentation.

CAM, while masking out everything outside this region. Zhai et al. [83] propose a two-stage weakly supervised learning framework called PASeg for annotating 3D medical images. In this approach, the annotator only needs to provide seven points: one inside the target object as a foreground seed and six outside as background seeds.

Contrastive Learning, a particular variant of SSL, is a powerful technique where the model learns to differentiate between similar and dissimilar image pairs [84]. For tumor segmentation, contrastive learning helps the model better understand the subtle differences between tumor and healthy tissues by learning effective representations of tumor features. This method is particularly useful when tumor heterogeneity is high, as it allows the model to focus on the most discriminative features for segmentation. Chaitanya et al. [85] extend contrastive learning for volumetric medical image segmentation with very limited annotations in a semi-supervised setting by exploiting domain- and problem-specific cues. They propose novel contrastive strategies that involve using structural similarities across volumetric images as a domain-specific cue and local contrastive loss to capture distinctive representations for per-pixel segmentation as a problem-specific cue. The method achieves an accuracy within 8% of benchmark performance using just two labeled MRI volumes, representing only 4% (for Automated Cardiac Diagnosis Challenge, ACDC) of the data used to train the benchmark. These emerging methods represent the next wave of advancements in medical image segmentation. By reducing reliance on large, labeled datasets and enhancing the model's ability to learn meaningful representations from the data, they hold great promise for improving the precision and efficiency of tumor and cancer segmentation in clinical practice. A brief comparison of the aforementioned four methods is presented in Figure 4.6 in terms of performance and complexity.

4.2.3 Feature Extraction

After tumor segmentation, features capturing various aspects of a lesion, such as shape, intensity, texture, and wavelet-based properties, are extracted and quantified. These features reflect both the morphological and biological behavior of the tumor and are essential for predicting treatment response and patient outcomes.

TABLE 4.1
Some Shape Features and Their Description

Shape Feature	Description
Volume	Represents the total number of voxels constituting the tumor. Tumor volume is a critical metric in radiation dose planning, with larger tumors often demanding more aggressive treatment regimens.
Surface area	The surface area of the tumor. Tumors with large surface areas relative to their volumes are typically more irregular and invasive, which may complicate treatment targeting.
Sphericity	Measures how closely the tumor approximates a sphere. Lower sphericity often correlates with irregular or infiltrative growth, particularly in aggressive malignancies.
Surface-to-volume ratio	This ratio quantifies the compactness of the tumor. A low ratio suggests a smooth, round lesion, while a higher ratio often indicates a spiculated or irregular lesion.
Compactness	Reflects the tumor's geometric compactness. Low compactness may indicate a more diffuse, irregular growth pattern, often observed in more aggressive tumors.
Elongation	Describes the extent to which a tumor is stretched or elongated along its principal axes. A higher elongation value indicates that the tumor is more elongated, while a value close to 1 suggests it is more spherical.
Maximum 3D diameter	Refers to the longest straight line that can be drawn through the tumor, capturing the largest dimension of the tumor. This feature is relevant for determining the extent of tumor spread and is often used in size-based analyses
Spherical harmonics	A spherical harmonic-based analysis captures complex 3D shape features by decomposing a tumor's structure into harmonics that represent both overall shape and fine irregularities.

4.2.3.1 Shape Features

Shape features are fundamental in radiomics [86], providing critical insights into a tumor's geometric properties, spatial structure, and morphological behavior (Table 4.1). Extracted from 3D reconstructions of segmented lesions, these features help assess tumor growth, invasiveness, and treatment response. Key metrics include tumor volume, which influences RT planning, as larger tumors may require higher doses or advanced techniques like IMRT or SBRT. The surface area, reflecting the tumor's outer boundary, indicates irregularity and invasiveness, often complicating targeting. Sphericity and compactness offer insights into tumor form, with lower sphericity values linked to more aggressive, irregular tumors. The surface-to-volume ratio further quantifies tumor compactness, with higher ratios suggesting more complex growth patterns. In tumor analysis, spherical harmonic-based analysis captures detailed 3D shape characteristics by breaking down the tumor's surface into a series of spherical harmonic functions, each representing different levels of shape complexity [26]. Lower frequencies capture the tumor's overall, symmetrical structure, while higher frequencies highlight irregularities like nodules or protrusions. This decomposition helps classify tumors by identifying unique shape features that correlate with malignancy, growth patterns, or aggressiveness, thus aiding in distinguishing between tumor types and potentially supporting diagnostic and treatment decisions based on shape-based biomarkers. While shape features are crucial for RT planning, especially for irregular tumors, they do not capture the tumor's molecular or cellular characteristics. Nonetheless, they are essential for optimizing radiation targeting, especially in asymmetrical tumors.

4.2.3.2 Intensity Features

Intensity features, or first-order statistical features, describe the distribution of voxel intensities within a tumor, providing a fundamental understanding of its signal intensity without considering spatial relationships [87]. These features, derived directly from pixel or voxel values, are typically represented by histograms and offer insights into tumor density, composition, and metabolic activity, which are key indicators of tumor aggressiveness and treatment response. For example, mean intensity reflects the average voxel intensity within a tumor. In CT scans, intensity is measured in Hounsfield Units (HU), where higher values indicate denser structures, while in PET imaging, it's expressed as standard uptake values (SUV), reflecting glucose metabolism. Tumors with high mean SUVs tend to be more metabolically active and aggressive, potentially requiring more targeted treatment. Standard deviation measures the variability of voxel intensities, with higher values suggesting heterogeneity, which can indicate complex tumors that may pose challenges in treatment planning. Additional features, such as skewness and kurtosis, provide deeper insights into the intensity distribution. Skewness measures the asymmetry of the intensity distribution, with positive skewness possibly indicating areas of necrosis or high metabolic activity. Kurtosis reflects the peakedness of the distribution, where high kurtosis indicates clustered intensities and low kurtosis suggests a more heterogeneous distribution. Entropy, a measure of complexity, is another key feature, with higher values often associated with heterogeneous tumors that may require more sophisticated RT approaches. In RT, intensity features help differentiate between aggressive and indolent tumors. High mean SUV in PET imaging may signal the need for dose escalation, while high standard deviation or entropy indicates radiosensitivity variations within the tumor, necessitating individualized treatment strategies like IMRT.

4.2.3.3 Texture Features

Texture features offer a detailed analysis of the spatial arrangement and relationships between voxel intensities within a tumor, providing critical insights into its internal heterogeneity [88]. These second-order statistical features reveal patterns often invisible to the naked eye and are essential for characterizing tumor aggressiveness, predicting treatment response, and determining clinical outcomes [89]. Unlike intensity features, which focus on voxel value distribution, texture features capture how voxel intensities are spatially organized, reflecting the tumor's structural complexity. A widely used method to quantify texture is the gray-level co-occurrence matrix (GLCM) [90], which measures the frequency of voxel pairs with specific intensities at a given distance and orientation. From the GLCM, features such as contrast, homogeneity, and entropy are derived. Contrast highlights local intensity variation, indicating regions like necrosis or rapid cell proliferation, while homogeneity measures intensity similarity, with lower values pointing to highly heterogeneous, aggressive tumors. The gray-level run length matrix (GLRLM) captures the length of consecutive voxel runs with the same intensity, where features like short-run emphasis indicate fine textures, and long-run emphasis reflects larger homogeneous regions, often corresponding to necrotic areas. Similarly, the gray-level size zone matrix (GLSZM) quantifies the size of uniform intensity zones, offering further insight into the tumor's architecture, such as areas with high cellular density or metabolic activity. Texture features (Table 4.2) are important in RT, as tumor heterogeneity is linked to poor prognosis and treatment resistance. Tumors with high contrast and low homogeneity often contain subclonal populations

TABLE 4.2
Some Texture Features and Their Description

Texture Feature	Description
GLCM	Measures the frequency of voxel pairs with specific intensity values occurring at a certain distance and orientation. GLCM features such as contrast and homogeneity quantify local intensity variations and smoothness.
GLRLM	Describes the length of consecutive runs of voxels with the same intensity, highlighting patterns of homogeneity or heterogeneity within the tumor. Short-run emphasis captures fine textures, while long-run emphasis reflects larger homogeneous regions.
GLSZM	Quantifies the size and number of homogeneous zones within the ROI, providing insights into tumor uniformity or complexity. Larger zones often suggest necrotic or less active regions, while small zones indicate fine texture patterns.
Entropy	Measures the randomness or complexity within a region of interest (e.g., tumor) by assessing the distribution of voxel intensities. In simple terms, it quantifies how heterogeneous or uniform the tissue structure is.

with varying radiosensitivity, complicating treatment. Texture analysis allows for more personalized approaches, such as dose painting, where higher radiation doses are delivered to more aggressive regions. These rich, complex features significantly enhance radiomics-based treatment planning.

Wavelet-based features provide a powerful method for analyzing tumors across multiple scales by decomposing image data into different frequency components [91]. Wavelet transforms capture both fine and coarse textures, offering multi-resolution analysis that reveals details missed by first- and second-order features. High-frequency components often correspond to aggressive, rapidly changing tumor regions, while low-frequency components capture broader, more homogeneous areas. This multi-scale characterization is valuable in adaptive RT, where treatment is adjusted based on tumor changes over time. Following feature extraction, radiomics analysis identifies patterns and correlations within the data, often involving thousands of features. Feature selection then narrows this down to the most relevant ones, which are fed into ML or DL models.

In literature, radiomics representations have shown significant promise in predicting patient outcomes, as they reflect various underlying physiological properties of tumors [35]. These representations can be harnessed in radiomic approaches to develop predictive biomarkers. For instance, image intensity-based values—such as attenuation values from CT scans and physiological data from FDG-PET scans—can be used to quantify the distribution of voxel intensity across a tumor, aiding in the identification of prognostic biomarkers [92] and tumor phenotypes [93]. Tumor heterogeneity is another key area of radiomic analysis, with textural heterogeneity features capturing spatial relationships between voxel intensities within a defined ROI [35,88]. This method allows for a deeper understanding of tumor composition and behavior. Similarly, shape radiomics, which refers to features that describe the three-dimensional structure of a tumor, enhances the assessment of tumor morphology and growth patterns. Recent trials have shown that tracking tumor volume changes throughout treatment can provide more accurate insights than traditional Response Evaluation Criteria in Solid Tumors (RECIST) measurements for monitoring cancer progression across various types [94]. Notably, greater complexity in tumor shape is often linked to poorer clinical outcomes [86]. Peritumoral radiomics, which extracts textural and statistical features from the surrounding tissue, has also shown significant prognostic value in various tumor types [89]. Including these peritumoral analyses enhances the predictive accuracy of radiomic signatures beyond what can be achieved by intra-tumoral analysis alone [89]. Additionally, radiomics of tumor vascularity, such as vessel tortuosity—a feature that characterizes the irregularity in tumor-associated vasculature—has demonstrated potential in predicting chemotherapy response in patients with breast cancer or malignant gliomas, as well as the response to targeted therapies in breast cancer brain metastases [95]. Moreover, vessel tortuosity measurements have been useful in identifying patients with non-small cell lung cancer (NSCLC) who are at risk for hyper-progression when treated with immune checkpoint inhibitors [96]. The commonly used features are summarized in Table 4.3.

4.3 METHODS OF RADIOMICS ANALYSIS

Radiomics analysis methodologies are broadly classified into two main categories: hand-crafted feature-based approaches and deep learning-based approaches, as shown in Figure 4.7.

4.3.1 Hand-Crafted Radiomics

Hand-crafted radiomics involves extracting predefined features, such as tumor shape, texture, and intensity distribution, to build predictive models for diagnosis, prognosis, and treatment planning. While widely used for its interpretability, this approach may miss complex patterns within the data and requires careful preprocessing. In contrast, Habitat Imaging identifies distinct tumor regions, or "habitats," each with unique cellular and genetic traits. By using multiregional spatial interaction (MSI) matrices, the interactions between these regions can be analyzed, revealing how various sections of a tumor influence each other [97]. Habitat detection involves two levels of clustering:

TABLE 4.3
Summary of the Widely Used Radiomics Features in the Literature

Radiomics Features	Description
Intensity-based	Quantifies values like attenuation from CT scans and physiological data from FDG-PET, used to assess voxel intensity distribution across the tumor, aiding in prognostic biomarker development.
Textural heterogeneity features [35,88]	Examines how the intensity values of image voxels relate to each other within a specific region of interest to quantify tumor heterogeneity and provide insights into tumor behavior.
Shape radiomics [86]	Analyzes 3D shape and volume of the tumor, offering insights into tumor morphology and growth patterns. Often, greater shape complexity correlates with poor outcomes.
Peritumoral radiomics [89]	Extracts textural and statistical features from the tissue surrounding the tumor, enhancing the predictive power of radiomic signatures beyond intra-tumoral analysis.
Tumor vascularity radiomics (vessel tortuosity) [96]	Measures the abnormal shape of tumor-associated vasculature. Vessel tortuosity has been linked to chemotherapy response and immune checkpoint inhibitor outcomes.

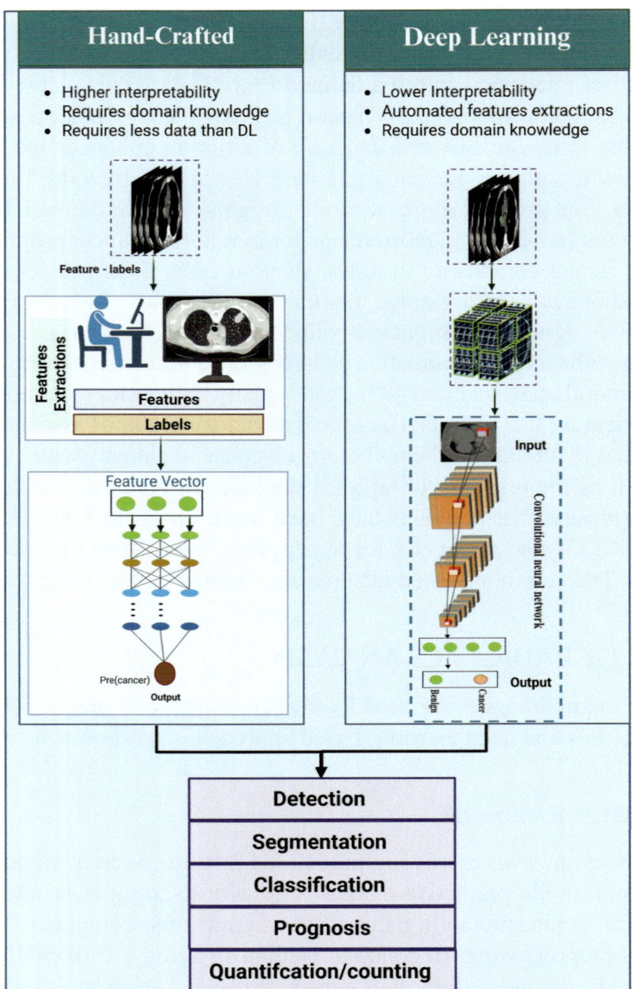

FIGURE 4.7 Traditional hand-crafted radiomics pipeline vs DL-based pipeline in cancer applications.

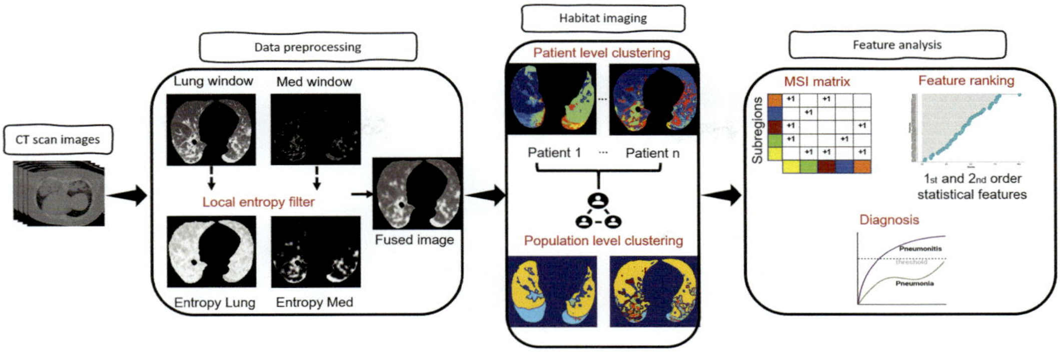

FIGURE 4.8 Pipeline of habitat imaging approach.

patient-level, using some algorithm such as simple linear iterative clustering for superpixel segmentation, and population-level, using hierarchical clustering to identify patterns across patients [98]. The habitat imaging pipeline is shown in Figure 4.8. Aminu et al. [97] conducted a study using AI-powered habitat imaging to predict COVID-19 severity and detection, with a specific focus on cancer patients. Leveraging multicenter datasets, the study demonstrated that habitat imaging models trained on the cancer cohort significantly outperformed traditional AI models, including DL approaches, that have been developed for use in the general population. Sujit et al. [99] utilized habitat imaging patterns from CT and FDG-PET scans to identify intrinsic radiological subtypes, which were then used to stratify NSCLC patients' risk of recurrence after surgery or radiotherapy in diverse, multi-institutional cohorts. Their study showed that these habitat imaging subtypes effectively categorized NSCLC patients by recurrence risk, offering valuable insights for personalized treatment planning.

4.3.2 Machine Learning Methods

ML- and DL-based methods in radiomics offer a more automated, data-driven approach. Rather than manually defining features, DL models, like CNNs, learn relevant patterns and representations directly from the imaging data [100]. This allows DL to capture more complex, nonlinear relationships within the images, often leading to improved performance in tasks like tumor segmentation [64,82], classification [101], and outcome prediction. However, these methods come with their own set of challenges, particularly in terms of interpretability and the need for large, annotated datasets for training. Each type of algorithm in Figure 4.9 plays a specific role in analyzing medical images, making predictions, and enhancing precision in RT. Supervised learning is the most common approach in DL, where the model learns from labeled data provided during training, meaning that the input data (medical images) are paired with known outcomes or labels (such as cancer or no cancer). The model learns the relationship between the input features and the outcomes, allowing it to make predictions on new, unseen data. For example, supervised learning models such as RFs [60], support vector machines [102], and neural networks (as seen in parts (a), (b), and (d) of Figure 4.9) are widely used to predict the presence of tumors or estimate survival rates based on radiomic features extracted from imaging. While unsupervised learning works with unlabeled data to find hidden patterns. The aim is to uncover patterns, groupings, or hidden structures within the data without having predefined labels. This approach can be useful in radiomics for discovering new imaging biomarkers or patient subgroups based on similar radiomic profiles. Algorithms such as GANs, as shown in Figure 4.9g, can be used to create realistic synthetic images for augmenting training data, which helps improve model robustness without needing large, labeled datasets.

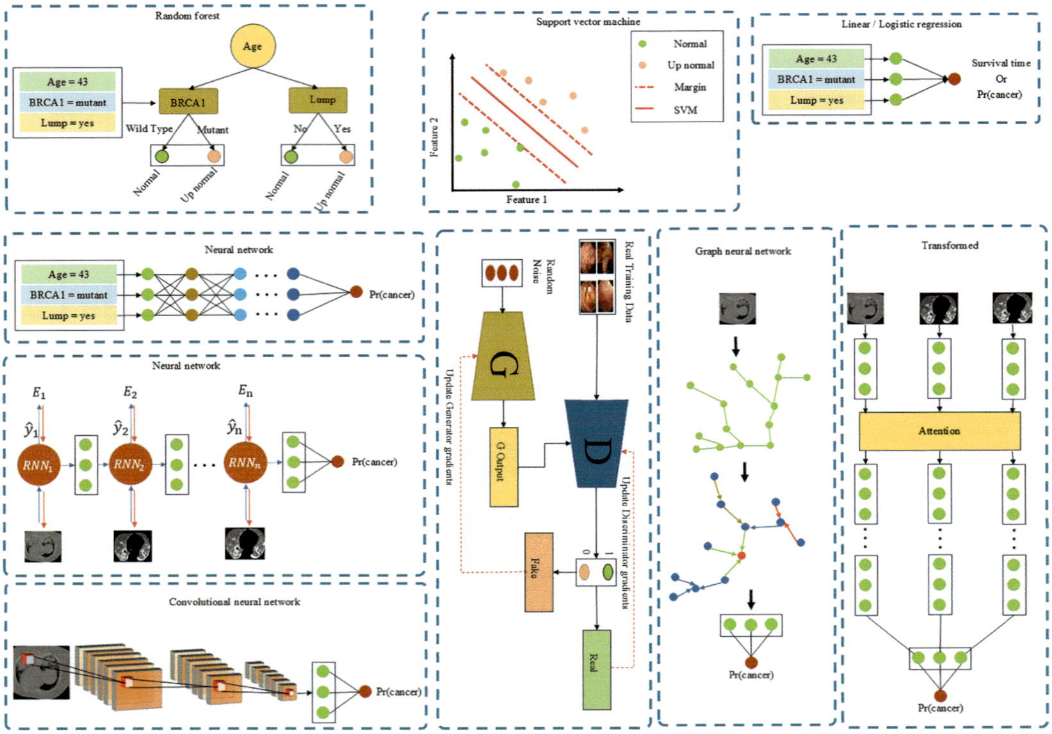

FIGURE 4.9 Commonly used ML models: (a) Random forest model: Constructs decision trees based on binary choices regarding input features to make predictions; (b) SVM: Learns a separating line or hyperplane in feature space with the maximum margin between two data classes; (c) Regression model: Employs input feature combinations to predict continuous (linear regression) or binary (logistic regression) labels; (d) Neural network: Utilizes neuron layers for sequential computation of linear combinations and nonlinear functions to predict outcomes, such as cancer probability; (e) RNN: Processes sequences by applying consistent neural network layers to each object and maintaining memory of processed elements; (f) CNN: Employs filter patches to scan images for patterns, identifying low-level (edges) and high-level (tumor morphology) features in layers; (g) GAN: Consists of a generator and discriminator network that compete to produce and evaluate data, used for tasks like image synthesis; (h) GNN: Suited for graph data like neighboring cell relationships, encoding node and edge features and propagating information across the graph for predictions. Each model class features various architectures, encompassing different neuron layer sizes and arrangements; and (i) Transformer: Analyzes sequences via repetitive attention operations, comparing and updating the internal sequence representation.

Graph neural networks (GNNs) and transformers are primarily used in supervised learning in cancer research, where labeled data such as tumor characteristics or patient outcomes are available. GNNs excel at modeling relationships and interactions between tumor regions, genes [103], or molecular markers. This makes them particularly useful for analyzing tumor heterogeneity, spatial relationships, and molecular interactions within cancer research [104]. For example, in lung cancer [105], GNNs can map the connections between different tumor nodules or molecular markers, helping to predict disease progression by understanding complex internal interactions [105] (Figure 4.9h). Similarly, transformers (Figure 4.9f) are employed in tasks like tumor segmentation, classification, and outcome prediction by focusing attention on the most relevant parts of medical images, such as highly metabolic tumor areas, enabling more precise diagnosis [106].

However, both GNNs and transformers can also be adapted for unsupervised or semi-supervised learning when labeled data is limited. In unsupervised learning, GNNs can uncover hidden structures, such as clustering different tumor regions, while transformers can use techniques like SSL to learn from large unlabeled datasets. This allows for pretraining on vast amounts of data, which can then be fine-tuned for specific supervised tasks [106]. Despite these possibilities, the most common use of GNNs and transformers in cancer research remains within a supervised learning framework. Table 4.4 provides a comprehensive summary of ML algorithms commonly applied in radiomics, highlighting both their key advantages and limitations.

4.4 AI AND RADIOMICS APPLICATION IN RADIATION THERAPY

The advent of AI and radiomics has greatly enhanced the potential for personalized medicine in radiation oncology. Numerous studies have demonstrated the application of AI-driven radiomics in the detection, characterization, and treatment response evaluation of various cancers, including lung cancer (LC) (Figure 4.10). In this section, we explore the contributions of AI and radiomics across three critical areas: detection, tumor characterization, and evaluation of treatment response.

4.4.1 Detection

Accurate and early detection of tumors is crucial for successful cancer treatment, particularly in RT, where treatment planning depends on the precise identification of target areas. AI-based models [22], including DL algorithms like CNNs and SVMs, have demonstrated superior performance in detecting various types of cancers by automatically analyzing medical imaging.

In LC detection, AI-based models have been instrumental in identifying early-stage malignancies that might be missed by traditional methods. For instance, authors in Ref. [101] introduced a new classifier based on a convolutional neural network utilizing CT imaging, which exhibited a true positive detection rate of 89% for lung nodules. The overall accuracy of the model was 77.6% and 84.58% for CNN and deep fully convolutional neural network (DFCNet), respectively. It performed well even when detecting small or low-density nodules—an area where manual detection typically struggles. One of the challenges associated with AI-based detection is the high false positive rate, which can lead to unnecessary interventions. However, radiomics has provided a promising solution to this issue. Radiomic approaches, by extracting and analyzing specific features from medical images, have been shown to effectively distinguish between true nodules and false positives. As a result, this method has led to a significant reduction in false positive rates, making the detection process more reliable and reducing unnecessary follow-up procedures [107].

Another noteworthy study by Weikert et al. [39] tested a faster R-CNN algorithm that demonstrated high detection rates for early-stage LC, with a detection rate of 90.4% for T1 tumors and 70.8% for T2 tumors. However, the detection rates dropped for more advanced stages, with the algorithm detecting only 29.4% of T3 tumors and 8.8% of T4 tumors. This discrepancy can be attributed to the design of the algorithm, which is primarily optimized for nodules smaller than 3 cm, and thus may struggle with larger or more complex tumor presentations.

AI-driven computer-aided detection (CAD) systems have been utilized not only in LC but also in breast, liver, and brain cancer detection. These systems excel at identifying abnormalities by learning complex patterns within the data, significantly reducing interobserver variability and increasing consistency. For instance, in breast cancer, CNN-based models have achieved sensitivity rates as high as 94% in detecting microcalcifications and small masses in mammograms. Such advancements in AI-driven detection allow for earlier diagnosis and intervention, which are critical for improving long-term outcomes in cancer treatment. Moreover, AI systems are now being integrated into clinical workflows, assisting radiologists by highlighting areas of concern, thus reducing the time and effort needed for manual reviews. The increased accuracy and efficiency in detecting tumors using AI models make them indispensable tools in modern radiological practice, paving the way for more timely and accurate RT planning.

TABLE 4.4
ML Algorithms Used in Radiomics, Along with Their Strengths and Limitations

Algorithm	Advantages	Limitations
Logistic regression	• Easy to interpret • Does not require input scaling • Low computational cost • Easy to implement and regularize	• Cannot handle nonlinear relationships • Assumes feature independence • Susceptible to overfitting when using many features
Support vector machine	• Effective in high-dimensional spaces • Can handle nonlinear data with kernel functions • Provides robust decision boundaries	• Sensitive to parameter tuning • Requires careful selection of kernel • Can be computationally expensive for large datasets
Random forest	• Handles large datasets well • Robust against overfitting • Can manage missing data • Provides feature importance insights	• Requires extensive computational resources for large datasets • May become difficult to interpret with too many trees
Convolutional neural network	• Excellent for image data • Automatically extracts spatial hierarchies of features • Outperforms traditional models in image recognition tasks	• Requires large, labeled datasets • Computationally expensive to train • Susceptible to overfitting, particularly with small datasets
Artificial neural network	• Highly flexible and powerful • Can learn complex nonlinear relationships • Distributed memory enables parallel processing	• Black-box nature makes results difficult to interpret • Tends to overfit without proper regularization • Requires significant tuning of hyperparameters
Recurrent neural network	• Ideal for sequential data • Can model temporal dependencies in datasets like time series or longitudinal imaging data	• Prone to vanishing/exploding gradients • Computationally intensive to train • May struggle with long-term dependencies without modifications (e.g., LSTM, GRU)
Graph neural network	• Capable of modeling relationships between connected data (e.g., biological networks) • Effective in analyzing non-Euclidean data structures	• Requires well-defined graph structures • Computationally demanding for large-scale graphs • Less mature and standardized than CNNs and RNNs for medical imaging applications
Bayesian networks	• Incorporates prior knowledge and uncertainty • Provides interpretable probabilistic predictions • Can manage incomplete data	• Computationally expensive • Requires careful selection of prior distributions • May struggle with high-dimensional data
Generative adversarial network	• Excellent for generating synthetic data • Can augment training data to improve model robustness • Effective for generating realistic medical images	• Difficult to train and prone to instability • Requires large amounts of data for training • Mode collapse is a frequent issue

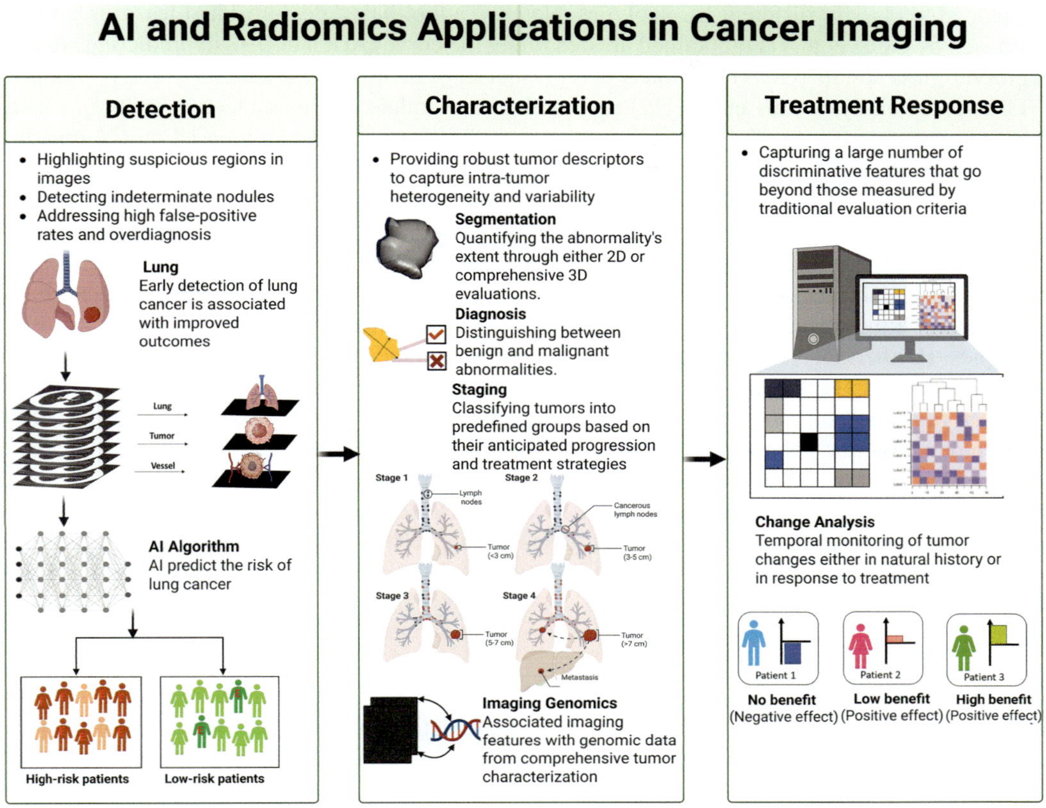

FIGURE 4.10 AI-driven radiomics applications in cancer imaging: Detection, where AI models process imaging data to identify lung tumors and differentiate them from normal structures; Characterization, where detailed radiomic analysis quantifies tumor biology, including molecular markers and heterogeneity, guiding personalized treatment strategies; and Treatment Response, where AI evaluates changes in tumor features over time, predicting the effectiveness of therapy and stratifying patients based on their response to RT.

4.4.2 Characterization

After detecting the tumor, accurate characterization is essential to determine its biological properties, aggressiveness, and potential mutational burden [22]. AI-based radiomics models have been highly effective in extracting complex, high-dimensional imaging features, which can then be linked to tumor biology and molecular markers, providing insights that extend beyond conventional imaging methods.

One of the key aspects of tumor characterization in radiomics is the quantification of tumor heterogeneity [108]. Tumor heterogeneity, which reflects variations in cellular composition, metabolism, and genetic mutations, is a significant predictor of treatment response and prognosis. AI-based models, such as those in Ref. [109], demonstrated the utility of the CNN-based method in characterizing lung nodules through heat maps, where color-coded CT values provided visual insights. Their study highlighted that internal heat within a nodule was a strong indicator of malignancy, whereas peripheral features such as satellite heat, a surrounding heat rim, and calcifications were more indicative of benignity. In radiomic models, Xu et al. [110] observed that malignancy classification for nodules smaller than 1 cm improved significantly. They found that texture features were more important for smaller nodules (T1a and T1b), while shape features played a greater role in classifying larger nodules (T1c). For both solid and ground-glass nodules, DL methods have been developed to classify different LC subtypes. Notably, a tool-based deep residual learning network proposed by Gong et al. [111] obtained an area under the curve (AUC) of 0.92 in predicting whether a ground-glass nodule (GGN) was likely to represent stage invasive adenocarcinoma (IA) or non-IA GGN. Additionally, Uthoff et al. [112] proposed a lung nodule ML classification technique using radiomic features from both the nodule and surrounding lung parenchyma based on CT imaging, achieving an AUC-ROC of 0.965 on the independent validation cohort.

Radiomics has also enabled the exploration of novel biomarkers for therapy response, particularly in the context of immunotherapies. Sun et al. [113] proposed a radiomic signature to assess immune phenotypes based on CD8 cell presence and location as a predictive biomarker on CT scans. This signature allowed for the differentiation between inflamed and immune-desert tumors, correlating with clinical outcomes in patients undergoing treatment with anti-PD-L1 or anti-PD-1 therapies. Furthermore, radiomic analysis can capture somatic mutations that reveal tumor phenotypes. Wang et al. [114], in a study of stage I lung adenocarcinoma patients, identified an association between tumor speculation and KRAS mutation. Similarly, the work in Ref. [115] examined the link among radiomic phenotypes and mutations in Epidermal Growth Factor Receptor (EGFR) and Kirsten Rat Sarcoma Viral Oncogene (KRAS). They observed that EGFR-positive tumors tend to be more heterogeneous, smaller, and lower in density on CT scans, whereas KRAS mutations could not be reliably discerned using volumetric data, despite KRAS tumors appearing more homogeneous. Their findings suggest that radiomic signatures may provide an avenue for distinguishing EGFR-positive from EGFR-negative cases.

4.4.3 Treatment Response

AI-driven radiomics has also proven valuable in predicting and monitoring treatment response [13,116]. Predicting how a tumor will respond to treatment early in the course of therapy is critical for adapting treatment plans and improving outcomes. AI models are now being used to analyze changes in radiomic features over time, a process known as delta-radiomics, to assess treatment efficacy [22].

Treatment with EGFR tyrosine kinase inhibitors (TKIs) often leads to an initial tumor shrinkage followed by a slow progression over months, which could suggest the tumor's sensitivity to EGFR inhibitors [117,118]. However, this slow progression might lead to an underestimation of the therapy's true efficacy when assessments rely solely on CT imaging. In response, the concept of delta-radiomics has been introduced, which evaluates changes in quantitative features captured through imaging during treatment, thereby adding a temporal dimension to the analysis. For instance, Bak et al. [119] found that changes in tumor density during treatment in advanced NSCLC patients correlated with improved survival rates, indicating that increased tumor homogeneity during therapy is a marker of a positive treatment response. The study showed that AUC2, a radiomic feature reflecting longitudinal tumor volume changes, was strongly correlated with overall survival. Their prediction model achieved impressive performance, with AUROC values of 0.948 at 1 year and 0.862 at 3 years. Key radiomic features, including kurtosis, surface area, and entropy, were identified as significant predictors of survival. Similarly, Trebeschi et al. [120] constructed ML models to predict treatment response in melanoma and NSCLC patients undergoing anti-PD-1 immunotherapy, discovering that lesions with greater morphological heterogeneity were associated with a better response to immunotherapy. The models achieved high predictive performance, where the radiomic biomarker demonstrated an AUC of up to 0.83. Showkatian et al. [121] developed a scalable multi-instance transformer (SMIT) model to noninvasively predict PD-L1 expression in stage IV NSCLC patients, using chest CT scans instead of invasive biopsies. Analyzing 746 patients split into training, validation, and testing groups, the SMIT model achieved high performance in predicting PD-L1 status with an AUC of 81%. The SMIT model's PD-L1 predictions were comparable to those obtained via biopsy and immunohistochemistry, also demonstrating strong alignment with IHC-based progression-free survival predictions.

Additionally, Fave et al. [122] examined pretreatment and delta-radiomics features to determine the prognostic value of these features in NSCLC patients receiving RT. While pretreatment imaging features were not found to be predictive of outcomes like local recurrence or distant metastases, significant radiomic changes during the course of RT allowed for stratification of patients into high- and low-risk groups based on texture changes, offering insights into tumor response following treatment. This demonstrates the value of monitoring radiomic feature changes during therapy to better predict patient outcomes. Table 4.5 summarizes the application of radiomics and AI in medical imaging.

4.5 FACTORS INFLUENCING RADIOMIC FEATURES

While radiomics has shown considerable promise, the robustness and reproducibility of extracted features can be influenced by several key factors, ranging from how features are defined to the processes used in image acquisition and analysis (Figure 4.11). Standardizing these factors is critical for ensuring reliable and clinically useful radiomic analyses. These factors are as follows.

4.5.1 Feature Definition

A key challenge in radiomics is the lack of standardized definitions for many radiomic features, leading to inconsistencies in their interpretation and application [22]. As noted in Ref. [123], different studies may use varying mathematical formulations for the same feature or label different features with the same name. For example, two studies may refer to "entropy" or "homogeneity," but their methods for calculating these features could differ significantly. In addition, some features are calculated from 2D slices of the tumor (2D texture) while others derive from the entire tumor volume (3D texture), as described in Refs. [124,125]. Such discrepancies complicate the comparison of results across studies and highlight the need for consensus on radiomic feature definitions.

Moreover, there are differences in how radiomic texture features are derived from the GLCM. Some studies, such as [126], compute the GLCM in individual directions, while others average the matrix across 13 different directions, leading to variability in texture feature extraction. To address these inconsistencies, the radiomics community has recognized the urgent need for standardization efforts, with calls for harmonization in feature extraction protocols from various groups, including [1,127,128]. Developing a consensus around feature definitions will not only improve reproducibility but also enhance the integration of radiomics into clinical workflows.

4.5.2 Image Acquisition and Processing

The reliability of radiomic features is also affected by how images are acquired and processed. Several studies, including [129,130], have shown that test–retest variations in imaging protocols can significantly impact the robustness of certain radiomic features. Changes in acquisition parameters such as slice thickness, contrast settings, and imaging modality (CT, PET, or MRI) can result in variations in extracted features. Fave et al. [125] demonstrated that even slight modifications to image reconstruction parameters can alter radiomic features and subsequently influence their predictive power. Similarly, Yan et al. [131] and Galavis et al. [132] found that differences in image reconstruction algorithms led to variability in feature reproducibility, underscoring the importance of harmonizing imaging protocols.

The segmentation of lesions also plays a key role in the reliability of radiomic analyses. Hatt et al. [133] observed that features extracted from manually segmented lesions can vary substantially between observers, which introduces bias into radiomic studies. To mitigate this issue, many researchers are advocating for the use of automated or semiautomated segmentation techniques, which offer greater consistency. For instance, Larue et al. [134] recommend automating as much

TABLE 4.5
Summary of Representative AI and Radiomics Studies in Cancer Applications

References	Tasks	Data Modality	Algorithm	Performance
Weikert et al. [39]	Lung Cancer Detection	FDG-PET/CT	Faster R-CNN	High detection performance for T1 tumors (90.4%), decreasing for T2 (70.8%), T3 (29.4%), and T4 (8.8%). Excellent segmentation performance for T1 tumors (r=0.908, p<0.001) and tumors without pleural contact (r=0.971, p<0.001). Algorithm struggles with larger tumors and pleural contact. False positives: 0.41 per exam
Masood et al. [101]	Lung Cancer Detection	CT	DFCNet (deep fully convolutional neural network)	DFCNet achieved an overall accuracy of 84.58%, compared to 77.6% for traditional CNNs
Gong et al. [111]	Characterization of Ground-Glass Nodules	CT	Deep residual learning network	AUC of 0.92±0.03, matching the performance of a senior radiologist and outperforming a junior radiologist (AUC 0.90±0.03)
Uthoff et al. [112]	Characterization	CT	ML-based radiomic Model	AUC-ROC: 0.965
Sun et al. [113]	Characterization	CT	ML method	AUC=0.67 in validation with The Cancer Genome Atlas (TCGA) dataset; discriminated inflamed from immune-desert tumors with AUC=0.76
Wang et al. [114]	Characterization	CT	Logistic regression	KRAS mutation, 41.77%. Spiculation is significantly associated with KRAS mutations (OR=2.99; 95% CI, 1.16–7.68). Pleural attachment revealed an increased risk of death (HR=2.46; 95% CI, 1.09–5.53). In addition, combined analysis improved survival prediction (p=0.014)
Velazquez et al. [115]	Characterization	CT and somatic mutation	ML-based methods	Radiomic signatures significantly outperformed traditional radiographic predictors. EGFR+/EGFR– signature achieved AUC=0.69 (AUC=0.75 when combined with clinical model). EGFR+/KRAS+ signature achieved AUC=0.80 (AUC=0.86 when combined with clinical model). KRAS+/KRAS– signature achieved AUC=0.63
Bak et al. [119]	Treatment Response	CT	Multivariate Cox regression	The prediction model achieved an AUROC of 0.948 at 1 year and 0.862 at 3 years.
Trebeschi et al. [120]	Treatment Response	CT	Machine learning model	Achieved AUC=0.83 for NSCLC lesions and AUC=0.64 for melanoma lymph nodes. Combined patient-level predictions yielded AUC=0.76. The biomarker was associated with mitosis-related pathways and a 1-year survival difference of 24%.
Fave et al. [122]	Treatment Response	CT	Linear mixed-effects models, multivariate Cox regression	Adding pretreatment compactness2 improved the prediction of overall survival, increasing the c-index from 0.597 to 0.672. For predicting distant metastases, the c-index rose from 0.539 to 0.632 with the addition of pretreatment compactness2. In the case of local recurrence, a change in the radiomics feature (texture strength) resulted in a c-index of 0.558 and showed significant patient stratification (p=0.0269)

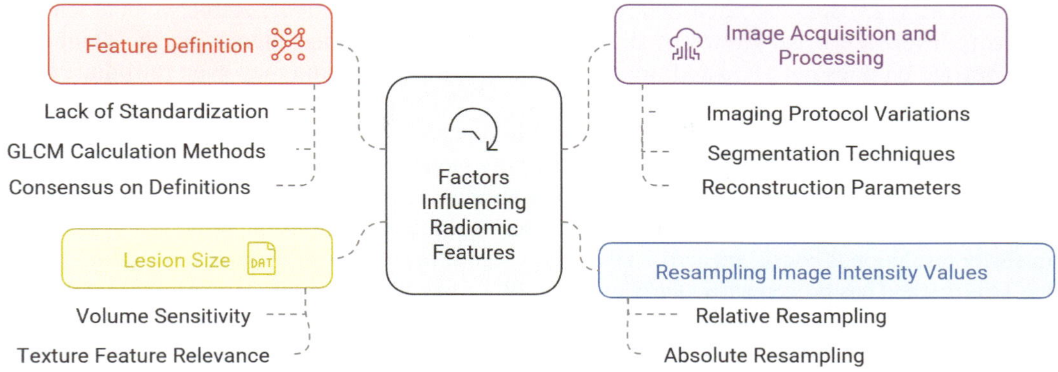

FIGURE 4.11 Factors influencing radiomics features, including inconsistencies in feature definitions, image acquisition and processing variations, lesion size, and image intensity resampling. These factors can significantly impact the extraction and interpretation of radiomic features from medical imaging, affecting the reliability of radiomics-based analyses and models.

of the image processing and segmentation pipeline as possible to enhance the reproducibility of radiomic analyses. Standardized and reproducible image acquisition and segmentation procedures are essential to ensure that radiomic features can be reliably applied in multi-institutional studies.

4.5.3 Lesion Size

Lesion size is another critical factor that influences radiomic features, particularly texture-based metrics. Brooks and Grigsby [135] studied the correlation between tumor volume (TV) and entropy derived from GLCM in a cohort of 70 cervical cancer patients. Their findings indicated that entropy is highly sensitive to volume differences, especially when the TV is less than 45 cm^3 (approximately 700 voxels). Below this threshold, entropy becomes five times more sensitive to volume changes, leading the authors to caution against using this feature in small tumors, as it could result in skewed analyses. Given that many early-stage tumors have small volumes, this limitation could exclude a significant number of patients from radiomic analyses in clinical oncology.

Further, authors in Ref. [126] explored the influence of TV on four texture features using PET imaging in a larger cohort of 555 cancer patients (including lung and breast cancers). Their study found that the correlation between radiomic features and TV tends to decrease as tumor size increases. This suggests that some texture features may be more relevant for characterizing smaller tumors, while larger tumors may present more homogenous textures that are less informative for radiomic analysis. These findings highlight the need to consider TV when selecting radiomic features for analysis, especially in cancers where tumor size is a key prognostic factor.

4.5.4 Resampling Image Intensity Values

Resampling of image intensity values, also known as discretization, is a fundamental preprocessing step in radiomic analysis. This process reduces the range of intensity levels (e.g., pixel or voxel values) in an image, grouping them into a smaller number of bins to streamline the calculation of texture features and reduce noise. However, this process comes at the cost of some loss of information, as noted by Tixier et al. [136]. Two primary approaches to resampling have been explored in the literature: relative and absolute resampling.

In the relative resampling approach, the intensity values are divided into a fixed number of discrete bins (e.g., 16, 32, or 64), irrespective of the tumor's specific intensity range.

Orlhac et al. [123] demonstrated that texture features remain relatively stable when at least 32 intensity levels are used. However, Hatt et al. [126] cautioned that increasing the number of bins beyond 64 does not yield additional predictive information and may even introduce noise into the analysis.

Recently, an absolute resampling method was introduced, where intensity values are resampled using a fixed bin size in units relevant to the imaging modality (e.g., SUV for PET scans). Studies such as those in Refs. [137,138] have shown that absolute resampling offers better predictive performance in PET imaging compared to relative resampling. Absolute resampling ensures that the intensity resolution is consistent across all images, regardless of the tumor's size or metabolic activity. This method has proven particularly useful in PET imaging, where tumor uptake of radiotracers can vary significantly between patients. As observed in Refs. [116,135,137], absolute resampling has become the preferred approach for maintaining a balance between computational efficiency and predictive power in radiomic analyses. The summary of studies investigating radiomic feature reproducibility across different modalities is presented in Table 4.6.

TABLE 4.6
Summary of Studies Investigating Radiomic Feature Reproducibility across Different Modalities

Disease	Modality Investigated	Sources of Variability	Statistical Analysis	Reproducibility Insights	References
NSCLC	CT	Acquisition parameters variations	Intraclass correlation coefficient (ICC)	Texture features are notably sensitive to reconstruction and acquisition parameters variations. Features such as shape descriptors tend to be more reproducible under consistent settings	[17]
Lung, liver, and kidney cancers	CT	Segmentation variability.	ICC	Shape features exhibit greater reproducibility compared to first-order features or GLCM features under differing segmentations.	[38]
NSCLC	CT	Imaging protocol variations, such as CT acquisition parameters, and test–retest conditions	ICC	Tested under variations caused by patient factors and different segmentation methods (manual vs. automated).	[129]
Malignancies, including adrenal gland carcinoma, lung cancer, epiglottis cancer, and esophagus cancer	PET	Acquisition modes, reconstruction parameter	Percentage difference (% Diff)	High reproducibility observed in entropy, first-order features, energy, and low gray-level run emphasis, though differences in feature definitions (e.g., entropy) may arise	[132]

(Continued)

TABLE 4.6 (*Continued*)
Summary of Studies Investigating Radiomic Feature Reproducibility across Different Modalities

Disease	Modality Investigated	Sources of Variability	Statistical Analysis	Reproducibility Insights	References
Esophageal cancer	FDG-PET	Tumor volume (TV) delineation strategies (adaptive threshold vs. FLAB)	Cox regression (univariate and multivariate analyses) and Kaplan–Meier survival analysis	FLAB was found to be important independent prognostic factors, emphasizing the need for reliable and precise PET tumor delineation tools in oncology.	[133]
Lung cancer	FDG-PET	SUV discretization methods (relative discretization vs. absolute resolution)	ICC	RB (constant intensity resolution) enables more consistent comparisons between and within patients, while RD (variable bin size) can add variability to how features are interpreted	[137]
Fibrosing interstitial lung disease	CT	Scanner differences, Reconstruction parameters (kernels, slice thickness)	ICC	Consistent reconstruction yields repeatable radiomic features, but slice thickness has a larger impact than reconstruction kernel differences.	[139]
Liver cancer	CT	Variability in CT radiation dose, reconstruction settings, including section thickness and algorithms.	Hierarchical clustering.	Shape features, including the maximum axial diameter and tumor volume, are more reproducible than other feature types.	[140]
Lung cancer (phantom study)	CT	CT acquisition parameters and scanner differences.	ICC and AUC	Variability in CT radiation dose, reconstruction settings, including section thickness and algorithms.	[141]

4.6 RADIOMIC FEATURES HARMONIZATION

Radiomic feature harmonization refers to the process of aligning and standardizing radiomic features across different datasets, imaging protocols, or acquisition settings to ensure that the extracted features are comparable and robust to variability. This harmonization is essential for building models that are generalizable and reproducible across different institutions and studies. The following subsections explore two key methods for radiomic feature harmonization: selecting features based on their reliability and applying batch effect correction techniques to mitigate technical variability.

4.6.1 Strategies for Feature Selection Based on Reliability

A crucial step in radiomic feature harmonization is selecting features that exhibit robustness against the variability introduced by acquisition and reconstruction processes. These variations can stem from differences in imaging devices, protocols, or reconstruction algorithms, leading to features that are unreliable and prone to capturing noise rather than meaningful biological signals. Removing such unreliable features has become a widely adopted strategy for improving the generalizability of models, especially when tested on external datasets [136,142–144]. The key benefit of this approach is a reduction in the number of features, simplifying both the statistical analysis and model development. Moreover, the retained features are more likely to maintain their predictive power when applied to datasets from different institutions or scanners. However, this method also presents challenges. First, it may result in the loss of clinically significant features that, despite being sensitive to technical variations, could hold valuable discriminative power. Additionally, determining the optimal subset of features that are both robust and informative is highly context-dependent, requiring careful selection for each combination of imaging modality, cancer type, and clinical task.

To this end, several advanced techniques reported in the literature can assist in identifying reliable features for radiomic analysis, as presented in Figure 4.12 (top part). Stability selection involves repeated subsampling of the data to identify features that are consistently selected across different subsamples, ensuring stability [145]. Recursive feature elimination (RFE) is a process that gradually removes the least important features, focusing on those that contribute most to model accuracy, while the variance threshold method filters out features with low variance across samples, deeming them uninformative [146]. Mutual information measures how dependent features are on the target variable, helping select those that offer the most useful information [147]. In contrast, random forest feature importance measures how frequently a feature contributes to decision splits within the model, identifying key contributors [148]. Lasso [149] and elastic net, both regularization techniques, penalize less informative features by driving their coefficients toward zero, focusing on the most important ones. Information gain (IG) quantifies the increase in information when a feature is used to split the data, helping in feature selection. Statistical tests like the T-test or ANOVA F-test are also useful for selecting features with significant differences between groups or conditions. Principal component analysis (PCA) ranks features based on their contribution to explaining the variance in the data, while Bayesian feature selection applies probabilistic models to assess the likelihood of feature relevance, helping to identify which features should be retained for further analysis. These methods collectively enhance the robustness and reliability of radiomic feature selection. Figure 4.12 summarizes the methods of radiomic feature harmonization.

4.6.2 Utilizing "Batch Effect" Correction Methods

Batch effects, a well-documented challenge in radiomic studies [144], arise from systematic technical variations unrelated to the biological phenomena under study. These effects can be caused by time-dependent changes in equipment, different acquisition settings, or variations between imaging batches. Definitions of batch effects vary, but they generally refer to the unintended, non-biological discrepancies introduced by differences in how and when data are collected [144,150,151]. The presence of batch effects can significantly undermine the comparability and reproducibility of results across studies. To mitigate this, various batch effect correction methods were developed, particularly in fields like genomics, where similar issues have long been encountered when combining data from multiple experiments. These methods fall into three main categories:

- Matrix Factorization Methods: These methods, such as singular value decomposition (SVD), surrogate variable analysis (SVA) and remove unwanted variation 2-step (RUV-2). SVD is used to factorize the input data matrix and reconstruct it while filtering out variations attributed to batch effects. This approach adjusts the data, ensuring that only biological variations are retained [88,102]. SVA identifies and removes unwanted batch variation by estimating residuals from the data. These residuals, assumed to contain batch effects, are adjusted using methods like SVD. By incorporating surrogate variables representing unmeasured confounding factors, SVA improves the accuracy of downstream analysis

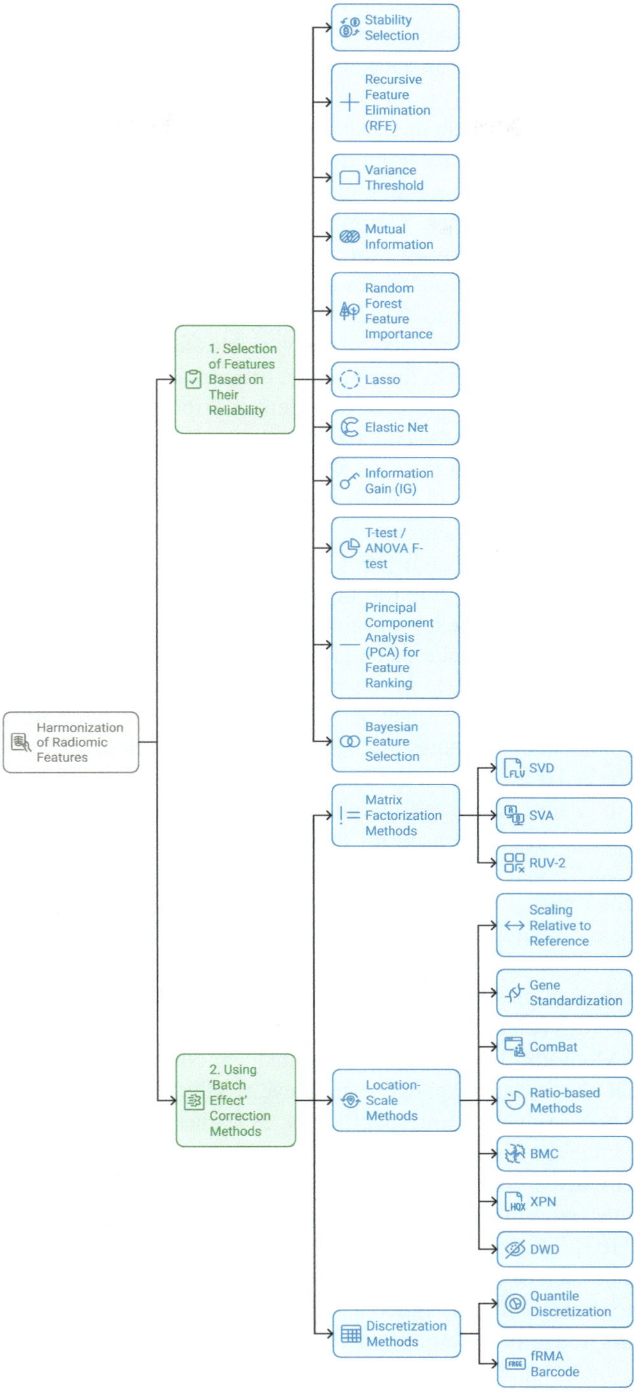

FIGURE 4.12 Methods for harmonization of radiomic features.

[152,153]. RUV-2 uses control variables to identify batch-related factors, assuming that these control variables are uncorrelated with the biological component of interest. This method is particularly useful for datasets where batch effects are significant but difficult to measure directly [154].

- Location-Scale Methods: These methods, such as ComBat [155], is a widely used method for correcting batch effects in imaging datasets. It works by using Bayesian estimation to adjust the location-scale (LS) parameters, specifically the mean and variance, for each variable across different batches. The method pools information from multiple variables within each batch that share similar expression characteristics, enabling a more robust estimation of batch effects and allowing for their removal [156]. Scaling relative to reference adjusts a variable's distribution to match that of the same variable in a reference dataset. As described in Ref. [157], the approach aligns variables across datasets, reducing inconsistencies by scaling them based on the reference distribution. Batch mean-centering (BMC) adjusts data based on the assumption of prevalent multiplicative batch effects [158]. It operates by subtracting the mean of each variable across all samples within a batch, helping to reduce batch-specific biases in the data. Gene standardization is a process of normalizing each variable by converting it to have a mean of 0 and a standard deviation of 1. This is achieved by subtracting the mean and dividing by the standard deviation of the variable across all samples within a batch [159]. Like BMC, this method assumes that in gene expression, each gene exhibits a multiplicative batch-specific effect. Ratio-based methods scale the expression values of each variable in a sample relative to a reference sample or set of reference samples within each batch [160]. When multiple reference samples are available, the arithmetic or geometric mean of their expression values can be used for scaling. More sophisticated approaches, such as XPN (cross-platform normalization) aims to find homogeneous clusters of variables and samples across different studies that share similar expression patterns [161]. This method aligns data from multiple platforms by focusing on these clusters to ensure comparability, and DWD (Distance Weighted Discrimination) is a modification of SVMs [102] used for batch effect correction. In this approach, samples from a single batch, considered to belong to a specific class, are classified using DWD to determine the optimal hyperplane that separates samples from different classes. Next, samples within each batch are projected along the direction of the normal vector by calculating the average distance of all batch samples to the hyperplane. This distance is then used to adjust the samples by subtracting the normal vector scaled by the mean distance, effectively removing batch effects.
- Discretization Methods: These techniques transform continuous expression data into specific categorical classes based on expression levels. This transformation simplifies the data by grouping expression values into specific ranges or classes, facilitating further analysis by treating these values as discrete categories rather than continuous variables [162]. Quantile discretization involves dividing data into equal-frequency bins. This process transforms expression values into bins based on quantiles, ensuring each bin contains an equal number of data points [163]. The central bins, containing values around the median, are merged into one interval, and each expression value is converted into an integer representing the bin it belongs to. The central bin is assigned a value of zero, and positive or negative integers are assigned to bins above or below the median. Frozen robust multi-array analysis (fRMA) [164] processes individual samples and combines them for future analysis. It achieves this by using a reference distribution for quantile normalization across new samples. This reference is based on a publicly available training set from a diverse population.

As widely acknowledged in the literature, integrating data from multiple centers presents a significant challenge for radiomic features [144,165–167], due to their sensitivity to variations in acquisition and reconstruction parameters, as well as scanner settings. These discrepancies make it difficult to directly compare feature values across different imaging protocols, hindering their applicability in multicenter studies. Several works have explored the effectiveness of ComBat harmonization in addressing variability in radiomics analyses across different imaging protocols. Orlhac et al. [165] explored the use of ComBat to correct for variations in CT radiomic features from scans collected across multiple centers. The study found that acquisition and reconstruction parameters significantly influenced all radiomic features. ComBat harmonization effectively reduced these differences, allowing for the reliable use of nearly all radiomic features after adjustment. Additionally, the authors reported enhanced performance metrics for radiomic signatures after applying ComBat, demonstrating its ability to improve the reliability and predictive power of the models. Another study [167] conducted a similar investigation into the use of ComBat for harmonizing radiomic features from PET scans acquired with varying protocols, reporting comparable results to those observed in the CT-scan study. This consistency across modalities highlights the robustness of ComBat as a harmonization tool in radiomics, reinforcing its importance in multicenter studies where variability in imaging practices can otherwise hinder the comparability of radiomic features. In addition to the standard ComBat method, Da-Ano et al. [166] assessed several modified versions—M-ComBat, B-ComBat, and BM-ComBat—and found that all these variations significantly improved the performance of radiomic signatures. These results suggest that ComBat and its variants are critical for ensuring the reliability and generalizability of radiomics-based models, specifically in multicenter or multimodal studies. The ability to harmonize data from different acquisition settings not only enhances the reproducibility of findings but also strengthens the clinical utility of radiomic models in real-world scenarios. These insights are particularly relevant to the discussion of developing robust and reproducible radiomic models for personalized cancer care.

4.7 CONCLUSION

To conclude, this chapter has highlighted both the promise and the challenges associated with radiomics in cancer care, especially when integrating AI to enhance diagnostic and treatment precision. We have explored how hand-crafted and DL-based radiomics approaches can extract valuable quantitative features from medical images, offering deep insights into tumor biology and patient outcomes. AI's ability to improve radiotherapy planning, refine treatment response predictions, and personalize cancer care has been underscored through the application of various ML models. The findings highlight the significant potential of AI in pushing beyond traditional boundaries, allowing for more accurate cancer detection and individualized treatment strategies. Despite the challenges in data quality, model interpretability, and reproducibility, the advances in AI-driven radiomics are undeniable, offering a powerful toolset for transforming oncology. As we look to the future, it's clear that continued development in AI and radiomics will pave the way for even more precise and predictive models, ultimately reshaping cancer care. The integration of these technologies holds the promise of not only improving patient outcomes but also fundamentally changing the way we approach cancer treatment and research.

REFERENCES

1. P. Lambin et al., "Radiomics: the bridge between medical imaging and personalized medicine," *Nature Reviews Clinical Oncology,* vol. 14, no. 12, pp. 749–762, 2017.
2. Z. Liu et al., "The applications of radiomics in precision diagnosis and treatment of oncology: opportunities and challenges," *Theranostics,* vol. 9, no. 5, p. 1303, 2019.
3. P. Lohmann et al., "Radiomics in neuro-oncology: basics, workflow, and applications," *Methods,* vol. 188, pp. 112–121, 2021.
4. M. M. Chen et al., "Artificial intelligence in oncologic imaging," *European Journal of Radiology Open,* vol. 9, p. 100441, 2022.
5. E. J. Limkin et al., "Promises and challenges for the implementation of computational medical imaging (radiomics) in oncology," *Annals of Oncology,* vol. 28, no. 6, pp. 1191–1206, 2017.

6. S. K. Zhou et al., "A review of deep learning in medical imaging: imaging traits, technology trends, case studies with progress highlights, and future promises," *Proceedings of the IEEE,* vol. 109, no. 5, pp. 820–838, 2021.
7. T. Xu, X. Liu, Y. Chen, S. Wang, C. Jiang, and J. Gong, "CT-based deep learning radiomics biomarker for programmed cell death ligand 1 expression in non-small cell lung cancer," *BMC Medical Imaging,* vol. 24, no. 1, p. 196, 2024.
8. J. Wu, K. K. Tha, L. Xing, and R. Li, "Radiomics and radiogenomics for precision radiotherapy," *Journal of Radiation Research,* vol. 59, no. suppl_1, pp. i25–i31, 2018.
9. J. M. Boone, "Radiological interpretation 2020: toward quantitative image assessment," *Medical Physics,* vol. 34, no. 11, pp. 4173–4179, 2007.
10. R. J. Gillies, P. E. Kinahan, and H. Hricak, "Radiomics: images are more than pictures, they are data," *Radiology,* vol. 278, no. 2, pp. 563–577, 2016.
11. Y.-P. Zhang et al., "Artificial intelligence-driven radiomics study in cancer: the role of feature engineering and modeling," *Military Medical Research,* vol. 10, no. 1, p. 22, 2023.
12. S. O. Osman et al., "Computed tomography-based radiomics for risk stratification in prostate cancer," *International Journal of Radiation Oncology, Biology, Physics,* vol. 105, no. 2, pp. 448–456, 2019.
13. M. R. Chetan and F. V. Gleeson, "Radiomics in predicting treatment response in non-small-cell lung cancer: current status, challenges and future perspectives," *European Radiology,* vol. 31, pp. 1049–1058, 2021.
14. F. Klemm and J. A. Joyce, "Microenvironmental regulation of therapeutic response in cancer," *Trends in Cell Biology,* vol. 25, no. 4, pp. 198–213, 2015.
15. S. Ramón y Cajal et al., "Clinical implications of intratumor heterogeneity: challenges and opportunities," *Journal of Molecular Medicine,* vol. 98, pp. 161–177, 2020.
16. Q. Al-Tashi et al., "Machine learning models for the identification of prognostic and predictive cancer biomarkers: a systematic review," *International Journal of Molecular Sciences,* vol. 24, no. 9, p. 7781, 2023.
17. H. J. Aerts et al., "Decoding tumour phenotype by noninvasive imaging using a quantitative radiomics approach," *Nature Communications,* vol. 5, no. 1, p. 4006, 2014.
18. J. Wu, A. T. Mayer, and R. Li, "Integrated imaging and molecular analysis to decipher tumor microenvironment in the era of immunotherapy," in *Seminars in Cancer Biology*, 2022, vol. 84: Elsevier, pp. 310–328.
19. C. Novelli, M. Taddeo, and L. Floridi, "Accountability in artificial intelligence: what it is and how it works," *Ai & Society,* vol. 39, no. 4, pp. 1871–1882, 2024.
20. S. Huang, J. Yang, S. Fong, and Q. Zhao, "Artificial intelligence in cancer diagnosis and prognosis: opportunities and challenges," *Cancer Letters,* vol. 471, pp. 61–71, 2020.
21. J. Wu et al., "Early-stage non–small cell lung cancer: quantitative imaging characteristics of 18F fluorodeoxyglucose PET/CT allow prediction of distant metastasis," *Radiology,* vol. 281, no. 1, pp. 270–278, 2016.
22. W. L. Bi et al., "Artificial intelligence in cancer imaging: clinical challenges and applications," CA*: A Cancer Journal for Clinicians,* vol. 69, no. 2, pp. 127–157, 2019.
23.] T. Jiang, J. L. Gradus, and A. J. Rosellini, "Supervised machine learning: a brief primer," *Behavior Therapy,* vol. 51, no. 5, pp. 675–687, 2020.
24. M. W. Berry, A. Mohamed, and B. W. Yap, *Supervised and Unsupervised Learning for Data Science.* Springer, 2019.
25. J. Wu et al., "Unsupervised clustering of quantitative image phenotypes reveals breast cancer subtypes with distinct prognoses and molecular pathways," *Clinical Cancer Research,* vol. 23, no. 13, pp. 3334–3342, 2017.
26. J. Wu et al., "Radiological tumour classification across imaging modality and histology," *Nature Machine Intelligence,* vol. 3, no. 9, pp. 787–798, 2021.
27. S. Shurrab and R. Duwairi, "Self-supervised learning methods and applications in medical imaging analysis: a survey," *PeerJ Computer Science,* vol. 8, p. e1045, 2022.
28. Z.-X. Cui et al., "Self-score: self-supervised learning on score-based models for mri reconstruction," *arXiv preprint arXiv:2209.00835,* 2022.
29. Q. Wei, M. T. Islam, Y. Zhou, and L. Xing, "Self-supervised deep learning of gene–gene interactions for improved gene expression recovery," *Briefings in Bioinformatics,* vol. 25, no. 2, p. bbae031, 2024.
30. Y. Li, "Deep reinforcement learning: an overview," *arXiv preprint arXiv:1701.07274,* 2017.

31. E. M. Tosca, A. De Carlo, D. Ronchi, and P. Magni, "Model-informed reinforcement learning for enabling precision dosing via adaptive dosing," *Clinical Pharmacology & Therapeutics,* vol. 116, no. 3, pp. 619–636, 2024.
32. C.-Y. Yang, C. Shiranthika, C.-Y. Wang, K.-W. Chen, and S. Sumathipala, "Reinforcement learning strategies in cancer chemotherapy treatments: a review," *Computer Methods and Programs in Biomedicine,* vol. 229, p. 107280, 2023.
33. R. Najjar, "Redefining radiology: a review of artificial intelligence integration in medical imaging," *Diagnostics,* vol. 13, no. 17, p. 2760, 2023.
34. Q. Al-Tashi et al., "SwarmDeepSurv: swarm intelligence advances deep survival network for prognostic radiomics signatures in four solid cancers," *Patterns,* vol. 4, no. 8, p. 100777, 2023.
35. K. Bera, N. Braman, A. Gupta, V. Velcheti, and A. Madabhushi, "Predicting cancer outcomes with radiomics and artificial intelligence in radiology," *Nature Reviews Clinical Oncology,* vol. 19, no. 2, pp. 132–146, 2022.
36. H. Tang et al., "Clinically applicable deep learning framework for organs at risk delineation in CT images," *Nature Machine Intelligence,* vol. 1, no. 10, pp. 480–491, 2019.
37. V. Kumar et al., "Radiomics: the process and the challenges," *Magnetic Resonance Imaging,* vol. 30, no. 9, pp. 1234–1248, 2012.
38. C. Haarburger, G. Müller-Franzes, L. Weninger, C. Kuhl, D. Truhn, and D. Merhof, "Radiomics feature reproducibility under inter-rater variability in segmentations of CT images," *Scientific Reports,* vol. 10, no. 1, p. 12688, 2020.
39. T. Weikert, T. Akinci D'Antonoli, J. Bremerich, B. Stieltjes, G. Sommer, and A. W. Sauter, "Evaluation of an AI-powered lung nodule algorithm for detection and 3D segmentation of primary lung tumors," *Contrast Media & Molecular Imaging,* vol. 2019, no. 1, p. 1545747, 2019.
40. R. Kohler, "A segmentation system based on thresholding," *Computer Graphics and Image Processing,* vol. 15, no. 4, pp. 319–338, 1981.
41. J. Zhang and J. Hu, "Image segmentation based on 2D Otsu method with histogram analysis," in *2008 International Conference on Computer Science and Software Engineering*, Wuhan, China, 2008, vol. 6: IEEE, pp. 105–108.
42. N. Shrivastava and J. Bharti, "Automatic seeded region growing image segmentation for medical image segmentation: a brief review," *International Journal of Image and Graphics,* vol. 20, no. 03, p. 2050018, 2020.
43. M. Padlia and J. Sharma, "Fractional Sobel filter based brain tumor detection and segmentation using statistical features and SVM," in Vijay Nath, Jyotsna Kumar Mandal (eds), *Nanoelectronics, Circuits and Communication Systems: Proceeding of NCCS 2017,* 2019: Springer, pp. 161–175.
44. R. Hemalatha, T. Thamizhvani, A. J. A. Dhivya, J. E. Joseph, B. Babu, and R. Chandrasekaran, "Active contour based segmentation techniques for medical image analysis," *Medical and Biological Image Analysis,* vol. 4, no. 17, p. 2, 2018.
45. H. Ng, S. Ong, K. Foong, P.-S. Goh, and W. Nowinski, "Medical image segmentation using k-means clustering and improved watershed algorithm," in *2006 IEEE Southwest Symposium on Image Analysis and Interpretation*, Denver, CO, USA, 2006: IEEE, pp. 61–65.
46. S. Beucher, "Watershed, hierarchical segmentation and waterfall algorithm," in *Mathematical Morphology and Its Applications to Image Processing,* Springer Netherlands, Dordrecht, pp. 69–76, 1994. https://doi.org/10.1007/978-94-011-1040-2_10
47. K. Held, E. R. Kops, B. J. Krause, W. M. Wells, R. Kikinis, and H.-W. Muller-Gartner, "Markov random field segmentation of brain MR images," *IEEE Transactions on Medical Imaging,* vol. 16, no. 6, pp. 878–886, 1997.
48. Y. Boykov and G. Funka-Lea, "Graph cuts and efficient ND image segmentation," *International Journal of Computer Vision,* vol. 70, no. 2, pp. 109–131, 2006.
49. W. Ju, D. Xiang, B. Zhang, L. Wang, I. Kopriva, and X. Chen, "Random walk and graph cut for co-segmentation of lung tumor on PET-CT images," *IEEE Transactions on Image Processing,* vol. 24, no. 12, pp. 5854–5867, 2015.
50. F. Xia, J. Liu, H. Nie, Y. Fu, L. Wan, and X. Kong, "Random walks: a review of algorithms and applications," *IEEE Transactions on Emerging Topics in Computational Intelligence,* vol. 4, no. 2, pp. 95–107, 2019.
51. N. Plath, M. Toussaint, and S. Nakajima, "Multi-class image segmentation using conditional random fields and global classification," in *Proceedings of the 26th Annual International Conference on Machine Learning*, Montreal, Quebec, Canada, 2009, pp. 817–824. https://doi.org/10.1145/1553374.1553479

52. X. Zhao, Y. Wu, G. Song, Z. Li, Y. Fan, and Y. Zhang, "Brain tumor segmentation using a fully convolutional neural network with conditional random fields," in *Brainlesion: Glioma, Multiple Sclerosis, Stroke and Traumatic Brain Injuries: Second International Workshop, BrainLes 2016, with the Challenges on BRATS, ISLES and mTOP 2016, Held in Conjunction with MICCAI 2016,* Athens, Greece, October 17, 2016, Revised Selected Papers 2, 2016: Springer, pp. 75–87.
53. T. A. Soomro et al., "Image segmentation for MR brain tumor detection using machine learning: a review," *IEEE Reviews in Biomedical Engineering,* vol. 16, pp. 70–90, 2022.
54. R. Ranjbarzadeh, A. Caputo, E. B. Tirkolaee, S. J. Ghoushchi, and M. Bendechache, "Brain tumor segmentation of MRI images: a comprehensive review on the application of artificial intelligence tools," *Computers in Biology and Medicine,* vol. 152, p. 106405, 2023.
55. R. Ayachi and N. Ben Amor, "Brain tumor segmentation using support vector machines," in *European Conference on Symbolic and Quantitative Approaches to Reasoning and Uncertainty, 10th European Conference, ECSQARU 2009,* Verona, Italy, July 1-3, 2009: Springer, pp. 736–747.
56. J. Amin, M. Sharif, M. Yasmin, and S. L. Fernandes, "A distinctive approach in brain tumor detection and classification using MRI," *Pattern Recognition Letters,* vol. 139, pp. 118–127, 2020.
57. Z. Zhang, "Introduction to machine learning: k-nearest neighbors," *Annals of Translational Medicine,* vol. 4, no. 11, p. 218, 2016.
58. N. E. A. Khalid, S. Ibrahim, and P. Haniff, "MRI brain abnormalities segmentation using k-nearest neighbors (k-NN)," *International Journal on Computer Science and Engineering,* vol. 3, no. 2, pp. 980–990, 2011.
59. R. Purwono, E. Purwanti, and R. Rulaningtyas, "Segmentation of cervical cancer CT-scan images using K-nearest neighbors method," in *The 2nd International Conference On Physical Instrumentation And Advanced Materials,* Surabaya, Indonesia, 2020, vol. 2314, no. 1: AIP Publishing.
60. F. Schroff, A. Criminisi, and A. Zisserman, "Object class segmentation using random forests," in *BMVC,* Leeds, UK, 2008, pp. 1–10.
61. D. Hartmann, D. Müller, I. Soto-Rey, and F. Kramer, "Assessing the role of random forests in medical image segmentation," *arXiv preprint arXiv:2103.16492,* 2021.
62. L. Cao, Y. Lu, C. Li, and W. Yang, "Automatic segmentation of pathological glomerular basement membrane in transmission electron microscopy images with random forest stacks," *Computational and Mathematical Methods in Medicine,* vol. 2019, no. 1, p. 1684218, 2019.
63. G. Du, X. Cao, J. Liang, X. Chen, and Y. Zhan, "Medical image segmentation based on U-Net: a review," *Journal of Imaging Science & Technology,* vol. 64, no. 2, pp. 020508-1–020508-12, 2020.
64. T. Hassanzadeh, D. Essam, and R. Sarker, "2D to 3D evolutionary deep convolutional neural networks for medical image segmentation," *IEEE Transactions on Medical Imaging,* vol. 40, no. 2, pp. 712–721, 2020.
65. K. Sailunaz, D. Bestepe, S. Alhajj, T. Özyer, J. Rokne, and R. Alhajj, "Brain tumor detection and segmentation: interactive framework with a visual interface and feedback facility for dynamically improved accuracy and trust," *Plos One,* vol. 18, no. 4, p. e0284418, 2023.
66. W. Gan et al., "Automatic segmentation of lung tumors on CT images based on a 2D & 3D hybrid convolutional neural network," *The British Journal of Radiology,* vol. 94, no. 1126, p. 20210038, 2021.
67. O. Ronneberger, P. Fischer, and T. Brox, "U-net: convolutional networks for biomedical image segmentation," in *Medical Image Computing and Computer-Assisted Intervention–MICCAI 2015: 18th International Conference,* Munich, Germany, October 5–9, 2015, proceedings, part III 18, 2015: Springer, pp. 234–241.
68. Z. Zhou, M. M. Rahman Siddiquee, N. Tajbakhsh, and J. Liang, "Unet++: a nested u-net architecture for medical image segmentation," in *Deep Learning in Medical Image Analysis and Multimodal Learning for Clinical Decision Support: 4th International Workshop, DLMIA 2018, and 8th International Workshop, ML-CDS 2018, Held in Conjunction with MICCAI 2018,* Granada, Spain, September 20, 2018, Proceedings 4, 2018: Springer, pp. 3–11.
69. Z. Zhou, M. M. R. Siddiquee, N. Tajbakhsh, and J. Liang, "Unet++: redesigning skip connections to exploit multiscale features in image segmentation," *IEEE Transactions on Medical Imaging,* vol. 39, no. 6, pp. 1856–1867, 2019.
70. A. Muneer, E. Showkatian, M. Altan, A. Sheshadri, and J. Wu, "PANDA: pneumonitis anomaly detection using attention U-net," in *Computational Mathematics Modeling in Cancer Analysis: Third International Workshop, CMMCA 2024,* Marrakesh, Morocco, October 6, 2024: Springer-Verlag, Berlin, Heidelberg, pp. 80–89. https://doi.org/10.1007/978-3-031-73360-4_9}
71. S. Xun et al., "Generative adversarial networks in medical image segmentation: a review," *Computers in Biology and Medicine,* vol. 140, p. 105063, 2022.

72. M. Salehjahromi et al., "Synthetic PET from CT improves diagnosis and prognosis for lung cancer: proof of concept," *Cell Reports Medicine,* vol. 5, no. 3, p. 101463, 2024.
73. A. Hatamizadeh et al., "Unetr: transformers for 3d medical image segmentation," in *2022 IEEE/CVF Winter Conference on Applications of Computer Vision (WACV)*, Waikoloa, HI, USA, 2022, pp. 574–584.
74. K. He, G. Gkioxari, P. Dollár, and R. Girshick, "Mask r-cnn," in *2017 IEEE International Conference on Computer Vision (ICCV)*, Venice, Italy, 2017, pp. 2961–2969.
75. V. Badrinarayanan, A. Kendall, and R. Cipolla, "Segnet: a deep convolutional encoder-decoder architecture for image segmentation," *IEEE Transactions on Pattern Analysis and Machine Intelligence,* vol. 39, no. 12, pp. 2481–2495, 2017.
76. X. Chen, Q. Duan, R. Wu, and Z. Yang, "Segmentation of lung computed tomography images based on SegNet in the diagnosis of lung cancer," *Journal of Radiation Research and Applied Sciences,* vol. 14, no. 1, pp. 396–403, 2021.
77. A. Dhere and J. Sivaswamy, "Self-supervised learning for segmentation," *arXiv preprint arXiv:2101.05456,* 2021.
78. C. Ouyang, C. Biffi, C. Chen, T. Kart, H. Qiu, and D. Rueckert, "Self-supervised learning for few-shot medical image segmentation," *IEEE Transactions on Medical Imaging,* vol. 41, no. 7, pp. 1837–1848, 2022.
79. W. Bai et al., "Self-supervised learning for cardiac mr image segmentation by anatomical position prediction," in *Medical Image Computing and Computer Assisted Intervention–MICCAI 2019: 22nd International Conference*, Shenzhen, China, October 13–17, 2019, Proceedings, Part II 22, 2019: Springer, pp. 541–549.
80. A. Taleb, C. Lippert, T. Klein, and M. Nabi, "Multimodal self-supervised learning for medical image analysis," in *Information Processing in Medical Imaging: 27th International Conference*, IPMI 2021, Virtual Event, June 28–June 30, 2021, Proceedings, 2021: Springer, Berlin, Heidelberg, pp. 661–673. https://doi.org/10.1007/978-3-030-78191-0_51
81. Z. Chen, Z. Tian, J. Zhu, C. Li, and S. Du, "C-cam: causal cam for weakly supervised semantic segmentation on medical image," in *2022 IEEE/CVF Conference on Computer Vision and Pattern Recognition (CVPR)*, New Orleans, LA, USA, 2022, pp. 11676–11685.
82. X. Feng, J. Yang, A. F. Laine, and E. D. Angelini, "Discriminative localization in CNNs for weakly-supervised segmentation of pulmonary nodules," in *Medical Image Computing and Computer Assisted Intervention– MICCAI 2017: 20th International Conference*, Quebec City, QC, Canada, September 11–13, 2017, Proceedings, Part III 20, 2017: Springer, pp. 568–576.
83. S. Zhai, G. Wang, X. Luo, Q. Yue, K. Li, and S. Zhang, "Pa-seg: learning from point annotations for 3D medical image segmentation using contextual regularization and cross knowledge distillation," *IEEE Transactions on Medical Imaging,* vol. 42, no. 8, pp. 2235–2246, 2023.
84. Y. Wu, D. Zeng, Z. Wang, Y. Shi, and J. Hu, "Distributed contrastive learning for medical image segmentation," *Medical Image Analysis,* vol. 81, p. 102564, 2022.
85. K. Chaitanya, E. Erdil, N. Karani, and E. Konukoglu, "Contrastive learning of global and local features for medical image segmentation with limited annotations," *Advances in Neural Information Processing Systems,* vol. 33, pp. 12546–12558, 2020.
86. E. J. Limkin et al., "The complexity of tumor shape, spiculatedness, correlates with tumor radiomic shape features," *Scientific Reports,* vol. 9, no. 1, p. 4329, 2019.
87. K. Fatania et al., "Intensity standardization of MRI prior to radiomic feature extraction for artificial intelligence research in glioma—a systematic review," *European Radiology,* vol. 32, no. 10, pp. 7014–7025, 2022.
88. P. Prasanna, P. Tiwari, and A. Madabhushi, "Co-occurrence of local anisotropic gradient orientations (CoLlAGe): a new radiomics descriptor," *Scientific Reports,* vol. 6, no. 1, pp. 1–14, 2016.
89. T. H. Dou, T. P. Coroller, J. J. van Griethuysen, R. H. Mak, and H. J. Aerts, "Peritumoral radiomics features predict distant metastasis in locally advanced NSCLC," *PloS One,* vol. 13, no. 11, p. e0206108, 2018.
90. R. M. Haralick, K. Shanmugam, and I. H. Dinstein, "Textural features for image classification," *IEEE Transactions on Systems, Man, and Cybernetics,* vol. SMC-3, no. 6, pp. 610–621, 1973.
91. V. K. Sudarshan et al., "Application of wavelet techniques for cancer diagnosis using ultrasound images: a review," *Computers in Biology and Medicine,* vol. 69, pp. 97–111, 2016.
92. J. W. Lee, S. Y. Kim, H. J. Lee, S. W. Han, J. E. Lee, and S. M. Lee, "Prognostic significance of CT-attenuation of tumor-adjacent breast adipose tissue in breast cancer patients with surgical resection," *Cancers,* vol. 11, no. 8, p. 1135, 2019.

93. T. Eguchi et al., "Tumor size and computed tomography attenuation of pulmonary pure ground-glass nodules are useful for predicting pathological invasiveness," *PLoS One,* vol. 9, no. 5, p. e97867, 2014.
94. E. A. Eisenhauer et al., "New response evaluation criteria in solid tumours: revised RECIST guideline (version 1.1)," *European Journal of Cancer,* vol. 45, no. 2, pp. 228–247, 2009.
95. V. Cheplygina, M. De Bruijne, and J. P. Pluim, "Not-so-supervised: a survey of semi-supervised, multi-instance, and transfer learning in medical image analysis," *Medical Image Analysis,* vol. 54, pp. 280–296, 2019.
96. P. Vaidya et al., "Novel, non-invasive imaging approach to identify patients with advanced non-small cell lung cancer at risk of hyperprogressive disease with immune checkpoint blockade," *Journal for Immunotherapy of Cancer,* vol. 8, no. 2, p. e001343, 2020.
97. M. Aminu et al., "Habitat imaging biomarkers for diagnosis and prognosis in cancer patients infected with COVID-19," *Cancers,* vol. 15, no. 1, p. 275, 2022.
98. J. Wu et al., "Tumor subregion evolution-based imaging features to assess early response and predict prognosis in oropharyngeal cancer," *Journal of Nuclear Medicine,* vol. 61, no. 3, pp. 327–336, 2020.
99. S. J. Sujit et al., "Enhancing NSCLC recurrence prediction with PET/CT habitat imaging, ctDNA, and integrative radiogenomics-blood insights," *Nature Communications,* vol. 15, no. 1, p. 3152, 2024.
100. X. Zhang et al., "Deep learning with radiomics for disease diagnosis and treatment: challenges and potential," *Frontiers in Oncology,* vol. 12, p. 773840, 2022.
101. A. Masood et al., "Computer-assisted decision support system in pulmonary cancer detection and stage classification on CT images," *Journal of Biomedical Informatics,* vol. 79, pp. 117–128, 2018.
102. N. Cristianini and J. Shawe-Taylor, *An Introduction to Support Vector Machines and Other Kernel-Based Learning Methods.* Cambridge University Press, 2000.
103. J. Gao, T. Lyu, F. Xiong, J. Wang, W. Ke, and Z. Li, "MGNN: a multimodal graph neural network for predicting the survival of cancer patients," in *Proceedings of the 43rd International ACM SIGIR Conference on Research and Development in Information Retrieval*, Xi'an, China, 2020, pp. 1697–1700.
104. G. Gogoshin and A. S. Rodin, "Graph neural networks in cancer and oncology research: emerging and future trends," *Cancers,* vol. 15, no. 24, p. 5858, 2023.
105. H. Ju, K. Kim, B. I. Kim, and S.-K. Woo, "Graph neural network model for prediction of non-small cell lung cancer lymph node metastasis using protein–protein interaction network and 18F-FDG PET/CT radiomics," *International Journal of Molecular Sciences,* vol. 25, no. 2, p. 698, 2024.
106. F. Shamshad et al., "Transformers in medical imaging: a survey," *Medical Image Analysis,* vol. 88, p. 102802, 2023.
107. J. Ma et al., "Computerized detection of lung nodules through radiomics," *Medical Physics,* vol. 44, no. 8, pp. 4148–4158, 2017.
108. E. Sala et al., "Unravelling tumour heterogeneity using next-generation imaging: radiomics, radiogenomics, and habitat imaging," *Clinical Radiology,* vol. 72, no. 1, pp. 3–10, 2017.
109. V. K. Venugopal et al., "Unboxing AI-radiological insights into a deep neural network for lung nodule characterization," *Academic Radiology,* vol. 27, no. 1, pp. 88–95, 2020.
110. Y. Xu et al., "Application of radiomics in predicting the malignancy of pulmonary nodules in different sizes," *American Journal of Roentgenology,* vol. 213, no. 6, pp. 1213–1220, 2019.
111. J. Gong et al., "A deep residual learning network for predicting lung adenocarcinoma manifesting as ground-glass nodule on CT images," *European Radiology,* vol. 30, pp. 1847–1855, 2020.
112. J. Uthoff et al., "Machine learning approach for distinguishing malignant and benign lung nodules utilizing standardized perinodular parenchymal features from CT," *Medical Physics,* vol. 46, no. 7, pp. 3207–3216, 2019.
113. R. Sun et al., "A radiomics approach to assess tumour-infiltrating CD8 cells and response to anti-PD-1 or anti-PD-L1 immunotherapy: an imaging biomarker, retrospective multicohort study," *The Lancet Oncology,* vol. 19, no. 9, pp. 1180–1191, 2018.
114. H. Wang et al., "Association between computed tomographic features and Kirsten rat sarcoma viral oncogene mutations in patients with stage I lung adenocarcinoma and their prognostic value," *Clinical Lung Cancer,* vol. 17, no. 4, pp. 271–278, 2016.
115. E. Rios Velazquez et al., "Somatic mutations drive distinct imaging phenotypes in lung cancer," *Cancer Research,* vol. 77, no. 14, pp. 3922–3930, 2017.
116. P. Desbordes et al., "Predictive value of initial FDG-PET features for treatment response and survival in esophageal cancer patients treated with chemo-radiation therapy using a random forest classifier," *PLoS One,* vol. 12, no. 3, p. e0173208, 2017.

117. M. Takeda, I. Okamoto, and K. Nakagawa, "Survival outcome assessed according to tumor response and shrinkage pattern in patients with EGFR mutation–positive non-small-cell lung cancer treated with gefitinib or erlotinib," *Journal of Thoracic Oncology,* vol. 9, no. 2, pp. 200–204, 2014.
118. A. Marchetti et al., "Early prediction of response to tyrosine kinase inhibitors by quantification of EGFR mutations in plasma of NSCLC patients," *Journal of Thoracic Oncology,* vol. 10, no. 10, pp. 1437–1443, 2015.
119. S. H. Bak, H. Park, I. Sohn, S. H. Lee, M.-J. Ahn, and H. Y. Lee, "Prognostic impact of longitudinal monitoring of radiomic features in patients with advanced non-small ell lung cancer," *Scientific Reports,* vol. 9, no. 1, p. 8730, 2019.
120. S. Trebeschi et al., "Predicting response to cancer immunotherapy using noninvasive radiomic biomarkers," *Annals of Oncology,* vol. 30, no. 6, pp. 998–1004, 2019.
121. E. Showkatian et al., "PD-L1 expression prediction using scalable multi instance transformer," in *Computational Mathematics Modeling in Cancer Analysis: Third International Workshop, CMMCA 2024, Marrakesh, Morocco, October 6, 2024, Proceedings,* Marrakesh, Morocco, 2024: Springer, Berlin, Heidelberg, pp. 61–69. https://doi.org/10.1007/978-3-031-73360-4_7
122. X. Fave et al., "Delta-radiomics features for the prediction of patient outcomes in non-small cell lung cancer," *Scientific Reports,* vol. 7, no. 1, p. 588, 2017.
123. F. Orlhac, M. Soussan, J.-A. Maisonobe, C. A. Garcia, B. Vanderlinden, and I. Buvat, "Tumor texture analysis in 18F-FDG PET: relationships between texture parameters, histogram indices, standardized uptake values, metabolic volumes, and total lesion glycolysis," *Journal of Nuclear Medicine,* vol. 55, no. 3, pp. 414–422, 2014.
124. F. Ng, R. Kozarski, B. Ganeshan, and V. Goh, "Assessment of tumor heterogeneity by CT texture analysis: can the largest cross-sectional area be used as an alternative to whole tumor analysis?," *European Journal of Radiology,* vol. 82, no. 2, pp. 342–348, 2013.
125. X. Fave et al., "Preliminary investigation into sources of uncertainty in quantitative imaging features," *Computerized Medical Imaging and Graphics,* vol. 44, pp. 54–61, 2015.
126. M. Hatt et al., "18F-FDG PET uptake characterization through texture analysis: investigating the complementary nature of heterogeneity and functional tumor volume in a multi–cancer site patient cohort," *Journal of Nuclear Medicine,* vol. 56, no. 1, pp. 38–44, 2015.
127. M. Sollini, L. Cozzi, L. Antunovic, A. Chiti, and M. Kirienko, "PET Radiomics in NSCLC: state of the art and a proposal for harmonization of methodology," *Scientific Reports,* vol. 7, no. 1, p. 358, 2017.
128. I. Buvat, F. Orlhac, and M. Soussan, "Tumor texture analysis in PET: where do we stand?," *Journal of Nuclear Medicine,* vol. 56, no. 11, pp. 1642–1644, 2015.
129. Y. Balagurunathan et al., "Reproducibility and prognosis of quantitative features extracted from CT images," *Translational Oncology,* vol. 7, no. 1, pp. 72–87, 2014.
130. M.-C. Desseroit et al., "Reliability of PET/CT shape and heterogeneity features in functional and morphologic components of non–small cell lung cancer tumors: a repeatability analysis in a prospective multicenter cohort," *Journal of Nuclear Medicine,* vol. 58, no. 3, pp. 406–411, 2017.
131. J. Yan et al., "Impact of image reconstruction settings on texture features in 18F-FDG PET," *Journal of Nuclear Medicine,* vol. 56, no. 11, pp. 1667–1673, 2015.
132. P. E. Galavis, C. Hollensen, N. Jallow, B. Paliwal, and R. Jeraj, "Variability of textural features in FDG PET images due to different acquisition modes and reconstruction parameters," *Acta Oncologica,* vol. 49, no. 7, pp. 1012–1016, 2010.
133. M. Hatt, D. Visvikis, N. M. Albarghach, F. Tixier, O. Pradier, and C. Cheze-le Rest, "Prognostic value of 18 F-FDG PET image-based parameters in oesophageal cancer and impact of tumour delineation methodology," *European Journal of Nuclear Medicine and Molecular Imaging,* vol. 38, pp. 1191–1202, 2011.
134. R. T. Larue, G. Defraene, D. De Ruysscher, P. Lambin, and W. Van Elmpt, "Quantitative radiomics studies for tissue characterization: a review of technology and methodological procedures," *The British Journal of Radiology,* vol. 90, no. 1070, p. 20160665, 2017.
135. F. J. Brooks and P. W. Grigsby, "The effect of small tumor volumes on studies of intratumoral heterogeneity of tracer uptake," *Journal of Nuclear Medicine,* vol. 55, no. 1, pp. 37–42, 2014.
136. F. Tixier, M. Hatt, C. C. Le Rest, A. Le Pogam, L. Corcos, and D. Visvikis, "Reproducibility of tumor uptake heterogeneity characterization through textural feature analysis in 18F-FDG PET," *Journal of Nuclear Medicine,* vol. 53, no. 5, pp. 693–700, 2012.
137. R. T. Leijenaar et al., "The effect of SUV discretization in quantitative FDG-PET radiomics: the need for standardized methodology in tumor texture analysis," *Scientific Reports,* vol. 5, no. 1, p. 11075, 2015.

138. F. Orlhac, M. Soussan, K. Chouahnia, E. Martinod, and I. Buvat, "18F-FDG PET-derived textural indices reflect tissue-specific uptake pattern in non-small cell lung cancer," *PLoS One,* vol. 10, no. 12, p. e0145063, 2015.
139. F. Prayer et al., "Variability of computed tomography radiomics features of fibrosing interstitial lung disease: a test-retest study," *Methods,* vol. 188, pp. 98–104, 2021.
140. M. Meyer et al., "Reproducibility of CT radiomic features within the same patient: influence of radiation dose and CT reconstruction settings," *Radiology,* vol. 293, no. 3, pp. 583–591, 2019.
141. L. Lu et al., "Identifying robust radiomics features for lung cancer by using in-vivo and phantom lung lesions," *Tomography,* vol. 7, no. 1, pp. 55–64, 2021.
142. X. Gao et al., "The method and efficacy of support vector machine classifiers based on texture features and multi-resolution histogram from 18F-FDG PET-CT images for the evaluation of mediastinal lymph nodes in patients with lung cancer," *European Journal of Radiology,* vol. 84, no. 2, pp. 312–317, 2015.
143. M. Hatt, F. Tixier, C. Cheze Le Rest, O. Pradier, and D. Visvikis, "Robustness of intratumour 18 F-FDG PET uptake heterogeneity quantification for therapy response prediction in oesophageal carcinoma," *European Journal of Nuclear Medicine and Molecular Imaging,* vol. 40, pp. 1662–1671, 2013.
144. R. Da-Ano, D. Visvikis, and M. Hatt, "Harmonization strategies for multicenter radiomics investigations," *Physics in Medicine & Biology,* vol. 65, no. 24, p. 24TR02, 2020.
145. N. Meinshausen and P. Bühlmann, "Stability selection," *Journal of the Royal Statistical Society Series B: Statistical Methodology,* vol. 72, no. 4, pp. 417–473, 2010.
146. X.-w. Chen and J. C. Jeong, "Enhanced recursive feature elimination," in *Sixth International Conference on Machine Learning and Applications (ICMLA 2007),* Cincinnati, OH, USA, 2007: IEEE, pp. 429–435.
147. H. Peng, F. Long, and C. Ding, "Feature selection based on mutual information criteria of max-dependency, max-relevance, and min-redundancy," *IEEE Transactions on Pattern Analysis and Machine Intelligence,* vol. 27, no. 8, pp. 1226–1238, 2005.
148. K. J. Archer and R. V. Kimes, "Empirical characterization of random forest variable importance measures," *Computational Statistics & Data Analysis,* vol. 52, no. 4, pp. 2249–2260, 2008.
149. H. Zou, "The adaptive lasso and its oracle properties," *Journal of the American Statistical Association,* vol. 101, no. 476, pp. 1418–1429, 2006.
150. J. A. Gagnon-Bartsch and T. P. Speed, "Using control genes to correct for unwanted variation in microarray data," *Biostatistics,* vol. 13, no. 3, pp. 539–552, 2012.
151. A. Scherer, *Batch Effects and Noise in Microarray Experiments: Sources and Solutions.* Wiley Online Library, 2009.
152. J. T. Leek, *Surrogate Variable Analysis.* University of Washington, 2007.
153. J. T. Leek and J. D. Storey, "A general framework for multiple testing dependence," *Proceedings of the National Academy of Sciences,* vol. 105, no. 48, pp. 18718–18723, 2008.
155. J. Maksimovic, J. A. Gagnon-Bartsch, T. P. Speed, and A. Oshlack, "Removing unwanted variation in a differential methylation analysis of Illumina HumanMethylation450 array data," *Nucleic Acids Research,* vol. 43, no. 16, pp. e106–e106, 2015.
155. W. E. Johnson, C. Li, and A. Rabinovic, "Adjusting batch effects in microarray expression data using empirical Bayes methods," *Biostatistics,* vol. 8, no. 1, pp. 118–127, 2007.
156. H. Horng et al., "Generalized ComBat harmonization methods for radiomic features with multi-modal distributions and multiple batch effects," *Scientific Reports,* vol. 12, no. 1, p. 4493, 2022.
157. K.-Y. Kim et al., "An attempt for combining microarray data sets by adjusting gene expressions," *Cancer Research and Treatment,* vol. 39, no. 2, pp. 74–81, 2007.
158. A. H. Sims et al., "The removal of multiplicative, systematic bias allows integration of breast cancer gene expression datasets–improving meta-analysis and prediction of prognosis," *BMC Medical Genomics,* vol. 1, pp. 1–14, 2008.
159. C. Li and W. H. Wong, "Model-based analysis of oligonucleotide arrays: expression index computation and outlier detection," *Proceedings of the National Academy of Sciences,* vol. 98, no. 1, pp. 31–36, 2001.
160. J. Luo et al., "A comparison of batch effect removal methods for enhancement of prediction performance using MAQC-II microarray gene expression data," *The Pharmacogenomics Journal,* vol. 10, no. 4, pp. 278–291, 2010.
161. A. A. Shabalin, H. Tjelmeland, C. Fan, C. M. Perou, and A. B. Nobel, "Merging two gene-expression studies via cross-platform normalization," *Bioinformatics,* vol. 24, no. 9, pp. 1154–1160, 2008.
162. S. Kotsiantis and D. Kanellopoulos, "Discretization techniques: a recent survey," *GESTS International Transactions on Computer Science and Engineering,* vol. 32, no. 1, pp. 47–58, 2006.
163. P. Warnat, R. Eils, and B. Brors, "Cross-platform analysis of cancer microarray data improves gene expression based classification of phenotypes," *BMC Bioinformatics,* vol. 6, pp. 1–15, 2005.

164. M. N. McCall and R. A. Irizarry, "Thawing frozen robust multi-array analysis (fRMA)," *BMC Bioinformatics,* vol. 12, pp. 1–7, 2011.
165. F. Orlhac, F. Frouin, C. Nioche, N. Ayache, and I. Buvat, "Validation of a method to compensate multicenter effects affecting CT radiomics," *Radiology,* vol. 291, no. 1, pp. 53–59, 2019.
166. R. Da-Ano et al., "Performance comparison of modified ComBat for harmonization of radiomic features for multicenter studies," *Scientific Reports,* vol. 10, no. 1, p. 10248, 2020.
167. F. Orlhac et al., "A postreconstruction harmonization method for multicenter radiomic studies in PET," *Journal of Nuclear Medicine,* vol. 59, no. 8, pp. 1321–1328, 2018.

5 Vision-Language Models for Medical Image Analysis

Mingzhe Hu, Zach Eidex, Feng Zhao, and Xiaofeng Yang

5.1 INTRODUCTION

Precision radiation therapy has long stood at the cutting edge of medical innovation, transforming how cancer and other conditions are treated through targeted applications of radiation. Its roots trace back to the early 20th century with the pioneering work in using radiation to selectively destroy malignant tissues. Over the decades, advancements such as the linear accelerator, intensity-modulated radiation therapy (IMRT), stereotactic radiosurgery, and proton therapy have significantly enhanced the precision, safety, and effectiveness of radiation treatments (Abshire and Lang, 2018). Each milestone has underscored the importance of precision in targeting tumors while sparing healthy tissues, a central goal of radiation therapy. Today, artificial intelligence (AI) represents a new frontier in this journey, with the potential to further refine imaging, diagnosis, and treatment planning. As such, the integration of AI-driven medical image analysis into precision radiation therapy holds promising potential to elevate patient outcomes and reshape clinical workflows.

Over the past decade, AI—mainly through computer vision models—has dramatically accelerated the capabilities of medical image analysis (Chen et al., 2022a). These models, which leverage deep learning and benefit from increasingly large, annotated datasets, have proven invaluable in performing complex imaging tasks like segmentation (Wang et al., 2022; Pan et al., 2023), registration (Fu et al., 2020), synthesis (Wang et al., 2021), and disease classification (Cai et al., 2020). By automating such processes, computer vision models have become essential in improving diagnostic accuracy and efficiency across various clinical applications, including radiology and oncology. However, despite their success, these models remain limited to visual data, which can constrain their ability to interpret contextual information provided in clinical notes, patient histories, and other text-based resources vital to comprehensive medical care.

In comparison, vision-language models (VLMs) have seen relatively limited use in the medical domain, primarily due to several unique challenges. Developing effective VLMs requires extensive multimodal datasets, where medical images are richly annotated with text. This resource has historically been scarce due to privacy regulations and the specialized expertise required for annotation (Gan et al., 2022). Furthermore, aligning visual and textual information in a way that reflects medical nuances demands highly sophisticated model architectures and computational resources. Recent advancements, however, have started to make VLMs surge. Innovations in transformer-based architectures, multimodal pretraining techniques, and access to diverse data sources have made training VLMs for specialized medical tasks feasible. As illustrated in Figure 5.1, VLMs can now perform various tasks in medical image analysis.

In this chapter, we explore VLMs in medical image analysis with a focus on applications in precision radiation therapy. While other imaging modalities, like microscopic and histopathology imaging, are also discussed, these insights can complement radiation therapy. Section 5.2 covers foundational concepts, including key terms, evaluation metrics, and pretraining strategies to provide the necessary background. Section 5.3, illustrated in Figure 5.2, delves into specific applications (5.3.1–5.3.6) of VLMs. Section 5.3.7 is dedicated to ChatGPT, one of the leading multimodal models, and Sections 5.3.8 and 5.3.9 focus on training and fine-tuning techniques for VLMs in

 DOI: 10.1201/9781003480365-6

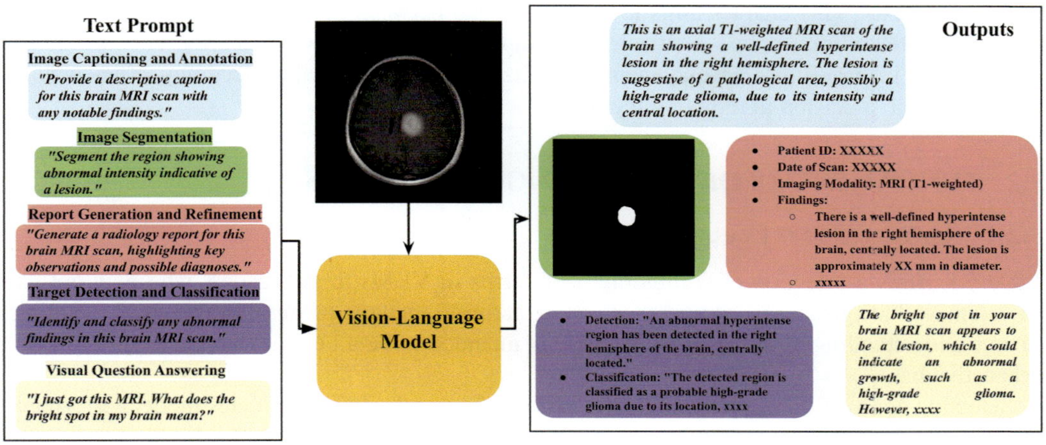

FIGURE 5.1 Example use case of VLMs for medical image analysis. Different tasks—such as image captioning and annotation, image segmentation, report generation and refinement, target detection and classification, and visual question answering—are illustrated for demonstration purposes only, showcasing the model's potential in interpreting and generating insights from brain MRI scans and text prompts to support diagnostic and patient communication needs.

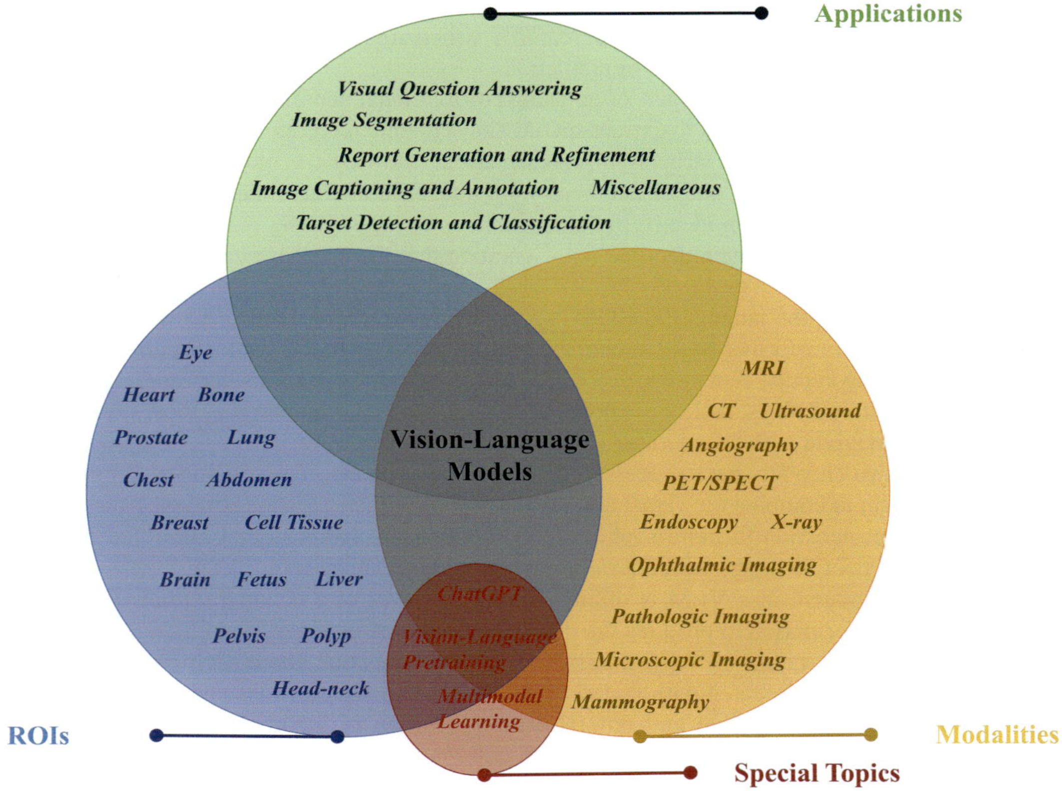

FIGURE 5.2 Overview of the scope of VLMs in this chapter, covering key applications, relevant anatomical regions of interest (ROIs), and imaging modalities. Special topics in vision-language pretraining, multimodal learning, and ChatGPT are also highlighted.

medical contexts. This chapter aims to bridge the gap between language and vision models and to inspire collaboration across medical and computer science fields. Furthermore, it serves as a launchpad to inspire future advancements in utilizing VLMs to enhance accuracy, efficiency, and patient-specific precision in radiation therapy.

5.2 FUNDAMENTALS OF VISION-LANGUAGE MODELS

5.2.1 Glossaries and Evaluation Metrics

Table 5.1 offers a selection of commonly used terms in VLMs to aid readers who may not have an extensive background in computer vision or natural language processing (NLP), facilitating a clearer understanding of our work. This table is intended to be a helpful reference, rather than an exhaustive list.

Selecting appropriate evaluation metrics is crucial, as each metric evaluates model performance from a unique perspective, ensuring a comprehensive assessment. Table 5.2 highlights essential metrics that collectively address various aspects of VLM effectiveness.

5.2.2 General Structure of Vision-Language Models

At their core, VLMs are designed to bridge the gap between visual and textual information, allowing for more nuanced interpretation and interaction with multimodal information. The general architecture of VLMs typically comprises two major components: (1) a visual encoder and (2) a language encoder, each responsible for processing data from its respective modality. These components work in tandem to extract meaningful features, which are then fused in a way that allows the model to generate informed responses or predictions.

The visual encoder takes in images, often using convolutional neural networks (CNNs) or more recent vision transformers (ViTs) to extract spatial and semantic features. This encoder transforms complex visual patterns into a structured representation, allowing the model to "see" and interpret specific regions, textures, and objects within an image. In medical imaging, for instance, the visual encoder might focus on identifying abnormalities or highlighting regions of interest, such as lesions or tumors, providing a detailed representation that the language component can further contextualize.

On the other hand, the language encoder is responsible for understanding textual information. Typically built on transformer-based architectures like BERT or GPT, capturing the nuances of language, including syntax, semantics, and context. In medical applications, the language encoder might interpret clinical notes, patient histories, or medical queries, transforming these into a format the model can integrate with visual data.

Once these two encoders have processed their respective inputs, the model uses a multimodal fusion mechanism to combine the visual and textual representations. Fusion strategies vary widely, from simple concatenation to more sophisticated attention mechanisms that allow the model to align specific parts of an image with relevant words or phrases in the text.

The final component in a VLM is often a prediction layer or a decoder, which synthesizes the multimodal information to produce the desired output. For instance, in a clinical setting, the model might output a radiology report, answer a patient's question about their scan, or classify an image based on the detected pathologies. This end-to-end structure (as shown in Figure 5.3) is designed to enable a flexible and powerful interpretation of medical images in ways that can enhance diagnostic workflows and facilitate communication with healthcare providers and patients alike.

TABLE 5.1
Key Terminologies and Definitions in VLMs

Term	Definition	Term	Definition	Term	Definition
VLM	A model designed to simultaneously process and interpret visual and textual data, enabling a deeper understanding of image content by leveraging contextual information from both modalities.	Cross-Modal Alignment	The process of linking and associating features across different data modalities (e.g., aligning text descriptions with visual elements), enabling the model to map related information across vision and language.	Multimodal Embedding	A shared representation space where features from different modalities (such as image and text) are mapped, allowing for seamless integration and retrieval across modalities.
Vision-Language Pretraining	The foundational training of VLMs on large datasets of paired images and text, equipping the model with generalizable knowledge across vision and language for downstream tasks.	Contrastive Learning	A learning approach where the model distinguishes between similar and dissimilar pairs (e.g., matching or mismatching image–text pairs), reinforcing the ability to link related information across modalities.	Prompt Engineering	The art of designing and refining prompts to guide model responses, particularly useful in VLMs to customize the model's focus on specific details or tasks within medical images.
Few-Shot Prompting	A technique where a model adapts to a new task with minimal labeled examples, using carefully crafted prompts to maximize performance in low-data scenarios, essential in specialized fields like medical imaging.	Prompt Fusion	The technique of combining multiple prompts to enhance model interpretability and task performance, allowing the integration of diverse contextual cues into VLM outputs.	Semantic Segmentation	A vision-language-driven segmentation technique where regions are divided based on semantic categories (e.g., organ vs. tumor), often using textual information to refine and classify segmentation boundaries.
Knowledge Distillation	A method of transferring knowledge from a larger, often multimodal model to a smaller, task-specific model, maintaining accuracy while reducing computational demands, particularly useful in resource-constrained medical environments.	Image–Text Joint Embedding	A unified representation where visual and textual information is co-embedded, enabling direct retrieval and matching between modalities, foundational for tasks like image-caption alignment and question answering.	Active Prompting	An iterative method where human feedback dynamically adjusts prompts to refine model outputs, commonly used in high-stakes fields like healthcare to improve precision and clinical relevance.

(Continued)

TABLE 5.1 ***(Continued)***
Key Terminologies and Definitions in VLMs

Term	Definition	Term	Definition	Term	Definition
Zero-Shot Transfer	The model's ability to generalize to tasks or datasets it has never seen before, based on its pretraining knowledge, enabling applications in new medical imaging contexts without additional retraining.	Task-Agnostic Pretraining	Pretraining that is not tailored to any specific downstream task, allowing the model to develop general features across multiple domains, making it adaptable to a variety of applications in medical imaging.	Modality-Specific Encoder	A component of the VLM designed to process one particular modality (either vision or language) before fusing the information, optimizing feature extraction specific to that modality.
Multimodal Fusion	The integration of multiple modalities (e.g., image and text) within a model's architecture, allowing for a cohesive understanding of both modalities in decision-making processes, critical for vision-language tasks.	Language-Conditioned Generation	A generative approach where language inputs guide the generation of outputs (e.g., captions, annotations) for visual data, tailoring responses based on linguistic context and ensuring relevance to medical imagery.	Spatial-Textual Attention	A mechanism that allows the model to focus on specific regions in an image in response to associated text, enabling precise localization of features like tumors or organs based on descriptive input.

TABLE 5.2
Key Evaluation Metrics for VLMs

Metric	Definition	Metric	Definition
Accuracy	Measures the proportion of correct predictions, used primarily in classification tasks to assess the model's overall performance in correctly identifying target classes.	Precision	The ratio of true positive predictions to all positive predictions (true positives + false positives), indicating the model's accuracy in identifying relevant items.
Recall	The ratio of true positive predictions to all actual positives (true positives + false negatives), measuring the model's ability to detect relevant instances.	F1 Score	The harmonic mean of precision and recall, balancing the trade-off between the two to provide a single measure of accuracy, especially useful for imbalanced datasets.
BLEU (Bilingual Evaluation Understudy)	A metric for evaluating text generation quality by comparing n-grams in the generated text to those in reference text, widely used in image captioning tasks.	ROUGE (recall-oriented understudy for gisting evaluation)	A set of metrics measuring overlap between generated and reference text, particularly used in summarization and report generation tasks.
CIDEr (consensus-based image description evaluation)	Measures the similarity between generated captions and reference captions by evaluating n-gram overlap, with an emphasis on consensus among references.	METEOR (metric for evaluation of translation with explicit ordering)	Evaluates text generation by matching stems, synonyms, and phrases between generated and reference captions, often used alongside BLEU.
SPICE (semantic propositional image caption evaluation)	A captioning metric focusing on the semantic content by comparing scene graphs of generated and reference captions to assess accuracy in meaning.	Mean reciprocal rank (MRR)	Used in retrieval tasks, calculates the average of the reciprocal ranks of correct answers in a list, assessing the model's ranking performance in multimodal retrieval.
Recall@K	Measures the proportion of relevant items found within the top-K retrieved results, widely used in image–text retrieval and matching tasks.	Visual question answering (VQA) accuracy	Measures the proportion of correct answers in VQA tasks, considering both exact match and partial match criteria based on question relevance and context.
IoU (intersection over union)	Commonly used in segmentation, calculates the overlap between predicted and actual segment regions, assessing how accurately the model delineates image areas.	mAP (mean average precision)	Measures the average precision across all classes and object locations, commonly used in object detection to evaluate how well the model locates and identifies targets.
Dice score	A metric used primarily in segmentation tasks, calculating the similarity between predicted and actual segmented regions. It ranges from 0 to 1, with 1 indicating perfect overlap.	KL divergence (Kullback–Leibler divergence)	Measures the difference between two probability distributions, often used to evaluate the model's predictive distribution against a reference distribution, assessing uncertainty and model calibration.

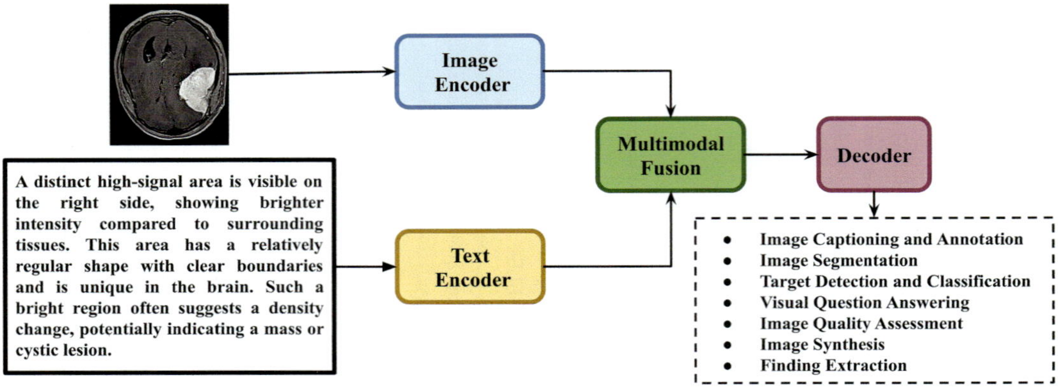

FIGURE 5.3 A typical structure of the VLM for medical image analysis.

5.2.3 Vision-Language Models Pretraining Strategies

Pretraining allows VLMs to understand and generate insights from visual and textual data before being fine-tuned on specific tasks (Gan et al., 2022). In the medical domain, where data availability, accuracy, and contextual relevance are essential, effective pretraining can significantly enhance a model's performance in specialized tasks such as report generation, anomaly detection, segmentation, and patient-specific diagnosis.

5.2.3.1 Cross-Modal Contrastive Learning

One widely adopted pretraining strategy for VLMs is cross-modal contrastive learning (Zhang et al., 2021), where the model learns to align visual and textual representations by distinguishing matching pairs from nonmatching ones. In this approach, pairs of images and text that describe the same content (e.g., an MRI image and a corresponding clinical note) are presented as positive, while mismatched (e.g., an MRI image paired with unrelated text) serve as negatives. This method helps the model learn relationships between visual and language elements, enhancing its capacity to retrieve or generate accurate information based on cross-modal cues.

5.2.3.2 Masked Image Modeling and Masked Language Modeling

Another practical approach is masked modeling, where certain parts of the input image or text are masked, and the model is trained to predict these missing pieces (Kwon et al., 2022). Masked image modeling (MIM) helps the visual encoder learn to reconstruct occluded sections of an image, improving its ability to capture fine-grained details where subtle features may indicate critical findings. Similarly, masked language modeling (MLM) requires the language encoder to predict masked words or phrases in a sentence, enhancing the model's linguistic comprehension.

5.2.3.2.1 Image–Text Matching (ITM)

Image–text matching (ITM) is another core pretraining technique, where the model learns to determine whether a given image and text description are contextually aligned (Abdullah and Rangarajan, 2021). Through ITM, VLMs can be trained to assess whether a textual input accurately describes an image, thus reinforcing their capability to validate and cross-reference information across modalities. This strategy is highly beneficial in applications that require generating diagnostic reports from images or verifying image–text pairs in automated workflows.

5.2.3.3 Multimodal Pretraining with Domain-Specific Data

In the medical imaging field, general-purpose VLMs often fail due to the specificity and technical complexity of the data. Therefore, pretraining with domain-specific data is crucial to bridge this gap. Using large-scale, curated medical datasets that include images (such as MRI, CT, or ultrasound scans) and corresponding clinical notes allows VLMs to develop a more specialized understanding of medical imaging. Pretraining on such datasets helps models capture unique medical terminology, recognize imaging features specific to certain conditions, and understand the context around diagnostic workflows.

5.2.3.4 Knowledge Distillation and Transfer Learning

Knowledge distillation and transfer learning are often applied to improve model performance on specific medical tasks without extensive pretraining (Wang and Yoon, 2021). Knowledge distillation allows a well-trained model (teacher) to pass on knowledge to a smaller, more efficient model (student), making it feasible to deploy VLMs in resource-constrained environments, such as clinical settings with limited computational resources. Transfer learning, meanwhile, allows VLMs to adapt from general-purpose pretraining to medical-specific tasks by fine-tuning on smaller, labeled datasets. This approach helps VLMs retain the foundational knowledge from large datasets while becoming more adept at handling specific medical image analysis tasks.

5.3 VISION-LANGUAGE MODELS FOR MEDICAL IMAGE ANALYSIS

5.3.1 Image Captioning and Annotation

Image captioning and annotation are critical processes in medical imaging, aimed at generating descriptive labels and structured information that accurately reflect the visual content of images. Image captioning involves the automatic generation of textual descriptions, while annotation includes marking regions of interest, labeling structures, or adding specific tags relevant to diagnosis or treatment. In radiation oncology, these tasks are traditionally performed through a combination of manual and semiautomated approaches. Radiologists and oncologists interpret different modalities such as CT, MRI, and PET scans, documenting findings and annotating critical anatomical landmarks, tumors, or other relevant structures. Although precise, these annotations are time-consuming and resource-intensive, relying on consistent expertise and thorough review. Semiautomated tools have been employed to assist specialists by suggesting regions of interest or labeling structures, yet these tools still demand verification and adjustments by clinicians.

VLMs offer promising enhancements to the image captioning and annotation tasks, automating and standardizing aspects of these processes by leveraging large-scale pretrained models capable of interpreting both visual and textual data. Through the integration of deep learning and NLP, VLMs can generate accurate captions, identify anatomical structures, and even suggest clinical findings based on visual information, significantly expediting the annotation process in radiation therapy. This not only helps to standardize documentation but also allows clinicians to focus more on complex decision-making, potentially improving accuracy by minimizing variability inherent in manual interpretation. By bringing efficiency, consistency, and scalability to image captioning and annotation, VLMs open up new possibilities for data-driven, personalized radiation therapy.

Allaouzi et al. conducted a pivotal study on automatic caption generation for medical images, examining both generative and retrieval-based approaches to alleviate medical experts' workload (Allaouzi et al., 2018). The study employed encoder–decoder architectures, specifically CNNs such as VGG-16 and Inception-V3 for encoding image features, coupled with RNNs (notably LSTMs) for textual decoding, enabling the generation of descriptive captions from visual data. Additionally, retrieval-based models were utilized to modify captions from similar images within extensive datasets when exact image-caption pairs were available, often aided by attention mechanisms to emphasize relevant visual features. Key datasets included IU X-Ray, PEIR Gross, BCIDR, and

ImageCLEF Caption, covering modalities like X-ray, CT, PET, MRI, and ultrasound. Although no new experimental results were presented, the study highlighted commonly used evaluation metrics, such as BLEU, ROUGE-L, METEOR, CIDEr, and SPICE, underscoring the importance of semantic content alignment with human judgment. The authors noted limitations in existing models, particularly in their adaptability to novel images outside preexisting datasets, emphasizing the need for expanded datasets and advanced generative methods.

Expanding on encoder–decoder architectures, another study turned attention to histopathological images (Elbedwehy et al., 2024). Elbedwehy et al. presented a significant advancement in descriptive captioning for histopathological images by combining the strengths of ConvNeXT-Large and PVT_v2_b5 as visual encoders with BioLinkBERT-Large for language processing, which allowed for more precise caption generation of complex tissue structures, particularly within stomach adenocarcinoma specimens. This framework first extracted detailed visual features via a concatenated model using ConvNeXT-Large and PVT_v2_b5, enhanced through data augmentation, and then processed these with BioLinkBERT-Large, which was fine-tuned alongside LSTM, RNN, and bidirectional-RNN variants to optimize the VLM pairing for descriptive captions. The model achieved superior results compared to prior approaches, evidenced by a BLEU4 score of 0.309, highlighting its effectiveness over simpler RNN-based architectures and demonstrating the considerable benefits of combining advanced vision and language models for specialized medical captioning tasks.

While detailed descriptive captioning in pathology has advanced, a separate exploration in echocardiography introduced EchoCLIP, a specialized model for cardiac interpretation (Christensen et al., 2024). By leveraging extensive echocardiogram video–text pairs and contrastive learning, this model achieves near-human diagnostic accuracy, showing the impact of targeted data in enhancing model performance. EchoCLIP employed ConvNeXt-Base as its image encoder and a CLIP-inspired transformer for text encoding, aligning echocardiographic frames with clinical report text through contrastive learning. This approach, alongside a specialized EchoCLIP-R variant incorporating a customized tokenizer, facilitated efficient text compression and improved text retrieval performance in echocardiography contexts. The model excelled in diverse zero-shot tasks, achieving a mean absolute error of 7.1% for left ventricular ejection fraction estimation and AUCs as high as 0.97 for identifying MitraClip devices, 0.92 for TAVR, and 0.84 for pacemakers. Moreover, EchoCLIP effectively distinguished patient-specific echocardiograms over time, with AUCs of 0.79 for post-transplant identification and 0.77 for post-cardiac surgery, highlighting its potential for longitudinal cardiac monitoring and robust clinical application in echocardiographic interpretation.

Unlike domain-specific applications, another research effort proposed a hybrid approach to improve captioning across a range of radiological datasets (Beddiar et al., 2023). By combining generative and retrieval-based techniques, this dual-model approach demonstrated a considerable boost in accuracy, highlighting the benefits of versatile architectures. The model architecture utilized ResNet50 as the CNN encoder to extract image features, which were then processed through an LSTM for text generation in a multistage setup. Additionally, a retrieval-based module was integrated, using TfIdf embeddings and cosine similarity to identify relevant captions from the training set, aiming to refine the generated captions for higher fidelity. A unique fusion process was implemented to select the optimal caption by evaluating both generated and retrieved captions against BLEU score criteria, allowing the model to leverage the strengths of generative text synthesis alongside refined similarity-based selection. This fused model achieved a BLEU-4 score of 18.61 on radiology images, considerably outperforming the multistage model (BLEU-4 of 7.89) and surpassing other state-of-the-art models like ODM. This dual approach enhanced the model's capability to generate more descriptive and contextually accurate captions for radiological data, particularly within the ROCO dataset.

Pushing further into the integration of language and vision, one study explored the infusion of enriched textual concepts directly into image encoding (Liu et al., 2020). This strategy not only enhances descriptive accuracy but also paves the way for models that understand both visual and contextual nuances across varied imaging scenes. The model employed a region-CNN for image

TABLE 5.3
Overview of VLMs for Image Captioning and Annotation

Reference	ROI	Modality	Dataset	Model Name	Backbone Model/ Module
Allaouzi et al. (2018)	Chest, bladder, and general diagnostic regions	X-ray, CT, PET, MRI, and ultrasound	IU X-Ray, PEIR Gross, BCIDR, and ImageCLEF	*	CNNs (VGG-16, Inception-V3), RNNs (LSTMs)
Liu et al. (2020)	*	*	MSCOCO	Flickr30k	Region-CNN, textual distilling module, textual association module
Elbedwehy et al. (2024)	Stomach adenocarcinoma tissue	Microscopic	PatchGastricADC22	*	ConvNeXT-large, PVT_v2_b5, BioLinkBERT-Large
Beddiar et al. (2023)	General	General	ROCO	*	CNN (ResNet50), LSTM, TfIdf embedding
Christensen et al. (2024)	Cardiac	Ultrasound	EchoNet-Dynamic	EchoCLIP	ConvNeXt-base, byte-pair encoding tokenizer, decoder-only transformer

The asterisks (*) indicate terms that are either not present in the original paper or do not apply in this context.

encoding, complemented by a textual distilling module (TDM) and a textual association module (TAM), which enriched visual features with contextual textual information. TDM used attention mechanisms to highlight key visual descriptors, while TAM linked these descriptors into cohesive textual phrases, which were then decoded into captions. Evaluated on the MSCOCO and Flickr30k datasets, this model significantly improved caption quality, achieving up to a 10% increase in CIDEr and a 9% rise in SPICE scores, outperforming previous benchmarks by enhancing descriptive accuracy and fluency across diverse scenes and objects.

The summary of works related to VLMs for image captioning and annotation is presented in Table 5.3.

5.3.2 Image Segmentation

Image segmentation has seen significant advancements through fully vision-based AI models, which have been widely applied in medical imaging to delineate anatomical structures and identify pathological regions with high precision. However, despite their accuracy, these models are limited in their ability to incorporate contextual or descriptive information beyond pixel-level data, which can be valuable in complex clinical scenarios. VLMs offer a complementary approach by integrating language inputs—such as anatomical labels, clinical descriptions, or specific diagnostic cues—alongside the visual data, enabling a more nuanced segmentation process that can align more closely with clinical requirements. This added context allows VLMs not only to recognize image features but also to understand relationships and hierarchies within anatomical regions, enhancing their interpretability and relevance to clinical workflows.

In radiation therapy, VLMs can be particularly advantageous by incorporating patient-specific or protocol-specific information as language inputs. For example, VLMs can utilize inputs such as organ names, tumor grading, prior clinical notes, or treatment planning details. This additional contextual information enables segmentation models to focus on clinically significant regions or adapt segmentation based on treatment intent, providing a level of customization not feasible with vision-only models. By combining visual and linguistic data, VLMs help bridge the gap between image features and clinical needs, making them highly valuable for personalized and precision-oriented approaches in radiation therapy.

Chen et al. introduced Bi-VLGM, a model that innovatively applies bi-level class-severity-aware vision-language graph matching to improve text-guided medical image segmentation (Chen et al., 2024b). The model integrates HRNetV2 for image segmentation with BioLinkBERT for encoding textual prompts, employing a graph-based strategy to align visual and textual features without relying on conventional contrastive techniques. This approach constructs two levels of graph matching: a word-level module that matches image features with class-specific text prompts using graph nodes to represent lesion classes, and a sentence-level module that aligns severity-encoded prompts with global image representations. By iteratively refining both local and global feature alignments, Bi-VLGM effectively preserves intra-modal relationships and captures subtle distinctions across complex lesion classes. The model demonstrated robust performance, achieving top mDice and mIoU scores of 86.39% on the BCSS dataset and 51.37% on the IDRiD dataset, respectively, and outperformed other models by 1%–3% on metrics like IoU and AUPR, especially excelling in differentiating similar lesion types across challenging datasets.

In their study on pneumothorax segmentation, Huemann et al. introduced ConTEXTual Net, a multimodal model that bridges vision and language domains to enhance segmentation precision in chest radiographs (Huemann et al., 2024). The model uses a U-Net for visual encoding, integrated with a pretrained RoBERTa-Large for text encoding, with cross-attention modules aligning the text and image features across the U-Net layers. By leveraging clinical reports from the CANDID-PTX dataset, the model was trained to capture subtle pneumothorax cases through supervised learning with cross-entropy loss. Through rigorous ablation studies and data augmentations, ConTEXTual Net's design was fine-tuned for optimal performance. It achieved an average Dice score of 0.716±0.016, outperforming standard models like the ResNet50 U-Net at 0.677±0.015 and closely aligning with expert-level consistency at 0.712±0.044. Furthermore, the model surpassed other multimodal approaches like LAVT (Dice score of 0.706±0.009), proving the value of clinical text integration in accurately identifying nuanced pneumothorax indicators while reducing false positives.

Similarly, Li et al. introduced LViT (Li et al., 2023), a model designed to integrate textual information with image data, advancing segmentation performance in medical imaging tasks. LViT combines a U-Net-based CNN for capturing detailed image features with a vision transformer (ViT) branch that merges text embeddings, bypassing a full language encoder to maintain efficiency. A double-U architecture facilitates deep image–text integration, with a pixel-level attention module (PLAM) enhancing feature retention at skip connections and an exponential pseudo-label iteration (EPI) method generating high-quality pseudo-labels in semi-supervised learning scenarios. Through a training approach combining Dice and cross-entropy losses, as well as a unique language-vision (LV) loss, LViT effectively leverages limited text annotations to enrich segmentation outcomes. Performance benchmarks were impressive: on the QaTa-COV19 dataset, it achieved a Dice score of 83.66% and mIoU of 75.11%, while on MosMedData+ and ESO-CT, it scored 74.57% Dice and 71.53% Dice, respectively, surpassing models like nnUNet and other CNN–transformer hybrids. This approach not only reduced dependency on annotated data but also proved highly effective in segmenting infection regions in COVID-19 cases and esophageal areas, marking a significant step forward in leveraging multimodal data for medical image analysis.

In their research on improving segmentation in echocardiography, Adhikari et al. examined the impact of pretraining vision-language segmentation models (VLSMs) with synthetic data on performance when fine-tuned with real echocardiographic data (Adhikari et al., 2023). The authors used models like CLIPSeg and CRIS, leveraging the dual-encoder structure of CLIP to separate image and text encodings, followed by a vision-language decoder. By generating synthetic echocardiography images via semantic diffusion models (SDMs), conditioned on anatomical masks, they created pretraining data with distributions similar to real-world echocardiography. This synthetic pretraining strategy, further enhanced by prompt engineering based on metadata (e.g., heart structure, view, patient age, and cardiac phase), was tested against real-only and synthetic-only training approaches. Their findings showed that models using the hybrid pretraining approach achieved the highest Dice scores, improving by approximately +0.34 over real-data-only training. Notably, the synthetic pretraining accelerated model convergence—CRIS converged 4.55 times faster, while CLIPSeg improved by 1.71 times. Overall, these results highlight the potential of synthetic pretraining to enhance segmentation accuracy and efficiency in VLSMs for echocardiographic applications, suggesting further gains may be achievable through refined synthetic data generation techniques.

For more general applications, Liu et al. introduced the Universal Model (Liu et al., 2024), an extensible framework integrating vision and language models to perform complex organ segmentation and tumor detection in CT scans. The model distinguishes itself by using a Swin UNETR-based vision backbone combined with CLIP and BioBERT embeddings, enabling it to adapt to new anatomical structures and handle partially labeled data without the need for retraining. The language-driven parameter generator (LPG) effectively translates linguistic descriptions into model parameters, while a class-specific segmentation head (CSH) employs a multilayer perceptron (MLP) for precise anatomical mapping. By utilizing binary cross-entropy and Dice loss, the Universal Model optimized segmentation across 25 organs and six tumor types, showing resilience in continually learning without memory overheads. Experimentally, it set new standards on organ segmentation benchmarks, with Dice scores reaching 95.42% for the liver and 67.15% for hepatic vessels, outperforming prior models with a remarkable 76.11% average Dice score across major organ tasks. Additionally, the Universal Model demonstrated efficiency by running 6 times faster than models tailored to specific datasets, underlining its robust adaptability across various clinical sites and datasets.

TABLE 5.4
Overview of VLMs for Image Segmentation

Reference	ROI	Modality	Dataset	Model Name	Backbone Model/Module
Chen et al. (2024b)	Tumor regions, stroma, lymphatic infiltration, necrosis, and retina	Pathology imaging, fundus images	BCSS, IDRiD, and DDR	Bi-VLGM	HRNetV2, BioLinkBERT
Huemann et al. (2024)	Lung (pneumothorax regions and surrounding structures)	X-ray	CANDID-PTX	ConTEXTual Net	U-Net, RoBERTa-Large
Li et al.,(2023)	Lung	CT, X-ray	MosMedData+, QaTa-COV19, ESO-CT	LViT	U-Net, ViT
Adhikari et al. (2023)	Heart	Ultrasound	CAMUS, synthetic echocardiography dataset	CLIPSeg, CRIS	CLIP
Liu et al. (2024)	Liver, spleen, pancreas, kidneys, lungs, and various associated tumors such as liver tumor, kidney tumor, and pancreatic tumor	CT	MSD, BTCV, Pancreas-CT, LiTS, KiTS, AMOS, AbdomenCT-1K, and CHAOS	*	Swin UNETR, CLIP and BioBERT

The asterisks (*) indicate terms that are either not present in the original paper or do not apply in this context.

The summary of works related to VLMs for image segmentation is presented in Table 5.4.

5.3.3 Report Generation and Refinement

VLMs have become increasingly valuable in the field of report generation and refinement, where they assist in creating structured, descriptive narratives based on medical images, and refining these narratives to enhance clarity and clinical relevance. By processing both visual data and accompanying clinical context, VLMs can generate preliminary reports that describe findings such as tumor characteristics, anatomical structures, and other clinically significant features, which can then be used as a foundation for final reports. These models go beyond simple transcription by incorporating clinical terminology and ensuring that descriptions align with standardized medical language, helping to maintain consistency and accuracy across reports. Additionally, VLMs are adept at refining existing reports, where they can identify ambiguities or inconsistencies and suggest improvements based on learned patterns from large medical datasets. In radiation therapy, this capability is crucial for producing precise and standardized reports that support effective communication among clinicians and enhance the quality of patient care.

Yan and Pei's Clinical-BERT (Yan and Pei, 2022) model represents a focused advance in radiographic vision-language tasks, delivering enhancements in both radiograph-based diagnosis and report generation. Built on DenseNet121 for image encoding and BERT-base for language processing, clinical-BERT leverages a set of domain-specific pretraining tasks tailored to medical diagnostics, including clinical diagnosis (CD), masked MeSH modeling (MMM), and image-MeSH matching (IMM). These tasks aim to align visual data with medical terminology, improving the relevance and precision of generated content. In practice, clinical-BERT demonstrated notable performance on key datasets: it achieved a BLEU-4 score of 0.170 and a CIDEr score of 0.432 on the IU X-Ray dataset, while on the COV-CTR dataset, it surpassed benchmarks with a BLEU-4 score of 0.641 and a CIDEr score of 1.218.

Building on clinical-BERT's advancements in aligning visual data with medical terminology, another approach leveraged specialized medical knowledge integration to enhance radiology report generation (Huang et al., 2023). This model, named KiUT, exemplifies how injecting clinical insights directly into vision-language interactions can improve interpretative depth. Leveraging a ResNet-101 as the visual encoder and MBERT for medical-specific language encoding, the model used a U-shaped transformer architecture, facilitating a continuous interaction between image features and generated text. Its core method integrates visual cues with clinical insights through a knowledge distiller, which draws from a graph of radiology findings to inject contextual and clinical information into the reports, thus enhancing the interpretive depth of generated texts. Experimentally, KiUT achieved impressive BLEU-1 scores of 0.525 on the IU-Xray dataset and 0.393 on MIMIC-CXR, surpassing other methods like XPRONET and R2GenCMN on clinical metrics, underscoring its potential for accurate, radiologist-level reporting.

While KiUT demonstrates the value of integrating clinical knowledge, the development of XRaySwinGen (Magalhães et al., 2024) further refines this cross-modal process by focusing on multilingual capability and robust hierarchical encoding. XRaySwinGen adeptly bridges visual and linguistic domains, handling both local and global features through a shifted window mechanism that preserves spatial detail. This cross-modal framework facilitates accurate report generation by aligning image data with textual descriptions via cross-attention layers. Trained on datasets in both English and Portuguese, including the NIH chest X-ray (CXR), IU X-Ray, and a private Brazilian hospital dataset, XRaySwinGen stands out in multilingual capability and adaptability. Experimentally, the model demonstrated substantial semantic relevance, achieving ROUGE-L and METEOR scores of 0.748 and 0.741 on the private dataset, and competitive ROUGE-L (0.404) and METEOR (0.393) scores on the NIH dataset. While its performance on the IU dataset was slightly lower on BLEU and ROUGE metrics compared to some baselines, it excelled in METEOR, highlighting its strength in generating coherent and contextually accurate reports.

Complementing the multilingual advances of XRaySwinGen, another study addressed universal medical report generation by aligning complex visual and semantic features through a novel interaction mechanism (Lin et al., 2023). They employed a ResNet-101 image encoder combined with a transformer-based decoder enhanced by a linear interaction multi-head attention (LIMHA) module, a novel addition designed to better capture intricate relationships between visual and semantic features. The approach leveraged a contrastive pretraining strategy, using MoCo v2, to align image features closely with medical report language, which proved instrumental in bridging the gap between multimodal data sources such as X-ray and retinal imaging. Through experiments on datasets like IU X-Ray, MIMIC-CXR, and Retina ImBank, the model showed impressive performance, improving the BLEU-1 score on IU X-Ray from 0.396 to 0.462 and achieving a BLEU-4 score of 0.456 on retinal datasets. These results underscore the model's versatility and effectiveness across various imaging modalities, marking a significant step forward in automated, accurate medical reporting.

Taking a distinct approach toward efficiency, a more recent model, MedEPT (Li, 2023), emphasizes computationally efficient architecture without sacrificing accuracy. This architecture combines a CLIP-based feature extractor with a vision transformer (ViT) for visual encoding, alongside language models like GPT-2 and T5 for text decoding. The method leverages parameter-efficient tuning strategies such as LoRA and BiTFiT and integrates soft semantic labels in its contrastive learning component to align image and text embeddings effectively. Key innovations include the MRGPID pipeline, which enables the model to synthesize captions even for image-only datasets, thus expanding the pool of usable data. Trained on diverse datasets like MIMIC-CXR, RSNA pneumonia, and COVID, MedEPT achieved impressive scores, including a BLEU-4 of 0.171 and CIDEr of 0.416 on the IU chest X-ray dataset. Notably, MedEPT accomplishes these results with only 10%

TABLE 5.5
Overview of VLMs for Report Generation and Refinement

Reference	ROI	Modality	Dataset	Model Name	Backbone Model/Module
Yan and Pei (2022)	Lung, thoracic region	X-ray	MIMIC-CXR, NIH ChestX-ray14, COV-CTR, IU X-Ray	Clinical-BERT	DenseNet121, BERT-base
Lin et al. (2023)	Chest, retina	X-ray, fundus photography, optical coherence tomography (OCT), fundus fluorescein angiography (FFA)	IU X-Ray, MIMIC-CXR, Retina ImBank, and Retina Chinese	*	ResNet-101, transformer
Li (2023)	Thoracic region	X-ray	MIMIC-CXR, RSNA pneumonia, COVID, and IU chest X-ray	MedEPT	CLIP, GPT-2, and T5
Huang et al. (2023)	Chest	X-ray	IU-Xray, MIMIC-CXR	KiUT	ResNet-101, MBERT
Magalhães et al. (2024)	Chest	X-ray	NIH chest X-ray, IU X-Ray	XRaySwinGen	Swin Transformer, GPT-2

The asterisks (*) indicate terms that are either not present in the original paper or do not apply in this context.

of the trainable parameters and 30% of the training time required by traditional models, underscoring its efficacy and scalability in large-scale medical applications.

The summary of works related to VLMs for report generation and refinement is presented in Table 5.5.

5.3.4 Target Detection and Classification

In the field of target detection and classification, VLMs offer unique advantages through human-in-the-loop workflows, active prompting, prompt learning, and prompt fusion techniques. These models allow clinicians to guide and refine the model's performance interactively, which is particularly valuable in radiation therapy where precision and adaptability are essential. By incorporating active prompting, VLMs can dynamically adjust their focus based on clinician input, aiding in the accurate identification and classification of specific lesions, tumors, or other critical structures. Prompt learning further enhances adaptability, allowing these models to apply new tasks or patient-specific details with minimal labeled data by using textual prompts that describe target regions or clinical risk factors. Additionally, prompt fusion combines multiple prompts to improve model performance in complex cases, enabling the model to synthesize multiple inputs for a more comprehensive understanding. This flexibility and interactivity make VLMs valuable tools for enabling efficient, context-aware detection and classification in radiation therapy workflows.

In their work on CXR diagnosis, Monajatipoor et al. presented BERTHop (Monajatipoor et al., 2022), a VLM specifically designed to bridge the gap between general V&L models and the unique demands of medical imaging. The model combined PixelHop++, an unsupervised visual model suitable for small datasets, with BlueBERT, a variant of BERT tailored for biomedical text. PixelHop++ extracted multifrequency visual features optimized through PCA, while BlueBERT encoded clinical text, both feeding into a transformer to establish meaningful image–text connections. By leveraging in-domain pretraining, BERTHop achieved robust performance without relying on general-domain data, proving highly data-efficient. Experimentally, BERTHop reached an impressive average AUC of 98.23%, surpassing the state-of-the-art model TieNet by 1.73% despite using a smaller dataset, and improving over similar V&L models by 14.37%, demonstrating its effectiveness in thoracic disease classification tasks.

Building on the strengths of models designed for radiographic classification, another study expanded into zero-shot and few-shot learning, examining the performance of large VLMs across varied imaging modalities (Van et al., 2024). They evaluated multiple VLMs, including BiomedCLIP, OpenCLIP, OpenFlamingo, LLaVA, and ChatGPT-4, each using distinct architectures tailored to handle image and language inputs, such as ViT-B/16 and ViT-G/14 for vision processing and models like GPT-4 for multimodal tasks. This research leveraged prompt engineering to tailor model responses to each dataset, employing unique prompts to emulate radiologist-like interpretations. In experiments, BiomedCLIP led with an average accuracy of 71.52%, while ChatGPT-4 followed closely at 66.09%. OpenFlamingo improved significantly with few-shot prompting, particularly on specific tasks, highlighting VLMs' adaptability across datasets without additional fine-tuning and providing valuable insights into their performance and limitations in medical image classification.

Further addressing the challenges of limited data availability, a new framework called MedPrompt (Zheng et al., 2024) introduced weakly supervised prompt learning to tackle low-resource medical image classification. This approach is groundbreaking in its ability to generate effective text prompts autonomously, reducing dependence on expert-designed prompts, which enhances the model's flexibility and cost-efficiency. MedPrompt operates through a two-stage process: an unsupervised pretrained VLM, reminiscent of CLIP, which captures image–text similarities, and a weakly supervised prompt generator that relies on class labels rather than detailed annotations. The system's vision encoder, based on ResNet or ViT, enables the prompt generator to create contextual class embeddings, which are subsequently used for image classification tasks. The model demonstrated exceptional zero-shot and few-shot learning capacities, performing impressively on datasets like CheXpert and COVID, where it achieved 0.6220 and 0.7997 accuracy in zero-shot settings, respectively. Moreover, in few-shot learning scenarios, MedPrompt nearly matched the accuracy of fully supervised models with minimal labeled data, marking a significant advancement in low-resource medical image classification.

While MedPrompt emphasizes prompt generation for low-resource classification, another approach (Guo et al., 2023) has explored enhancing lesion detection through a fusion of multiple prompts. This ensemble strategy applies different textual prompts describing lesion attributes to improve zero-shot detection accuracy across diverse datasets. Built on the GLIP vision-language framework, their method incorporated various textual prompts that described lesion attributes, such as shape and size, and passed these through GLIP's vision encoder to generate candidate regions. A step-wise clustering approach filtered these candidates by location, size, and other attributes, refining predictions to ensure that only the most relevant lesion candidates were retained. Testing the model on diverse datasets, including ISIC 2016, CVC-300, and BCCD, they employed fusion strategies based on attribute, category, and equal weighting to optimize performance. The model achieved notable improvements, recording average precision (AP) scores of 19.8% for skin lesions on ISIC 2016, 36.1% for polyps on CVC-300, and 15.8% for blood cells on BCCD, with corresponding AP50 scores of 30.9%, 47.9%, and 32.6%, respectively. This outperformed both single-prompt and other ensemble models, showcasing the robustness of their multi-prompt fusion strategy in enhancing lesion detection across varying medical imaging modalities.

Complementing the improvements in lesion detection, an investigation into AutoML Vision (Wan et al., 2021) for breast ultrasound classification demonstrated how automated architecture search can achieve near-CNN performance levels, providing an accessible solution for clinical settings without requiring extensive programming expertise. For the method, AutoML Vision leveraged Google's neural architecture search, allowing a fully automated model-building process, while traditional machine learning models like random forest (RF) and K-nearest neighbors (KNN) employed manually extracted radiomic features, including Haralick texture and Hu moments, to classify breast lesions. AutoML Vision reached an accuracy of 86%, sensitivity of 84%, and specificity of 88%, closely matching CNN's performance, which recorded a 91% accuracy. Statistical tests further confirmed no significant difference in outcomes, underscoring AutoML Vision's viability as a reliable, automated solution for medical imaging tasks.

The summary of works related to VLMs for target detection and classification is presented in Table 5.6.

5.3.5 Visual Question Answering

Visual question answering (VQA) represents a sophisticated application within VLMs, merging image analysis with NLP to provide answers based on visual content. In this task, the model is presented with an image alongside a natural language question regarding that image to generate an accurate and contextually appropriate response. This capability necessitates the model's understanding of visual elements—such as objects, textures, and spatial relationships—alongside its ability to interpret the question's intent and identify which visual details are pertinent for forming an answer.

In the realm of medical imaging, VQA models offer significant potential for both healthcare professionals and patients. For clinicians, including radiologists and oncologists, VQA can deliver rapid, data-driven responses to clinical inquiries about an image, thereby facilitating diagnosis and treatment planning. For example, when asked, "Is there evidence of tumor recurrence in this CT scan?" the model can scrutinize the image for indications of abnormal growth and provide an evidence-based reply. This capability is precious in high-stakes environments like radiation therapy, where swift and precise decision-making is crucial.

For patients, VQA models can demystify complex medical information, making it more accessible. By answering questions about their medical images in clear and comprehensible terms, VQA

TABLE 5.6
Overview of VLMs for Target Detection and Classification

Reference	ROI	Modality	Dataset	Model Name	Backbone Model/ Module
Monajatipoor et al. (2022)	Chest	X-ray	Open-I	BERTHop	PixelHop++, BlueBERT
Wan et al. (2021)	Breast	Ultrasound	BUSI, Mendeley Breast Ultrasound Image dataset	AutoML, Random Forest, K-Nearest Neighbors, and CNN	*
Zheng et al. (2024)	Chest	X-ray	CheXpert, MIMIC-CXR, COVID, and RSNA	MedPrompt	CLIP
Guo et al. (2023)	Skin lesions, polyps, and blood cells	Dermatoscopy, endoscopic, cytology	ISIC 2016, CVC-300, BCCD	*	GLIP
Van et al. (2024)	Brain, blood cells, and chest	MRI, Microscopy, and X-ray	BTD, ALL-IDB2, CX-Ray	BiomedCLIP, OpenCLIP, OpenFlamingo, LLaVA, ChatGPT-4	BiomedCLIP (ViT-B/16), OpenCLIP (ViT-G/14), OpenFlamingo (ViT-L/14 with INCITE-3B), LLaVA (ViT-L/14, LLaMA-2-7B), ChatGPT-4 (GPT-4)
Kandiyana et al. (2024)	Microglia cells	Microscopy imaging	*	GPT-4V	*
Qu et al. (2024)	Pathology slides	Whole slide imaging (WSI)	Camelyon 16 Dataset, TCGA-Lung Cancer Dataset	TOP	CLIP
Nazih et al. (2023)	Stomach tissues	Histopathology imaging	*	*	SWIN-Large, ConvNexT-Large, and PVT_v2_b5, BioLinkBERT-Large, and LSTM
Lu et al. (2023a)	Breast carcinoma, non-small cell lung carcinoma, renal cell carcinoma	Histopathology imaging	*	MI-Zero	CTransPath, HistPathGPT

The asterisks (*) indicate terms that are either not present in the original paper or do not apply in this context.

technology enables patients to better understand their diagnosis and treatment plans. This empowerment through information not only enhances patient engagement but can also alleviate anxiety, as individuals gain insights into their conditions without having to wait for follow-up consultations.

Liu et al. presented the MQAT (medical question answering transformer) (Liu et al., 2022), a simplified yet effective transformer-based model tailored for medical visual question answering (Med-VQA). This model integrates ResNet-10 to capture localized visual features while using a transformer encoder to handle global visual features and question fusion. The MQAT's design includes modal-type and positional embeddings to distinguish text from image tokens, enabling seamless feature fusion through transformer layers, with predictions generated by a multilayer perceptron (MLP) followed by batch normalization. The model was trained using cross-entropy loss, which facilitated efficient convergence and stable performance. On the SLAKE dataset, MQAT achieved a leading accuracy of 82.8%, marking a 0.7% improvement over previous models, while on VQA-RAD, it attained a competitive accuracy of 65.7%, excelling particularly in closed-ended question accuracy. This performance underscores the model's potential in simplifying and enhancing Med-VQA applications within radiology.

Building on MQAT's effective approach to Med-VQA through simplified transformer integration, a subsequent development utilized multimodal pretraining with extensive radiology datasets. This approach, seen in MMBERT (Khare et al., 2021), emphasizes the impact of large-scale data on enhancing model interpretability and performance in VQA tasks. This work illustrates how multimodal pretraining on the large ROCO dataset, consisting of over 81,000 radiology images, can significantly enhance model accuracy and provide improved interpretability through attention maps that highlight relevant anatomical regions. The model's methodology integrates visual features extracted by a ResNet-152 backbone with text embeddings from a BERT-based language model, comprising 4 BERT layers and 12 attention heads. During pretraining, MMBERT employed MLM, focusing on context prediction of masked medical terms within captions, thereby strengthening the model's ability to capture image–text dependencies. In the fine-tuning phase, pretrained weights were adapted to medical VQA-specific tasks, efficiently addressing both closed and open-ended questions. Experimental results highlight that MMBERT achieved a 5% accuracy boost on VQA-Med 2019, reaching 67.2% accuracy, and improved VQA-RAD accuracy to 72.0%, underscoring the model's capability to address complex medical queries with substantial gains in BLEU scores and overall accuracy.

While MMBERT achieved substantial gains with a multimodal BERT framework, another model pushed further into fine-grained alignment, integrating cross-attention mechanisms to better capture nuanced interactions between medical images and text. Wu et al.'s study on FGCVQA (fine-grained cross-attention for medical VQA) (Wu et al., 2023b) offers a substantial advancement in medical visual question answering by tackling the limitations of general VQA models in capturing nuanced visual-text alignment essential for clinical applications. Leveraging a ResNet-152 architecture for image encoding, the model extracts high-resolution, localized features from radiographic images, which are subsequently processed by a cross-modality encoder that utilizes self- and cross-attention mechanisms. This setup facilitates intricate feature fusion between image regions and text, enhancing the semantic alignment needed for accurate interpretation. Evaluated on the VQA-RAD dataset, FGCVQA demonstrated significant gains, achieving an overall accuracy of 77.4%, with improvements over MMBERT of 3.4% in open-ended and 6.7% in closed-ended question accuracy, underscoring its effectiveness in addressing the specialized needs of medical VQA tasks.

Complementing FGCVQA's detailed cross-attention strategy, an innovative model called VQAMix (Gong et al., 2022) took a novel approach to enhance data diversity in training, even in the absence of large external datasets. Gong et al. developed VQAMix to enhance medical VQA by introducing a conditional triplet mixup (CTM) strategy, which augments training diversity in the absence of external datasets. Leveraging this approach, VQAMix combines visual features extracted by CNN backbones like VGG or ResNet with linguistic embeddings from LSTM or GloVe. The model applies CTM by linearly blending image-question-answer triplets to improve robustness, employing techniques such as learning with missing labels (LML) and learning with conditional-mixed labels (LCL) to generate meaningful mixed samples while maintaining label relevance. Experimental results revealed a substantial performance boost, with VQAMix achieving around 7% accuracy improvement on the VQA-RAD dataset and 5% on Path-VQA, outperforming baselines in calibration metrics such as expected calibration error (ECE) and maximum calibration error (MCE), thereby strengthening its reliability for practical medical VQA applications.

In parallel to VQAMix's data augmentation technique, another study sought to improve question generation itself. Zhu et al. (2023) presented a novel approach to visual question generation (VQG) in medical imaging by introducing a multi-latent space diversity learning framework, aimed at enhancing the informativeness and variability of generated questions—a significant step forward from traditional models. Their methodology combined a CNN for extracting image features with an LSTM for language generation, structured around multiple latent spaces to capture diverse data aspects. Each latent space contributed unique information, managed by a maximal information coefficient (MIC) loss function, which maximized information discrepancy across spaces. This setup, along with a category-conditioned question generation process, used cross-entropy, MIC, and Kullback–Leibler divergence losses to ensure robust and varied question generation. Experimentally, the model outperformed existing VQG models, achieving a BLEU-4 score of 16.0, a METEOR score of 19.6, and a CIDEr score of 78.6, with improved diversity validated through a newly introduced similarity metric, underscoring its effectiveness in generating context-rich, varied questions.

In terms of accuracy, an additional step forward was achieved with the Greedy Soup model fusion, which integrates the top-performing models' parameters for VQA. This approach delivered state-of-the-art accuracy in Med-VQA benchmarks (Al-Hadhrami et al., 2023), demonstrating the potential of ensemble learning to address imbalanced datasets in medical applications. Their approach integrates the SWIN transformer for visual feature extraction—capturing both local and global information of retinal images—and ELECTRA-base for text processing, using contrastive estimation for refined language feature extraction. These extracted features were consolidated through a multilayer perceptron (MLP), enabling effective multimodal data fusion for classification. Additionally, they used Best-Value Model Selection and Greedy Soup fusion, which averaged top-performing model parameters, achieving significant accuracy. With an accuracy of 87.41%

TABLE 5.7
Overview of VLMs for Visual Question Answering

Reference	ROI	Modality	Dataset	Model Name	Backbone Model/Module
Liu et al. (2022)	Chest	X-ray	SLAKE, VQA-RAD, and ImageCLEF 2019	MQAT	ResNet-10, transformer
Al-Hadhrami et al. (2023)	Retina	Retinal imaging	DME	Med-VQA	SWIN-base-patch4-window7-224, ELECTRA-base transformer
Zhu et al. (2023)	Lung, chest, abdomen	X-ray	VQA-RAD, Slake	*	CNN, LSTM
Wu et al. (2023b)	Chest	X-ray	VQA-RAD	FGCVQA	ResNet-152, Cross-Modality Encoder
Khare et al. (2021)	General	MRI, ultrasound	VQA-Med 2019, VQA-RAD	MMBERT	ResNet-152, BERT
Gong et al. (2022)	Abdominal, brain, chest, cellular region	CT, MRI, X-ray, pathology imaging (FFPE)	VQA-RAD, Path-VQA	VQAMix	VGG, ResNet, LSTM, and GloVe

The asterisks (*) indicate terms that are either not present in the original paper or do not apply in this context.

and improved weighted metrics, this approach demonstrated substantial progress over the previous state-of-the-art accuracy of 83.49%, showing particular efficacy on imbalanced datasets.

The summary of works related to VLMs for VQA is presented in Table 5.7.

5.3.6 Miscellaneous

5.3.6.1 Text Detection

Li et al. developed an efficient approach for text detection in medical images, addressing unique challenges such as dense text areas and complex aspect ratios (Li et al., 2024b). Their method incorporated a modified ResNet-50 with deformable convolutions and a VLM inspired by CLIP, enhancing cross-modal feature learning. Key architectural components, the efficient feature enhancement module (EFEM) and multiscale feature fusion module (MSFM), were introduced to optimize feature extraction and segmentation. The model was pretrained on general text datasets (e.g., SynthText) and fine-tuned on the MEBI-2000 medical text dataset, which enabled robust performance on medical text detection tasks. In evaluations, the system outperformed prior models such as DBNet++ and PSE-Net, achieving an F-measure of 88.3% on the MEBI dataset with a processing speed of 23.9 FPS, and demonstrated improved accuracy on ICDAR2015 with an F-measure of 89.1%, offering a 1.8%–2.3% increase over other baseline methods. This balance of high accuracy and fast inference makes it ideal for real-time text detection in medical settings.

5.3.6.2 Image Quality Assurance

Luan et al. addressed a critical need in radiotherapy contouring by developing the CQA-AO pipeline for contour quality assurance and adaptive optimization, focusing on real-time error detection and precise error localization (Luan et al., 2024). The model, structured in three stages—contour QA, error categorization, and adaptive correction—leveraged a residual-U-net with ResNet-based vision encoding alongside a frozen ALBERT model to process language prompts. Initially, the model classified contours as acceptable or unacceptable, then performed multi-label classification to identify specific errors, with Grad-CAM providing spatial error visualization. Finally, adaptive correction aligned visual features with clinical language prompts to optimize the contours according to clinical standards. Performance evaluation demonstrated notable improvements, with Dice similarity coefficients for the brainstem, parotid gland, and mandible increasing by 9.4%, 25.9%, and 13.5%, respectively, alongside significant reductions in Hausdorff distance by 62%, 70.6%, and 81.6%. Radiologists' observer-blinded assessments showed contour acceptance improved by 11.9% for junior and 21.3% for senior evaluators, underscoring CQA-AO's potential in enhancing accuracy and efficiency in clinical contouring workflows.

5.3.6.3 Image Synthesis

Bluethgen et al.'s work represents a significant leap in synthetic CXR generation, leveraging a VLM called RoentGen, which uses the latent diffusion model (LDM) framework adapted specifically for radiological applications (Bluethgen et al., 2024). This model combines a U-Net architecture with CLIP-based cross-attention, further refined with domain-specific text encoders such as RadBERT and SapBERT, to accurately interpret and synthesize CXRs from medical prompts. Using the MIMIC-CXR dataset for training and CheXpert and VinDr-CXR for evaluation, RoentGen translates textual radiology descriptions into high-fidelity images of thoracic structures, focusing on abnormalities like pleural effusion, pneumothorax, and cardiomegaly. The synthetic images achieved strong diagnostic alignment with a Fréchet inception distance (FID) of 3.6, while maintaining diversity with a low MS-SSIM score. Classification tasks run on synthetic CXRs achieved an AUROC comparable to real data, around 0.82, and a combined real-synthetic training set outperformed models trained only on real data by up to 3.2% in AUROC on out-of-distribution samples, underlining RoentGen's effectiveness in augmenting datasets with realistic, diagnostically valuable synthetic CXRs.

5.3.6.4 Adversarial Robustness

Wu et al. explored the susceptibility of MedCLIP, a VLM based on CLIP, to backdoor attacks, specifically targeting unpaired medical image–text datasets (Jin et al., 2024). Leveraging datasets like MIMIC, COVIDX, and RSNA, this study underscored MedCLIP's vulnerability by employing two distinct attack strategies: BadMatch and BadDist. BadMatch introduced mislabeled data into unpaired image–text pairs, subtly altering model behavior, while BadDist further optimized this approach by adjusting embedding distances to intensify the attack's effectiveness without compromising the model's performance on clean data. Impressively, this dual approach achieved a backdoor success rate of up to 99% with only 0.05% misalignment, illustrating MedCLIP's high susceptibility to data poisoning attacks despite retaining baseline accuracy on clean datasets. This work significantly advances our understanding of security risks in medical AI, emphasizing the need for robust defenses against such covert attacks in clinical models.

5.3.6.5 Human-in-the-Loop Supervision

Kim et al. introduced a human-in-the-loop approach that leverages radiologists' eye fixation data (FIX1) to enhance the diagnostic capabilities of large multimodal models (LMMs) for CXR interpretation (Kim et al., 2024). By incorporating eye-tracking data from the MIMIC-Eye dataset, they were able to focus on clinically significant areas within the CXRs, enabling two key tasks: disease recommendation and report verification. The disease recommendation task allowed models like LLaVA-Med to provide diagnoses informed by eye fixation prompts, using ICD alignment and disease recognition techniques, while the report verification task enabled LLaVA-ERR to detect synthetic errors in radiology reports. In their results, fixation-enhanced prompts led to significant improvements in diagnostic precision. For instance, the LLaVA-ERR model achieved a near-perfect F1 score of 99.86% in report error identification with fixation data. Additionally, for disease recommendation, LLaVA-Med's F1 score increased from 2.27 to 18.67 with limited fixation data (FIX1), though excess fixation prompts could slightly reduce model accuracy, highlighting the importance of a balanced approach to incorporating fixation inputs.

5.3.6.6 Speech-to-Text Generation

Huh et al. developed the multimodal medical speech module (MMSM), which leverages visual information to improve medical speech-to-text accuracy by aligning visual and textual representations (Huh et al., 2023). The model integrates a vision transformer (ViT-S/16) as the visual encoder and a 12-layer transformer for textual encoding and multimodal fusion, with chest X-rays from the MIMIC-CXR dataset serving as the primary visual input. This system enhances medical transcription accuracy by utilizing visual cues from CXRs to clarify ambiguous terms and correct speech-to-text output errors. Through cross-modal contrastive learning and X-shaped cross-attention, MMSM aligns visual features with textual inputs to resolve transcription errors in clinical settings. Results demonstrated a substantial reduction in word error rate (WER) by approximately 0.05–0.08 compared to leading text-only STT models, along with improved BLEU, METEOR, and ROUGE scores, indicating better contextual alignment with medical terminology even under noisy conditions.

5.3.6.7 Interpretable Diagnosis

Zhang et al.'s study on MDNet establishes a semantically and visually interpretable framework specifically tailored for medical image diagnosis, distinguishing itself by offering transparency in its diagnostic outputs (Zhang et al., 2017). MDNet integrates an enhanced ResNet for image processing with an LSTM network that leverages attention mechanisms to bridge image features with diagnostic text, particularly benefiting pathology images, such as those in the BCIDR bladder cancer dataset. The model's architecture supports multiscale feature capture and aligns specific textual components to visual features using an auxiliary attention sharpening (AAS) module, improving alignment precision. Experimentally, MDNet achieved a 78.4% diagnostic conclusion accuracy

TABLE 5.8
Overview of VLMs for Miscellaneous Topics

Reference	ROI	Modality	Dataset	Model Name	Backbone Model/ Module
Li et al. (2024b)	*	*	MEBI-2000, SynthText, Total-Text, CTW1500, ICDAR2015, and MSRA-TD500	*	ResNet-50, CLIP, efficient feature enhancement module (EFEM), and multiscale feature fusion module (MSFM)
Li et al. (2024a)	*	*	SynthText, Total-Text, CTW1500, ICDAR2015, and MSRA-TD500	oCLIP	ResNet-50, efficient feature enhancement module (EFEM), and multiscale feature fusion module
Singh et al. (2021)	Chest	X-ray	IU-CXR	*	Inception-v3 CNN, LSTM, and Bi-LSTM
Luan et al. (2024)	Head–neck	Ct	TCIA Head–Neck Cetuximab, HGJ, CHUS, HMR, and CHUM	CQA-AO	Residual-UNet, ALBERT
Bluethgen et al. (2024)	Lung	X-ray	MIMIC-CXR, CheXpert and VinDr-CXR	RoentGen	Stable diffusion (SD), CLIP, RadBERT and SapBERT
Jin et al. (2024)	Thoracic region	X-ray	MIMIC, COVIDX, and RSNA	MedCLIP	CLIP
Oura et al. (2024)	*	General	Japanese Diagnostic Radiology (JDR) tests, Japanese Nuclear Medicine (JNM) tests, and Japanese Interventional Radiology (JIR) tests	GPT-4o, GPT-4V, Claude-3 Sonnet, and Claude-3 Opus	*
Kim et al. (2024)	Lung, chest	X-ray	MIMIC-Eye, MIMIC-CXR-VQA	LLaVA-Med, CXR-LLaVA, LLaVA-ERR, and LLaVA-1.5	*
Huh et al. (2023)	Thoracic	X-ray	MIMIC-CXR	MMSM	ViT-S/16, transformer
Zhang et al. (2017)	Bladder tissue, urothelial cell nuclei	pathology imaging	BCIDR, CIFAR	MDNet	ResNet, LSTM

The asterisks (*) indicate terms that are either not present in the original paper or do not apply in this context.

(DCA) on the BCIDR dataset, surpassing baselines in both diagnostic accuracy and alignment with pathologically significant regions, demonstrating its capability to provide interpretable and reliable diagnostic support.

The summary of works related to VLMs for miscellaneous topics is presented in Table 5.8.

5.3.7 ChatGPT for Medical Image Analysis

ChatGPT is an advanced language model developed by OpenAI, based on the transformer architecture that has driven remarkable advancements in NLP. From its early iteration in GPT-2 to the powerful GPT-4, ChatGPT has evolved significantly, with each version improving its ability to understand and generate contextually rich, human-like text. The latest version of ChatGPT, featuring multimodal capabilities, can process both language and images, making it a transformative tool for applications across various fields, including healthcare.

The multimodal functionality of ChatGPT-4, along with its widespread popularity and easy accessibility, has captured the attention of the medical imaging community. Researchers are increasingly motivated to leverage its advanced capabilities in applications such as image-guided diagnostics, automated report generation, and interactive diagnostic support. The combination of language and vision processing in a single model offers unique advantages, particularly within precision radiation therapy, where streamlined documentation, enhanced patient communication, and clinical decision support are critical.

Given the model's appeal, it is essential for researchers to approach its application in medical imaging with a balanced understanding. While ChatGPT's power and accessibility offer vast potential, they also necessitate a careful examination of its strengths and limitations within complex medical contexts. This section is dedicated to providing a comprehensive perspective on ChatGPT, aiming to equip researchers with the insight needed to apply it responsibly and effectively in radiation therapy, ensuring it is integrated thoughtfully to enhance clinical workflows and patient outcomes.

Suh et al. (2024) conducted a comparative evaluation of large multimodal models, GPT-4V from OpenAI and Gemini Pro Vision from Google DeepMind, assessing their diagnostic capabilities against human radiologists using complex radiologic cases from the Diagnosis Please series in Radiology. The study covered multiple image modalities, including CT, MRI, ultrasound, radiography, PET/CT, and fluoroscopy, and addressed various anatomical regions such as neuroradiology, gastrointestinal, and musculoskeletal areas, providing insights into the potential role of multimodal language models in radiologic assistance. The methodology involved a retrospective analysis across 190 cases where the models were prompted to generate differential diagnoses based on both images and brief patient histories. Diagnoses were produced under different temperature settings (0, 0.5, and 1) to gauge the impact of randomness on diagnostic breadth and accuracy, with preprocessing involving image downsizing as needed, and prompts encouraging creative yet clinically relevant responses. Results indicated that model accuracy improved at higher temperature settings, with GPT-4V achieving up to 49% accuracy at temperature 1 and Gemini Pro Vision reaching 39%, though neither consistently matched the radiologists' accuracy of 61%. Accuracy also varied by modality, as GPT-4V attained higher performance on ultrasound (54%–68%), compared to 38%–48% on CT and 34%–42% on radiography, highlighting differences in model effectiveness depending on image type and complexity.

GPT4MIA (Zhang and Chen, 2023) is an innovative application of GPT-3 as a transductive inference model for medical image analysis, aiming to improve classification accuracy in specialized medical imaging tasks (Zhang et al., 2023). GPT4MIA harnessed GPT-3's attention-based architecture by crafting prompts that map medical image features to class labels, effectively allowing it to integrate with vision-based models like ResNet. This approach facilitated classification by arranging feature similarities and reference data to enhance inference on unseen samples. Key applications included prediction error detection and classification accuracy enhancement, with GPT4MIA demonstrating robust performance on tasks such as RetinaMNIST, where it achieved an F-score of 0.693 and balanced accuracy of 0.679, surpassing conventional classifiers like SVM and KNN.

A hybrid VLM was designed to enhance CT image quality assessment by merging image analysis with language generation. IQAGPT (Chen et al., 2024d) incorporates a vision transformer (ViT-S/16) for image encoding and BERT-base as both text encoder and multimodal decoder, alongside ChatGPT, to produce comprehensive quality evaluations that include both quantitative scores and qualitative, human-like reports. The model was fine-tuned on CT-IQA, a dataset of abdominal

CT scans, with a focus on encoding both visual quality markers and textual annotations. By leveraging cross-modal attention, IQAGPT effectively fused visual and textual data, outputting assessments through a prompt-based template that translated radiologist-assigned scores into detailed descriptive captions. In evaluation, IQAGPT demonstrated substantial improvements over existing models, achieving a mean classification accuracy of 0.702 compared to ViT-C's 0.512 and outperformed CLIP-IQA in regression tasks, with higher PLCC and SROCC scores at 0.754 and 0.748, respectively, highlighting its capability to provide accurate and robust quality assessments across multiple metrics.

Hayden et al. explored GPT-4 with Vision (GPT-4V) as a diagnostic tool in radiology, particularly assessing its efficacy on the American College of Radiology (ACR) diagnostic radiology in-training examination (DXIT) questions, covering both text and image-based formats (Hayden et al., 2024). This research underscored the model's potential in medical education, notably achieving high accuracy on text-only questions but revealing limitations with complex radiologic image interpretation. GPT-4V was tested on 377 DXIT questions, including 195 text-only and 182 image-based questions, using a variety of zero-shot prompting strategies such as basic, short instruction, and chain-of-thought prompts to determine their impact on diagnostic accuracy. Chain-of-thought prompting notably improved accuracy on text-based questions to 83.8%, a 6.8% increase over basic prompting, while image-based question accuracy remained consistent across prompting styles. Overall, GPT-4V achieved a 65.3% accuracy rate, excelling with text-based questions at 81.5% but scoring lower at 47.8% on image-based questions, highlighting areas for improvement in vision-based diagnostic capabilities.

ChatGPT, even with the latest version, will not guarantee promising results (Shifai et al., 2024). GPT-4V, developed by OpenAI as an advanced multimodal extension of GPT-4, was tested against convolutional

TABLE 5.9
Overview of GPTs for Medical Image Analysis

References	ROI	Modality	Dataset	Model Name	GPT Version
Suh et al. (2024)	Neuroradiology, gastrointestinal, genitourinary, musculoskeletal, chest, cardiovascular, pediatric, and breast	CT, MRI, US, radiography, fluoroscopy, PET/CT, and digital subtraction angiography	"Diagnosis Please" cases from the *Radiology* journal	*	GPT-4V
Zhang and Chen (2023)	Retina, bone	MRI, CT	RetinaMNIST, FractureMNIST3D	GPT4MIA	GPT-3
Chen et al. (2024d)	Abdomen	CT	CT-IQA	IQAGPT	GPT-4
Hayden et al. (2024)	Breast, chest, genitourinary, and gastrointestinal	*	retired questions from the American College of Radiology Diagnostic Radiology In-Training Examination	*	GPT-4V
Shifai et al. (2024)	Skin	Dermatoscopy	*	*	GPT-4V
Chen et al. (2024a)	Pulmonary region	*	Taiwan Pulmonology and Critical Care Specialist Board Exams (2013–2023)	*	GPT-4, Gemini, and GPT-3.5
Hirano et al. (2024)	General	General	Japan Diagnostic Radiology Board Examination (JDRBE)	*	GPT-4TV

The asterisks (*) indicate terms that are either not present in the original paper or do not apply in this context.

CNNs optimized for melanoma detection, with results demonstrating that GPT-4V's performance significantly lagged behind these specialized models. The method involved using GPT-4V to interpret skin lesion images, relying heavily on descriptive prompts to elicit diagnostic insights. This approach underscored the model's limitations in direct pattern recognition, which is central to dermatological diagnostics. While GPT-4V showed proficiency in text-based tasks, its capacity to accurately analyze clinical visual information was limited, as shown by its lower diagnostic accuracy compared to CNNs, indicating the ongoing challenge of integrating VLMs effectively into image-centric diagnostic workflows.

Table 5.9 summarizes works using ChatGPT models for medical image analysis.

5.3.8 Multimodal Learning

Multimodal learning is an approach in machine learning that involves integrating information from multiple data modalities to enhance the understanding and interpretation of complex data. In medical image analysis, these modalities often include both visual data (e.g., images) and textual data (e.g., clinical notes, reports), each offering unique but complementary insights. The goal of multimodal learning is to enable a system to analyze and synthesize information across these diverse data types, leading to more robust and comprehensive models. This approach is particularly valuable in medical contexts where visual details in imaging studies and textual clinical documentation provide essential, interlinked information critical for accurate diagnosis and treatment.

In the realm of VLMs, multimodal learning is at the core, as these models are specifically designed to process and fuse image and text data, capturing the complex relationships between visual and linguistic features. Unlike other sections, which are more application-specific, this section delves into the technical innovations of how these modalities are extracted and integrated within the models. For example, advanced techniques such as masked modeling, contrastive learning, and prompt fusion have been applied to align and jointly embed image and text data within a shared feature space, enabling better cross-modal understanding. In radiation therapy, leveraging these multimodal integration techniques allows VLMs to comprehend contextual details—such as lesion location, staging information, and treatment intent—by effectively blending both visual patterns and clinical context, thus providing a foundation for improved, context-aware analysis in precision medical imaging. Figure 5.4 shows different fusion strategies for multimodal learning.

Chen et al. introduced the M3AE (multimodal masked autoencoder) (Chen et al., 2024c), a sophisticated model crafted for mapping medical images and corresponding texts into a shared

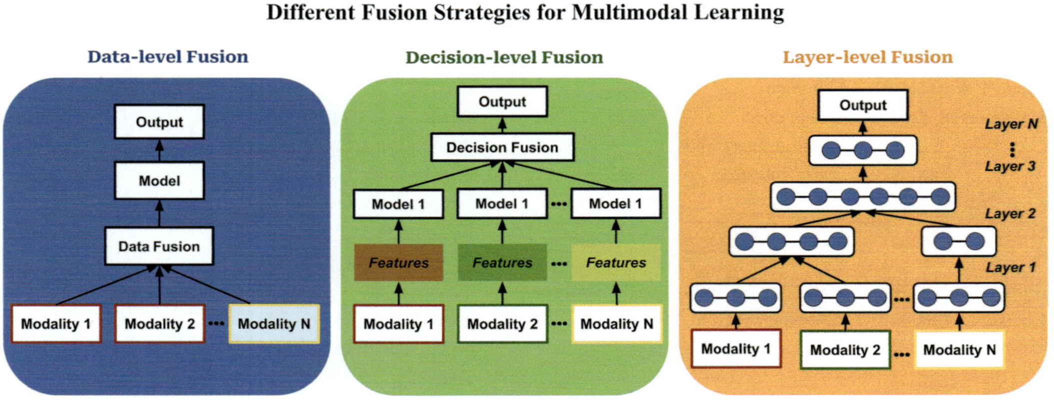

FIGURE 5.4 Overview of fusion strategies used in multimodal learning, highlighting three main approaches: data-level (early) fusion, which merges inputs from various modalities at the outset; layer-level (intermediate) fusion, where integration occurs within the model's intermediate layers; and decision-level (late) fusion, where information from each modality is combined at the final output stage.

latent space, highlighting an innovative approach to combining medical image and text data through masked modeling. This method leveraged ViTs for image encoding and RoBERTa-base for textual data, applying distinct masking strategies—75% for images and 15% for text—to optimize information extraction from each modality. The model employed a co-attention multimodal fusion mechanism that facilitated alignment between visual and textual features, allowing for effective cross-modal learning that enhanced downstream applications like Med-VQA and image–text retrieval. M3AE achieved notable performance improvements across various datasets; it reached an impressive 77.01% accuracy in Med-VQA, outperforming previous approaches by over 10%. Additionally, it excelled in medical image–text classification on MELINDA with a 78.5% accuracy and achieved a Recall@10 of 66.65% on the ROCO dataset in retrieval tasks, demonstrating its robust capabilities in both zero-shot and fine-tuned applications.

While M3AE has shown substantial success in integrating masked modeling for effective cross-modal learning, a different approach has been developed to address a major challenge in medical imaging: limited labeled data (Windsor et al., 2023). They crafted a dual-encoder model that leverages ResNet50, adapted with SimCLR for CXR imaging, paired with a domain-specific CXR-BERT for handling medical text. This setup incorporated both global and local contrastive loss (InfoNCE and GLoRIA) to improve spatial and semantic alignment between images and text, alongside synthetic data augmentation via the DeCLIP framework, which proved instrumental for working with limited data. Impressively, the model achieved robust performance, with its retrieval capabilities on par with models trained on 10 times more data, reaching over 95% of full-dataset performance even when trained on only 10% of the data. In classification tasks, especially those involving CXR disease detection, it outperformed competitive models like CLIP and BioVIL, achieving a balanced accuracy of 74.5% in linear probing and showing marked improvements in both zero-shot and data-efficient training setups.

Building on the innovations in handling low-data environments, a new model incorporates federated learning, allowing distributed datasets to collaboratively train a unified model—FedMedVLP (Lu et al., 2023b). By employing ResNet as the vision encoder, initially pretrained on CheXpert, and BERT-BASE as the language encoder, the model establishes a robust two-stream framework aligned through cross-modal transformer layers. The training methodology leveraged federated averaging (FedAvg) to optimize the model across distributed datasets, including public sources like ROCO, VQA-RAD, SLAKE, Med-VQA-2019, and MIMIC-CXR, in addition to a unique multi-institutional dataset, COVID-Fed. Core pretraining tasks—MLM and Image–text matching (ITM)—were implemented to enhance cross-modal embeddings while preserving data privacy. Evaluation demonstrated FedMedVLP's capabilities, achieving an R@1 of 28.1% on image-to-text retrieval for ROCO and 39.8% on COVID-Fed, with impressive accuracies on Med-VQA tasks—84.2% on VQA-RAD, 91.5% on SLAKE, and 86.8% on Med-VQA-2019. These results outperformed previous models by up to 8%, highlighting FedMedVLP's strong potential in large-scale medical AI applications.

While FedMedVLP showcases the benefits of federated learning, few-shot learning techniques have also been adapted for medical multimodal tasks. In their exploration of medical multimodal learning, Moor et al. presented Med-Flamingo (Moor et al., 2023), a novel model that leverages few-shot learning for enhanced VQA in clinical applications. By building on OpenFlamingo, Med-Flamingo integrates CLIP-ViT/L-14 as its vision model and the LLaMA-7B as its language backbone, effectively blending visual and text data. This architecture was further strengthened with training on paired medical image–text datasets like PMC-OA and the Visual USMLE set, emphasizing practical case vignettes. The model's key strength lies in its in-context few-shot learning, which allowed it to perform sophisticated VQA tasks, including rationale generation, setting it apart from previous medical VLMs that lacked such adaptability. Clinical evaluations, conducted through a bespoke app, underscored Med-Flamingo's capabilities, revealing a notable 20% boost in clinical evaluation scores over existing baselines, with an average rank of 1.67 versus 2.33. Impressively, the model achieved a clinical score of 5.61 on VQA-RAD, illustrating its superior performance in addressing complex medical queries and in preference evaluations on Visual USMLE, where it outshined its predecessors in few-shot VQA tasks.

Extending beyond few-shot learning, other recent advancements have focused on enriching contextual understanding through anatomy- and pathology-specific prompts. The MCPL (multi-modal collaborative prompt learning) (Wang et al., 2024) model is specifically crafted to enhance CLIP's performance on medical imaging tasks. The MCPL framework extends CLIP's capabilities by embedding anatomy- and pathology-specific prompts directly within the transformer's attention layers, allowing the model to grasp complex contextual details in medical text and images. Central to MCPL is its graph-guided prompt collaboration module (GPCM), which facilitates multi-way interactions among text, image, and anatomy- and pathology-specific prompts, resulting in a multi-modal representation that is both refined and interpretable, tailored to the medical field. Evaluated on datasets like MIMIC-CXR, CheXpert, and COVIDx, MCPL demonstrated notable performance, achieving a high 94.3% accuracy on COVIDx, all while maintaining a lean parameter footprint compared to full model fine-tuning. Additionally, in object detection tasks on the RSNA dataset, MCPL surpassed models such as BiomedCLIP, achieving a mAP of 25.4, underscoring its potential to elevate multimodal medical image analysis with efficiency and domain-specific precision.

Lastly, further innovations in 3D VLMing have targeted the need for detailed anatomical interpretation in modalities like CT imaging (Blankemeier et al., 2024). Merlin's robust integration of 3D imaging with radiology-specific text highlights the model's versatility in complex clinical scenarios, paving the way for high-precision multimodal analysis. Merlin's vision component was built on 3D ResNet152 with I3D initialization, while its language component utilized the Clinical Longformer, designed to handle lengthy radiology text. The training leveraged binary cross-entropy for phenotype classification and InfoNCE for contrastive learning, utilizing ICD codes from structured EHR data alongside unstructured radiology reports. The multitask training setup included zero-shot classification and cross-modal retrieval, with anatomical report sections enhancing the contrastive learning effectiveness. Merlin achieved an F1 score of 0.741 in zero-shot classification on internal data and 0.647 on external data, surpassing OpenCLIP and BioMedCLIP. For phenotype classification, Merlin achieved an AUROC of 0.812 across 692 phenotypes, with exceptional accuracy for 15% of these (AUROC > 0.9). Additionally, Merlin's cross-modal retrieval capabilities significantly outpaced baseline models, showing a 5–7 times improvement in zero-shot scenarios. In predicting chronic disease risk over a 5-year period, the model attained an AUROC of 0.757. For 3D semantic segmentation tasks, Merlin surpassed baselines by up to 11% in label-scarce situations, underscoring its versatility and efficacy in low-data environments.

Table 5.10 summarizes works that explored different multimodal learning strategies for VLMs on medical datasets.

5.3.9 Vision-Language Pretraining

Vision-language pretraining is a specialized subset of multimodal learning that focuses on building robust, transferable models specifically designed to handle both visual and language data in tandem. Unlike general multimodal learning, which aims to integrate information from multiple modalities, vision-language pretraining is centered on creating foundational models that deeply understand and relate visual and textual information. This process involves training on large datasets of paired images and text descriptions, enabling models to capture nuanced relationships between visual features and language cues. Vision-language pretrained models are optimized to recognize and interpret visual data in ways that are directly informed by textual context, making them uniquely suited for complex, information-dense tasks like medical image analysis.

In medical applications, particularly in radiation therapy, vision-language pretraining establishes a solid foundation for models to be fine-tuned for various domain-specific tasks, such as report generation, target detection, segmentation, and classification. By incorporating medical-specific knowledge during pretraining, these models gain an understanding of medical terminology and

TABLE 5.10
Overview of Multimodal Learning Strategies for Training VLMs

Reference	ROI	Modality	Dataset	Model Name	Backbone Model/ Module
Chen et al. (2024c)	General	CT, X-ray	ROCO, MedICaT	M3AE	ViT, RoBERTa-base
Wang et al. (2024)	Chest	X-ray	MIMIC-CXR, CheXpert, COVIDx, RSNA, and Object-CXR	MCPL	CLIP
Moor et al. (2023)	General	X-ray, pathology imaging	PMC-OA, Visual USMLE	Med-Flamingo	CLIP-ViT/L-14, LLaMA-7B
Blankemeier et al. (2024)	Abdomen	CT	VerSe, TotalSegmentator	Merlin	ResNet152 3D, Clinical Longformer
Lu et al. (2023b)	Chest	X-ray	ROCO, VQA-RAD, SLAKE, Med-VQA-2019, and MIMIC-CXR	FedMedVLP	ResNet, BERT
Windsor et al. (2023)	Thoracic region	X-ray	MIMIC-CXR-JPG	*	ResNet50, BERT
Li et al. (2020)	Thoracic region	X-ray	MIMIC-CXR, Open-I	VisualBERT, UNITER, LXMERT, and PixelBERT	*
Arnaout (2024)	Cardiac structure	Ultrasound	*	EchoCLIP	CLIP
Xie et al. (2024)	Thoracic region	X-ray	MIMIC-CXR-JPG	MedIM	ViT, BioClinicalBERT
Zhan et al. (2024)	Chest, thoracic spine, lungs, and heart	CT, X-ray, and pathology imaging	ROCO, MIMIC-CXR, VQA-RAD, SLAKE, Path-VQA, IU X-Ray, MIMIC-CXR, MELINDA, ROCO, CheXpert, RSNA Pneumonia, SIIM Pneumothorax, RSNA, MedNLI, PubMedQA, and BioAsq	UniDCP	CLIP-ViT, RoBERTa

The asterisks (*) indicate terms that are either not present in the original paper or do not apply in this context.

visual patterns relevant to clinical workflows. This pretraining process allows for rapid adaptation with minimal labeled data, as the model already possesses a baseline understanding of how to relate anatomical structures, diagnostic labels, and imaging patterns. Consequently, vision-language pretraining is invaluable in creating models that not only perform well in medical settings but also provide more interpretable and contextually aware outputs, enhancing their utility in radiation therapy and beyond.

Naseem et al. developed BioMedBLIP (Naseem et al., 2024), an adaptation of the BLIP framework tailored specifically for medical imaging tasks, which achieved significant improvements across tasks such as VQA, image captioning, and classification. The model leverages a vision transformer (ViT) as its vision encoder and a BERT-based language encoder, fine-tuned for medical applications by employing domain-specific cross-modal data and binary classification layers that integrate image–text pairs. This approach allowed BioMedBLIP to achieve specialized representations ideal for medical data interpretation, using extensive datasets like ROCO and MIMIC-CXR to enhance its performance on complex multimodal tasks. Experimental results demonstrated BioMedBLIP's robust capabilities, with it achieving an 82% accuracy on SLAKE-Overall and 90.87% on SLAKE-Close for VQA tasks, and in open-ended VQA-RAD tasks, it outperformed baseline models with a score of 46.37. In image captioning, the model's BioMedBLIP-ROCO-50 variant recorded a BLEU-1 score of 25.1, marking a 1.2% improvement over the original BLIP model.

While BioMedBLIP set new benchmarks in task-specific accuracy for vision-language integration, a different approach has taken a multitask strategy to boost cross-modal alignment. The MPMA (Zhang et al., 2023a) framework enhances interaction between images and text, incorporating joint reconstruction and alignment techniques to strengthen adaptability in clinical applications. The model utilizes a vision transformer (ViT) as its image encoder and a BERT-based model for language processing, employing global and local alignment (GLA) alongside memory-augmented cross-modal fusion (MA-CMF) to strengthen its adaptability in medical contexts. The MPMA framework approaches image and text tasks with a multitask strategy, applying masked image modeling (MIM) for image reconstruction and MLM for text, both with high masking ratios to deepen feature extraction. The model achieved superior performance over previous methods, with an AUC of 90.6% on the CheXpert dataset and higher BLEU-4 scores on MIMIC-CXR, demonstrating its effectiveness in image classification and report generation.

The challenge of limited labeled data for CXR VLMs by converting traditional image–label pairs into image–text pairs using radiologist-informed prompt templates, significantly enhancing model versatility. The CXR-CLIP (You et al., 2023) model adopted a dual-stream architecture, employing ResNet-50 or Swin-Tiny as image encoders and BioClinicalBERT for text encoding. To reinforce multimodal alignment, they introduced two novel contrastive loss functions—image contrastive loss (ICL) and text contrastive loss (TCL)—to optimize study-level feature learning, applying multi-view supervision (MVS) across multiple views and text sections per study. In experiments, CXR-CLIP delivered strong zero-shot and few-shot performance, achieving AUCs above 78% on datasets like VinDR-CXR and RSNA. Notably, in image-to-text retrieval, the ResNet-50 variant outperformed existing models, recording Recall@1 of 21.4% on MIMIC-CXR and 3.8% on Open-I, underscoring CXR-CLIP's robust retrieval and classification capabilities.

While CXR-CLIP addresses data scarcity through creative pairing techniques, M-FLAG (Liu et al., 2023b) optimizes computational efficiency with its parameter-efficient architecture. By freezing the language model and focusing on alignment within a shared latent space, M-FLAG achieves high accuracy with reduced resource requirements. This approach included an innovative orthogonality loss, designed to maintain a balanced latent space and prevent collapse, resulting in highly stable embeddings while requiring 78% fewer parameters than conventional models. The model processed image and language embeddings separately, aligning them within a shared latent space using an alignment loss, and only trained the vision component, thereby reducing computational costs. Experimental results demonstrated M-FLAG's exceptional performance across multiple tasks: achieving up to an 80.2% AUC on classification tasks (MIMIC, CXP, NIH datasets), a 64.8% Dice score in segmentation (SIIM dataset), and a mean average precision of 25.4% for detection tasks (RSNA dataset), even with limited data fine-tuning.

In addition to efficiency gains, another model, PTUnifier (Chen et al., 2023), advances flexibility in handling single, cross-modal, and multimodal inputs seamlessly. Its prompt-based structure and dual-fusion encoding enable it to generalize across a wide array of medical tasks, demonstrating strong adaptability and performance gains in vision-language applications. The model applied a prompt-based system, allowing it to adapt flexibly to various input types—images alone, text alone, or combined image–text pairs—by dynamically selecting from a pool of visual and textual

TABLE 5.11
Overview of VLMs Pretraining Strategies

Reference	ROI	Modality	Dataset	Model Name	Backbone Model/ Module
Naseem et al. (2024)	General	CT, MRI, X-ray, ultrasound, fluoroscopy, PET, and mammography	ROCO, MIMIC-CXR, SLAKE, VQA-RAD, Path-VQA, and ImageCLEF	BioMedBLIP	BLIP, ViT, BERT
You et al. (2023)	Thoracic region	X-ray	MIMIC-CXR, CheXpert, ChestX-ray14, RSNA, SIIM, VinDR-CXR, and Open-I	CXR-CLIP	ResNet-50, Swin-Tiny, BioClinicalBERT
Liu et al. (2023b)	Chest	X-ray	MIMIC-CXR	M-FLAG	ResNet50, CXR-BERT
Zhang et al. (2023a)	Thoracic region	X-ray	MIMIC-CXR, ROCO datasets	MPMA	ViT, BERT
Chen et al. (2023)	Chest	general	ROCO, MedICaT, and MIMIC-CXR	PTUnifier	CLIP-ViT-B, RoBERTa-base
Chen et al. (2022b)	Chest	general	MedICaT, MIMIC-CXR	*	ViT, RoBERTa
Tung et al. (2024)	Thoracic region	X-ray	MIMIC-CXR, ChestX-ray14, and RSNA Pneumonia	MVLP	CLIP, BioClinicalBERT, MedPALM
Liu et al. (2023a)	Thoracic region	X-ray	MIMIC-CXR	SAT	ResNet-50, BioClinicalBERT
Zhang et al. (2023b)	Lung, heart and pleura	X-ray	MIMIC-CXR, PadChest, NIH ChestXray14, CheXpert, and ChestX-Det10	KAD	ResNet-50, BERT
Wu et al. (2023a)	Lung and thoracic region	X-ray	MIMIC-CXR, ChestX-ray14, RSNA Pneumonia, SIIM-ACR Pneumothorax, COVIDx CXR-2, COVID Rural, and EdemaSeverity	MedKLIP	ResNet-50, Clinical-BERT
Moon et al. (2022)	Chest	X-ray	MIMIC-CXR, Open-I	MedViLL	ResNet-50, BERT-base

The asterisks (*) indicate terms that are either not present in the original paper or do not apply in this context.

prompts. This setup optimized performance through a combined training strategy that leveraged image–text contrast (ITC) and fusion-encoder tasks, such as MLM and image–text matching (ITM). PTUnifier achieved impressive results, outperforming previous benchmarks with an increase of +2% in AUROC for image classification, +2.2% in text classification accuracy, +7.5% in Recall@1 for image-to-text retrieval, +9.5% in text-to-image retrieval, and a +3.4% boost in multimodal VQA accuracy. This substantial improvement underscores PTUnifier's strong generalization and adaptability across diverse medical vision-language tasks.

Table 5.11 concludes various medical image VLMs pretreating strategies.

5.4 DISCUSSION

While VLMs have shown significant promise in advancing medical image analysis, as reviewed in the preceding sections, numerous challenges hinder the full integration of VLMs into clinical workflows, as they face considerable obstacles related to data quality, privacy, safety, and interpretability. In this section, we address these critical challenges and explore potential solutions to ensure that VLMs can meet the stringent requirements of precision radiation therapy and other high-stakes medical applications.

5.4.1 Data Quality, Accessibility, and Clinical Representation

In medical image analysis, the performance and trustworthiness of VLMs are deeply rooted in the quality and diversity of the data on which they are trained. Precision radiation therapy, which requires accurate and patient-specific imaging, accentuates these requirements. High-quality, meticulously annotated datasets ensure that VLMs can provide clinically relevant and accurate interpretations. However, achieving this level of quality takes time and effort. Medical data often vary in resolution, protocol, and annotation quality, which may lead to inconsistencies undermining model performance and generalizability across diverse clinical scenarios.

Another significant barrier is data accessibility. Due to privacy regulations such as HIPAA and GDPR, access to large, varied datasets is often restricted, limiting the model's exposure to a broad range of clinical cases. These constraints create bottlenecks in training robust VLMs, as limited data diversity can impede the model's ability to generalize across different patient populations, imaging techniques, and pathologies (Hu et al., 2024). Consequently, solutions like synthetic data generation, federated learning, and standardized protocols for data sharing have become essential to enhance data access while respecting patient privacy.

Addressing these data challenges supports the development of more accurate and reliable VLMs and pushes the field closer to realizing AI-driven advancements in patient care. Integrating collaborative efforts among medical institutions to create accessible, anonymized datasets and establishing rigorous data curation protocols can significantly elevate the capability of VLMs to handle the complexities inherent in precision radiation therapy.

5.4.2 Privacy and Security Concerns

VLMs process sensitive patient information, including images and diagnostic histories, creating risks of unauthorized access and data breaches. Due to the large-scale data requirements for training VLMs, data aggregation from multiple sources heightens these risks, making patient confidentiality a pressing concern. Protecting privacy in this context requires strategies like differential privacy and strict compliance with regulations such as HIPAA and GDPR to maintain patient trust (Cai, 2023).

On the security front, VLMs face vulnerabilities from adversarial attacks (Qiu et al., 2019), where slight alterations in input data can lead to incorrect diagnoses or expose sensitive embedded information. Given the sensitivity of medical imaging, even minimal modifications to an image could mislead the model's interpretation. A comprehensive approach that includes advanced adversarial defenses, regular audits, and ethical oversight is essential to counteract these risks. This layered strategy fortifies model integrity and aligns with regulatory standards, reinforcing both security and public confidence in the technology.

5.4.3 Interpretability and Trustworthiness in Clinical Settings

The interpretability of VLMs is crucial in clinical applications, where understanding the "why" behind a model's predictions is often as important as the predictions themselves. Medical imaging for precision radiation therapy demands transparency, as clinicians must be able to validate and trust model outputs before integrating them into high-stakes decision-making. However, VLMs often operate as "black boxes," producing results without explaining how specific image features contributed to their interpretations (Zhang et al., 2024a). This opacity can create hesitancy among clinicians, especially when patient care and treatment planning decisions are on the line.

Integrating interpretability-focused techniques—such as attention maps, SHAP values, and layer-wise relevance propagation (LRP)—can offer insights into the model's decision-making pathways (Ben Melech Stan et al., 2024; Palit et al., 2023). These methods help clinicians see which image regions the model prioritizes, enabling a more transparent and trustworthy workflow.

5.4.4 Clinical Collaboration and Human-in-the-Loop Design

VLMs' effectiveness can be significantly enhanced when coupled with the expertise of clinicians, radiologists, and medical physicists (Kim et al., 2024; Kandiyana et al., 2024). In the complex environment of precision radiation therapy, human oversight is essential to refine VLM outputs, ensuring they align with each patient case's unique details. This human-in-the-loop (Wu et al., 2022) approach mitigates the risk of errors that may arise from fully automated processes, reinforcing the model's reliability by contextualizing its outputs within clinical realities (Budd et al., 2021).

Moreover, clinical collaboration facilitates the integration of VLM insights into practical decision-making, where expert interpretation and validation add a layer of ethical and diagnostic rigor. This synergy between human expertise and AI-driven analysis improves diagnostic accuracy and workflow efficiency and ensures that VLMs are used as responsible and supportive tools in patient care.

5.4.5 Model Generalization and Adaptation

Achieving robust generalization in VLMs is crucial in precision radiation therapy, where model reliability across diverse clinical scenarios is critical. VLMs trained on limited or homogeneous datasets often need help to perform consistently when faced with new imaging modalities, variations in patient anatomy, or rare pathologies. This limitation can lead to performance discrepancies, especially in underrepresented populations, ultimately affecting diagnostic reliability. Techniques like domain adaptation (Li, 2024), transfer learning, and fine-tuning on domain-specific datasets (Zhang et al., 2024b) are being explored to help VLMs bridge the gap between controlled training environments and real-world clinical diversity. In addition to these approaches, data augmentation strategies—such as synthetic data generation (Liu et al., 2023c)—have emerged as valuable tools to expose VLMs to a broader range of scenarios, enhancing their resilience and adaptability.

5.4.6 Bias, Hallucination, and Diagnostic Reliability

Biases in these VLMs often stem from imbalanced training data, where specific demographics, pathologies, or imaging types may need more representation. This can lead to skewed predictions that may inadvertently favor or disadvantage specific patient groups, potentially affecting the fairness and accuracy of medical diagnoses. Ensuring diverse, representative datasets and incorporating fairness-focused training approaches are essential to mitigate these biases.

Hallucinations—outputs generated by the model that appear plausible but lack a factual basis—pose another significant risk in clinical applications (Wang et al., 2023). In medical contexts, a hallucinated output could result in an inaccurate diagnosis or treatment recommendation, endangering patient outcomes (Gu et al., 2024). Addressing this issue requires alignment between visual and textual components and rigorous validation mechanisms to ensure that the model's responses are firmly grounded in medical evidence (Jiang et al., 2024).

5.4.7 Evaluation Metrics and Clinical Validation Standards

Evaluating VLMs for medical image analysis requires metrics beyond traditional performance indicators to capture the nuanced demands of clinical applications. Standard metrics often fall short, as they may need to fully account for the complexity of medical imaging tasks, such as recognizing subtle diagnostic markers in radiation therapy imaging. Specialized benchmarks that reflect real-world clinical challenges are essential to effectively assessing VLMs in these high-stakes contexts (Royer et al., 2024; Xia et al., 2024). Such benchmarks ideally include diverse patient populations, a wide array of imaging modalities, and a range of clinical scenarios to understand model performance comprehensively.

Clinical validation is equally critical to ensure that VLM outputs are accurate and meaningful in practice. This validation process involves rigorous clinical testing, where models are exposed to real-world data and conditions that differ from those in experimental setups. By establishing clear, clinically relevant standards for VLM validation, researchers can better gauge a model's readiness for deployment, minimizing the risk of misdiagnoses or other adverse outcomes.

REFERENCES

Abdullah T and Rangarajan L. 2021. Image-text matching: Methods and challenges. In V. Suma, Joy Iong-Zong Chen, Zubair Baig, Haoxiang Wang (eds), *Inventive Systems and Control: Proceedings of ICISC 2021*, Coimbatore, India, 213–22.

Abshire D and Lang M K. 2018. *Seminars in Oncology Nursing,* vol. Series 34: Elsevier. pp. 151–7.

Adhikari R, Dhakal M, Thapaliya S, Poudel K, Bhandari P and Khanal B. 2023. Synthetic boost: Leveraging synthetic data for enhanced vision-language segmentation in echocardiography. In Bernhard Kainz, Alison Noble, Julia Schnabel, Bishesh Khanal, Johanna Paula Müller, Thomas Day (eds), *4th International Workshop, ASMUS 2023, Held in Conjunction with MICCAI 2023*, Vancouver, BC, Canada, 89–99.

Al-Hadhrami S, Menai M E B, Al-Ahmadi S and Alnafessah A. 2023. An effective med-VQA method using a transformer with weights fusion of multiple fine-tuned models. *Applied Sciences* **13**: 9735.

Allaouzi I, Ben Ahmed M, Benamrou B and Ouardouz M. 2018. Automatic caption generation for medical images. *Proceedings of the 3rd International Conference on Smart City Applications,* Tetouan, Morocco, 1–6. https://doi.org/10.1145/3286606.3286863

Arnaout R. 2024. Adapting vision–language AI models to cardiology tasks *Nature Medicine* **30**: 1245–1246.

Beddiar D R, Oussalah M and Seppanen T. 2023. Retrieved generative captioning for medical images. *Proceedings of the 20th International Conference on Content-Based Multimedia Indexing*, 48–54.

Ben Melech Stan G, Aflalo E, Rohekar R Y, Bhiwandiwalla A, Tseng S-Y, Olson M L, Gurwicz Y, Wu C, Duan N and Lal V. 2024. An interpretability tool for large vision-language models. In: Proceedings of the IEEE/CVF. *Conference on Computer Vision and Pattern Recognition (CVPR) Workshops*. pp. 8182–8187 (2024) Seattle WA, USA

Blankemeier L, Cohen J P, Kumar A, Van Veen D, Gardezi S J S, Paschali M, Chen Z, Delbrouck J-B, Reis E and Truyts C. 2024. Merlin: A vision language foundation model for 3D computed tomography. *arXiv preprint arXiv:2406.06512*.

Bluethgen C, Chambon P, Delbrouck J-B, van der Sluijs R, Połacin M, Zambrano Chaves J M, Abraham T M, Purohit S, Langlotz C P and Chaudhari A S. 2024. A vision–language foundation model for the generation of realistic chest X-ray images. *Nature Biomedical Engineering* **9**: 1–13.

Budd S, Robinson E C and Kainz B. 2021. A survey on active learning and human-in-the-loop deep learning for medical image analysis. *Medical Image Analysis* **71**: 102062.

Cai L, Gao J and Zhao D. 2020. A review of the application of deep learning in medical image classification and segmentation. *Annals of Translational Medicine* **8**: 713.

Cai W. 2023. Feasibility and prospect of privacy-preserving large language models in radiology. *Radiological Society of North America* **309**: e232335.

Chen C-H, Hsieh K-Y, Huang K-E and Lai H-Y. 2024a. Comparing vision-capable models, GPT-4 and gemini, with GPT-3.5 on Taiwan's pulmonologist exam. *Cureus* **16**: e67641.

Chen W, Liu J, Liu T and Yuan Y. 2024b. Bi-VLGM: Bi-level class-severity-aware vision-language graph matching for text guided medical image segmentation *International Journal of Computer Vision* **133**: 1375–1391.

Chen X, Wang X, Zhang K, Fung K-M, Thai T C, Moore K, Mannel R S, Liu H, Zheng B and Qiu Y. 2022a. Recent advances and clinical applications of deep learning in medical image analysis. *Medical Image Analysis* **79**: 102444.

Chen Z, Diao S, Wang B, Li G and Wan X. 2023. Towards unifying medical vision-and-language pre-training via soft prompts. *Proceedings of the IEEE/CVF International Conference on Computer Vision*, Paris, France, 23403–13.

Chen Z, Du Y, Hu J, Liu Y, Li G, Wan X and Chang T-H. 2024c. Mapping medical image-text to a joint space via masked modeling. *Medical Image Analysis* **91**: 103018.

Chen Z, Hu B, Niu C, Chen T, Li Y, Shan H and Wang G. 2024d. IQAGPT: Computed tomography image quality assessment with vision-language and ChatGPT models. *Visual Computing for Industry, Biomedicine, and Art* **7**: 20.

Chen Z, Li G and Wan X. 2022b. Align, reason and learn: Enhancing medical vision-and-language pre-training with knowledge. *Proceedings of the 30th ACM International Conference on Multimedia*, Lisboa, Portugal, 5152–61. https://doi.org/10.1145/3503161.3547948

Christensen M, Vukadinovic M, Yuan N and Ouyang D. 2024. Vision–language foundation model for echocardiogram interpretation. *Nature Medicine* **30**: 1481–8.

Elbedwehy S, Medhat T, Hamza T and Alrahmawy M F. 2024. Enhanced descriptive captioning model for histopathological patches. *Multimedia Tools and Applications* 83: 36645–64.

Fu Y, Lei Y, Wang T, Curran W J, Liu T and Yang X. 2020. Deep learning in medical image registration: A review. *Physics in Medicine & Biology* **65**: 20TR01.

Gan Z, Li L, Li C, Wang L, Liu Z and Gao J. 2022. Vision-language pre-training: Basics, recent advances, and future trends. *Foundations and Trends® in Computer Graphics and Vision* 14: 163–352.

Gong H, Chen G, Mao M, Li Z and Li G. 2022. Vqamix: Conditional triplet mixup for medical visual question answering. *IEEE Transactions on Medical Imaging* 41: 3332–43.

Gu Z, Yin C, Liu F and Zhang P. 2024. MedVH: Towards systematic evaluation of hallucination for large vision language models in the medical context. *arXiv preprint arXiv:2407.02730.*

Guo M, Yi H, Qin Z, Wang H, Men A and Lao Q. 2023. Multiple prompt fusion for zero-shot lesion detection using VLMs. *Medical Image Computing and Computer Assisted Intervention – MICCAI 2023: 26th International Conference*, Vancouver, BC, Canada, October 8–12, 2023, Proceedings, Part V, Vancouver, BC, Canada, 283–92. https://doi.org/10.1007/978-3-031-43904-9_28

Hayden N, Gilbert S, Poisson L M, Griffith B and Klochko C. 2024. Performance of GPT-4 with vision on text-and image-based ACR diagnostic radiology in-training examination questions. *Radiology* **312**: e240153.

Hirano Y, Hanaoka S, Nakao T, Miki S, Kikuchi T, Nakamura Y, Nomura Y, Yoshikawa T and Abe O. 2024. GPT-4 Turbo with vision fails to outperform text-only GPT-4 Turbo in the Japan diagnostic radiology board examination. *Japanese Journal of Radiology* **42**: 918–926.

Hu M, Qian J, Pan S, Li Y, Qiu R L and Yang X. 2024. Advancing medical imaging with language models: Featuring a spotlight on ChatGPT. *Physics in Medicine & Biology* 69: 10TR01.

Huang Z, Zhang X and Zhang S. 2023. Kiut: Knowledge-injected u-transformer for radiology report generation. *2023 IEEE/CVF Conference on Computer Vision and Pattern Recognition (CVPR)*, Vancouver, BC, Canada, 19809–18.

Hüemann Z, Tie X, Hu J and Bradshaw T J. 2024. ConTEXTual net: A multimodal VLM for segmentation of pneumothorax. *Journal of Imaging Informatics in Medicine* **37**(4):1652–1663. https://doi.org/10.1007/s10278-024-01051-8. Epub 2024 Mar 14. PMID: 38485899; PMCID: PMC11300752

Huh J, Park S, Lee J E and Ye J C. 2023. Improving medical speech-to-text accuracy using vision-language pre-training models. *IEEE Journal of Biomedical and Health Informatics* **28**: 1692–1703.

Jiang Y, Chen J, Yang D, Li M, Wang S, Wu T, Li K and Zhang L. 2024. MedThink: Inducing medical large-scale visual language models to hallucinate less by thinking more. *arXiv preprint arXiv:2406.11451.*

Jin R, Huang C-Y, You C and Li X. 2024. Backdoor attack on unpaired medical image-text foundation models: A pilot study on MedCLIP. *2024 IEEE Conference on Secure and Trustworthy Machine Learning (SaTML)*, Toronto, ON, Canada, 272–85.

Kandiyana A, Mouton P R, Hall L O and Goldgof D. 2024. Active prompting of vision language models for human-in-the-loop classification and explanation of microscopy images *2024. IEEE 37th International Symposium on Computer-Based Medical Systems (CBMS)*, Guadalajara, Mexico, 205–12.

Khare Y, Bagal V, Mathew M, Devi A, Priyakumar U D and Jawahar C. 2021. MMBERT: Multimodal BERT pretraining for improved medical VQA. *2021 IEEE 18th International Symposium on Biomedical Imaging (ISBI)*, Nice, France, 1033–6.

Kim Y, Wu J, Abdulle Y, Gao Y and Wu H. 2024. Human-in-the-loop chest X-ray diagnosis: Enhancing large multimodal models with eye fixation inputs. *In Trustworthy Artificial Intelligence for Healthcare: Second International Workshop, TAI4H 2024*, Jeju, South Korea, August 4, 2024, Proceedings. Springer-Verlag, Berlin, Heidelberg, 66–80.

Kwon G, Cai Z, Ravichandran A, Bas E, Bhotika R and Soatto S. 2022. Masked vision and language modeling for multi-modal representation learning. *arXiv preprint arXiv:2208.02131.*

Li L. 2024. Adapting pretrained VLMs in medical domains.

Li Q. 2023. Harnessing the power of pre-trained VLMs for efficient medical report generation. *Proceedings of the 32nd ACM International Conference on Information and Knowledge Management (CIKM '23)*, Birmingham, United Kingdom, 1308–17.

Li T, Bai J and Wang Q. 2024a. Enhancing medical text detection with vision-language pre-training and efficient segmentation. *Complex & Intelligent Systems* **10**: 1–13.

Li T, Bai J, Wang Q and Xu H. 2024b. Efficient medical images text detection with vision-language pre-training approach. *Asian Conference on Machine Learning*, Istanbul, Turkey, 755–70.

Li Y, Wang H and Luo Y. 2020. A comparison of pre-trained vision-and-language models for multimodal representation learning across medical images and reports. *2020 IEEE International Conference on Bioinformatics and Biomedicine (BIBM)*, Seoul, Korea (South), 1999–2004.

Li Z, Li Y, Li Q, Wang P, Guo D, Lu L, Jin D, Zhang Y and Hong Q. 2023. LViT: Language meets vision transformer in medical image segmentation. *IEEE Transactions on Medical Imaging* **43**: 96–107.

Lin Z, Zhang D, Shi D, Xu R, Tao Q, Wu L, He M and Ge Z. 2023. Contrastive pre-training and linear interaction attention-based transformer for universal medical reports generation. *Journal of Biomedical Informatics* 138: 104281.

Liu B, Lu D, Wei D, Wu X, Wang Y, Zhang Y and Zheng Y. 2023a. Improving medical vision-language contrastive pretraining with semantics-aware triage. *IEEE Transactions on Medical Imaging* **42**: 3579–89.

Liu C, Cheng S, Chen C, Qiao M, Zhang W, Shah A, Bai W and Arcucci R. 2023b. M-flag: Medical vision-language pre-training with frozen language models and latent space geometry optimization *International Conference on Medical Image Computing and Computer-Assisted Intervention* – MICCAI 2023: 26th International Conference, Vancouver, BC, Canada, October 8–12, 2023, 637–47.

Liu C, Shah A, Bai W and Arcucci R. 2023c. Utilizing synthetic data for medical vision-language pre-training: Bypassing the need for real images. *arXiv preprint arXiv:2310.07027.*

Liu F, Wu X, Ge S, Zhang X, Fan W and Zou Y. 2020. Bridging the gap between vision and language domains for improved image captioning. *Proceedings of the 28th ACM International Conference on Multimedia (MM '20)*, Seattle WA USA, 4153–61.

Liu J, Zhang Y, Wang K, Yavuz M C, Chen X, Yuan Y, Li H, Yang Y, Yuille A and Tang Y. 2024. Universal and extensible language-vision models for organ segmentation and tumor detection from abdominal computed tomography. *Medical Image Analysis* **97**: 103226.

Liu L, Su X, Guo H and Zhu D. 2022. A transformer-based medical visual question answering model. *2022 26th International Conference on Pattern Recognition (ICPR)*, Montreal, QC, Canada, 1712–8.

Lu M Y, Chen B, Zhang A, Williamson D F, Chen R J, Ding T, Le L P, Chuang Y-S and Mahmood F. 2023a. Visual language pretrained multiple instance zero-shot transfer for histopathology images. *Proceedings of the IEEE/CVF Conference on Computer Vision and Pattern Recognition (CVPR)*, Vancouver, BC, Canada, 19764–75.

Lu S, Liu Z, Liu T and Zhou W. 2023b. Scaling-up medical vision-and-language representation learning with federated learning. *Engineering Applications of Artificial Intelligence* 126: 107037.

Luan S, Ou-Yang J, Yang X, Wei W, Xue X and Zhu B. 2024. A multi-modal vision-language pipeline strategy for contour quality assurance and adaptive optimization. *Physics in Medicine & Biology* **69**: 065005.

Magalhães G V, Santos R L d S, Vogado L H, de Paiva A C and dos Santos Neto P d A. 2024. XRaySwinGen: Automatic medical reporting for X-ray exams with multimodal model. *Heliyon* **10**: e27516.

Monajatipoor M, Rouhsedaghat M, Li L H, Jay Kuo C-C, Chien A and Chang K-W. 2022. Berthop: An effective vision-and-language model for chest x-ray disease diagnosis. In *Medical Image Computing and Computer Assisted Intervention – MICCAI 2022: 25th International Conference*, Singapore, 725–34.

Moon J H, Lee H, Shin W, Kim Y-H and Choi E. 2022. Multi-modal understanding and generation for medical images and text via vision-language pre-training. *IEEE Journal of Biomedical and Health Informatics* 26: 6070–80.

Moor M, Huang Q, Wu S, Yasunaga M, Dalmia Y, Leskovec J, Zakka C, Reis E P and Rajpurkar P. 2023. Med-flamingo: A multimodal medical few-shot learner. *Machine Learning for Health (ML4H)* **225**: 353–67.

Naseem U, Thapa S and Masood A. 2024. Advancing accuracy in multimodal medical tasks through bootstrapped language-image pretraining (BioMedBLIP): Performance evaluation study. *JMIR Medical Informatics* **12**: e56627.

Nazih W, Aseeri A O, Atallah O Y and El-Sappagh S. 2023. Vision transformer model for predicting the severity of diabetic retinopathy in fundus photography-based retina images. *IEEE Access* 11: 117546–61.

Oura T, Tatekawa H, Horiuchi D, Matsushita S, Takita H, Atsukawa N, Mitsuyama Y, Yoshida A, Murai K and Tanaka R. 2024. Diagnostic accuracy of VLMs on Japanese diagnostic radiology, nuclear medicine, and interventional radiology specialty board examinations. *Japanese Journal of Radiology* **42**: 1392–8.

Palit V, Pandey R, Arora A and Liang P P. 2023. Towards Vision-Language Mechanistic Interpretability: A Causal Tracing Tool for BLIP. *2023 IEEE/CVF International Conference on Computer Vision Workshops (ICCVW), Paris, France*, 2856–61.

Pan S, Chang C W, Wang T, Wynne J, Hu M, Lei Y, Liu T, Patel P, Roper J and Yang X. 2023. Abdomen CT multi-organ segmentation using token-based MLP-mixer. *Medical Physics* **50:** 3027–38.

Qiu S, Liu Q, Zhou S and Wu C. 2019. Review of artificial intelligence adversarial attack and defense technologies. *Applied Sciences* **9**: 909.

Qu L, Fu K, Wang M and Song Z. 2024. The rise of ai language pathologists: Exploring two-level prompt learning for few-shot weakly-supervised whole slide image classification. In *Proceedings of the 37th International Conference on Neural Information Processing Systems (NIPS '23)*, New Orleans LA USA.

Royer C, Menze B and Sekuboyina A. 2024. Multimedeval: A benchmark and a toolkit for evaluating medical VLMs. *arXiv preprint arXiv:2402.09262.*

Shifai N, van Doorn R, Malvehy J and Sangers T E. 2024. Can ChatGPT vision diagnose melanoma? An exploratory diagnostic accuracy study. *Journal of the American Academy of Dermatology* 90: 1057–9.

Singh S, Karimi S, Ho-Shon K and Hamey L. 2021. Show, tell and summarise: Learning to generate and summarise radiology findings from medical images. *Neural Computing and Applications* 33: 7441–65.

Suh P S, Shim W H, Suh C H, Heo H, Park C R, Eom H J, Park K J, Choe J, Kim P H and Park H J. 2024. Comparing diagnostic accuracy of radiologists versus GPT-4V and Gemini Pro Vision using image inputs from diagnosis please cases. *Radiology* **312**: e240273.

Tsuneki M and Kanavati F. 2022. Inference of captions from histopathological patches. In *International Conference on Medical Imaging with Deep Learning*, Zürich, Swiss, vol. Series: PMLR, 1235–50.

Tung C, Lin Y, Yin J, Ye Q and Chen H. 2024. Exploring vision language pretraining with knowledge enhancement via large language model. *International Workshop on Trustworthy Artificial Intelligence for Healthcare,* Second International Workshop, TAI4H 2024, Jeju, South Korea, 81–91.

Van M H, Verma P and Wu X. 2024. On large visual language models for medical imaging analysis: An empirical study. *2024 IEEE/ACM Conference on Connected Health: Applications, Systems and Engineering Technologies (CHASE)*, Wilmington, DE, USA, 172–6.

Wan K W, Wong C H, Ip H F, Fan D, Yuen P L, Fong H Y and Ying M. 2021. Evaluation of the performance of traditional machine learning algorithms, convolutional neural network and AutoML Vision in ultrasound breast lesions classification: A comparative study. *Quantitative Imaging in Medicine and Surgery* **11**: 1381.

Wang J, Zhou Y, Xu G, Shi P, Zhao C, Xu H, Ye Q, Yan M, Zhang J and Zhu J. 2023. Evaluation and analysis of hallucination in large VLMs. *arXiv preprint arXiv:2308.15126.*

Wang L and Yoon K-J. 2021. Knowledge distillation and student-teacher learning for visual intelligence: A review and new outlooks. *IEEE Transactions on Pattern Analysis and Machine Intelligence* 44: 3048–68.

Wang P, Zhang H and Yuan Y. 2024. MCPL: Multi-modal collaborative prompt learning for medical VLM. *IEEE Transactions on Medical Imaging* 43: 4224–35.

Wang R, Lei T, Cui R, Zhang B, Meng H and Nandi A K. 2022. Medical image segmentation using deep learning: A survey. *IET Image Processing* 16: 1243–67.

Wang T, Lei Y, Fu Y, Wynne J F, Curran W J, Liu T and Yang X. 2021. A review on medical imaging synthesis using deep learning and its clinical applications. *Journal of Applied Clinical Medical Physics* **22**: 11–36.

Windsor R, Jamaludin A, Kadir T and Zisserman A. 2023. VLMling for radiological imaging and reports in the low data regime. *arXiv preprint arXiv:2303.17644*.

Wu C, Zhang X, Zhang Y, Wang Y and Xie W. 2023a. Medklip: Medical knowledge enhanced language-image pre-training for x-ray diagnosis. *2023 IEEE/CVF International Conference on Computer Vision (ICCV)*, Paris, France, 21372–83.

Wu X, Xiao L, Sun Y, Zhang J, Ma T and He L. 2022. A survey of human-in-the-loop for machine learning. *Future Generation Computer Systems* 135: 364–81.

Wu Z, Shu X, Yan S and Lu Z. 2023b. FGCVQA: Fine-grained cross-attention for medical VQA. *2023 IEEE International Conference on Image Processing (ICIP)*, Kuala Lumpur, Malaysia, 975–9.

Xia P, Chen Z, Tian J, Gong Y, Hou R, Xu Y, Wu Z, Fan Z, Zhou Y and Zhu K. 2024. CARES: A comprehensive benchmark of trustworthiness in medical vision language models. *arXiv preprint arXiv:2406.06007*.

Xie Y, Gu L, Harada T, Zhang J, Xia Y and Wu Q. 2024. Rethinking masked image modelling for medical image representation. *Medical Image Analysis* **98**: 103304.

Yan B and Pei M. 2022. Clinical-bert: Vision-language pre-training for radiograph diagnosis and reports generation. *Proceedings of the AAAI Conference on Artificial Intelligence* 36: 2982–90.

You K, Gu J, Ham J, Park B, Kim J, Hong E K, Baek W and Roh B. 2023. Cxr-clip: Toward large scale chest x-ray language-image pre-training. In *Medical Image Computing and Computer Assisted Intervention – MICCAI 2023: 26th International Conference*, Vancouver, BC, Canada,, 101–11.

Zhan C, Zhang Y, Lin Y, Wang G and Wang H. 2024. Unidcp: Unifying multiple medical vision-language tasks via dynamic cross-modal learnable prompts. *IEEE Transactions on Multimedia* **26**: 9736–48.

Zhang H, Koh J Y, Baldridge J, Lee H and Yang Y. 2021. Cross-modal contrastive learning for text-to-image generation. *2021 IEEE/CVF Conference on Computer Vision and Pattern Recognition (CVPR)*, Nashville, TN, USA,, 833–42.

Zhang J, Huang J, Jin S and Lu S. 2024a. VLMs for vision tasks: A survey. *IEEE Transactions on Pattern Analysis and Machine Intelligence* **46**: 5625–44.

Zhang K, Yang Y, Yu J, Jiang H, Fan J, Huang Q and Han W. 2023a. Multi-task paired masking with alignment modeling for medical vision-language pre-training. *IEEE Transactions on Multimedia* 26: 4706–21.

Zhang K, Zhou R, Adhikarla E, Yan Z, Liu Y, Yu J, Liu Z, Chen X, Davison B D and Ren H. 2024b. A generalist vision–language foundation model for diverse biomedical tasks. *Nature Medicine* **30**: 3129–41.

Zhang X, Wu C, Zhang Y, Xie W and Wang Y. 2023b. Knowledge-enhanced visual-language pre-training on chest radiology images. *Nature Communications* **14**: 4542.

Zhang Y and Chen D Z. 2023. GPT4MIA: Utilizing generative pre-trained transformer (GPT-3) as a plug-and-play transductive model for medical image analysis. In *Medical Image Computing and Computer Assisted Intervention – MICCAI 2023 Workshops : ISIC 2023, Care-AI 2023, MedAGI 2023, DeCaF 2023*, Held in Conjunction with MICCAI 2023, Vancouver, BC, Canada, 151–60.

Zhang Z, Xie Y, Xing F, McGough M and Yang L. 2017. Mdnet: A semantically and visually interpretable medical image diagnosis network. *2017 IEEE Conference on Computer Vision and Pattern Recognition (CVPR)*, Honolulu, HI, USA, 6428–36.

Zheng F, Cao J, Yu W, Chen Z, Xiao N and Lu Y. 2024. Exploring low-resource medical image classification with weakly supervised prompt learning. *Pattern Recognition* **149:** 110250.

Zhu H, Togo R, Ogawa T and Haseyama M. 2023. Diversity learning based on multi-latent space for medical image visual question generation. *Sensors* **23:** 1057.

6 AI-driven Image-Guided Radiation Therapy

Yunxiang Li, Jiacheng Xie, and You Zhang

6.1 INTRODUCTION

Image-guided radiation therapy (IGRT) represents a significant advancement in the field of radiation oncology, aiming to enhance the precision and effectiveness of cancer treatment through integrating advanced imaging techniques into the whole clinical workflow. Imaging now has been seamlessly integrated into key radiotherapy components, including pre-treatment simulation, intra-treatment delivery, and post-treatment follow-ups. In this section, we offer an overview of recent advancements in harnessing artificial intelligence (AI) within IGRT, highlighting its transformative potential in improving precision and efficacy across the entire IGRT continuum.

6.2 SIMULATION IN IMAGE-GUIDED RADIATION THERAPY

In radiation therapy, the simulation phase serves as the cornerstone of the entire treatment process, primarily aimed at providing precise and detailed imaging support for treatment planning. Specifically, during this phase, imaging techniques, such as magnetic resonance imaging (MRI) [1], computed tomography (CT), or positron emission tomography (PET), are typically used [2]. MRI provides high-contrast soft-tissue anatomical information, making it particularly suitable for treatment sites where the boundaries between the tumor and surrounding soft tissues are less distinct for other modalities, such as the brain, prostate, and abdominal cases [3]. CT, on the other hand, offers high spatial-resolution imaging with excellent geometric integrity and is particularly useful to capture and locate bony structures and air cavities. It is also the primary source of electron density information required for radiation dose calculations [4]. PET provides information on the metabolism of tumors, helping to identify areas of high metabolic activity, which is especially useful for defining treatment target volumes and stratifying dose prescriptions for treatment plans of complex tumors such as those in the head and neck regions [5,6]. Using different imaging data, clinicians can design an optimal radiation dose distribution that ensures the tumor receives a sufficient dose while protecting the surrounding healthy tissues.

However, each imaging modality faces its challenges in clinical practice. For example, in CT, which uses X-ray beams, artifacts caused by high-attenuation metal objects or patient movement can significantly reduce the image quality [7]. While MRI offers excellent soft-tissue contrast, its lengthy acquisition makes it prone to motion artifacts [8]. It also suffers from geometric distortions due to factors including the inhomogeneity of magnetic fields. PET, dependent on radiotracers, has relatively low spatial resolution and may not accurately describe specific anatomical details due to the limitations of tracer metabolism. Given these challenges, and with the rapid development of AI in the medical field, numerous AI technologies have been gradually introduced into the simulation phase of radiation therapy to address these issues [9]. These AI technologies are primarily applied in applications, including image reconstruction, image synthesis, multimodal image registration, and image segmentation. For instance, AI-driven image reconstruction techniques can effectively reduce noise and artifacts through network-learned imaging priors, improving image quality and enabling more accurate delineations of the target area and normal tissues. It can significantly improve the quality of reconstructed images from under-sampling scenarios to allow fast imaging.

DOI: 10.1201/9781003480365-7

Image synthesis techniques, particularly those based on generative adversarial networks (GANs), can synthesize MRI data into CT images to provide the electron density information necessary for radiation dose calculations and offer complementary information from different imaging modalities [10]. Multimodal image registration techniques use AI-based algorithms to precisely align images from different modalities, correcting spatial discrepancies and merging the anatomical and functional information provided by different imaging modalities. AI-based automatic segmentation techniques can significantly reduce the time and errors associated with manual target delineation by clinicians, increasing clinical efficiency, safety, and accuracy.

6.2.1 The Development of Generative Models for Applications in RT Simulation

The applications of AI in the simulation phase of RT are closely tied to advancements in various cutting-edge generative model techniques. Therefore, we first introduce several common model types used in these applications, including GANs [11], Variational Autoencoders (VAEs) [12], and diffusion models [13]. In Figure 6.1, we present a schematic diagram of these models along with their emergence timeline.

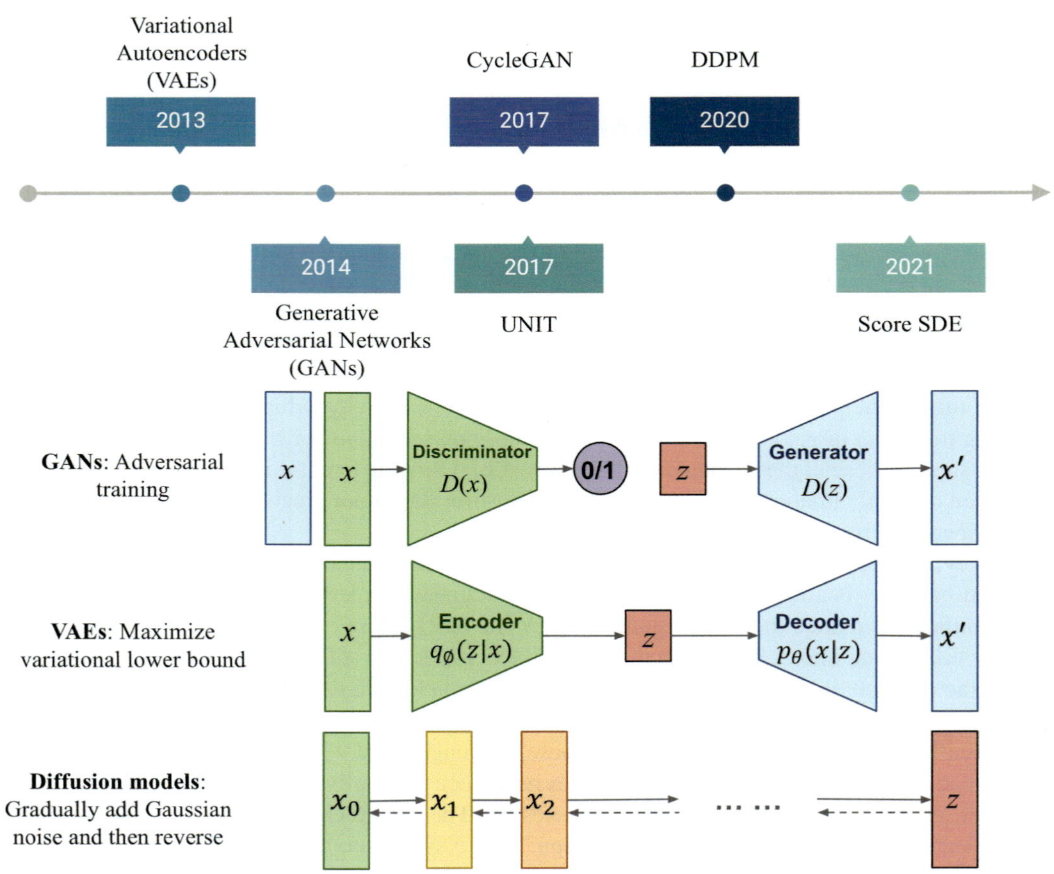

FIGURE 6.1 The timeline of the development of different generative models, along with a schematic diagram of the structure of these generative models, where x represents the image and z represents the latent variable.

6.2.1.1 Generative Adversarial Networks

GANs are one of the most widely applied generative models in the field of radiation therapy. GANs operate through adversarial interactions between two networks: a generator and a discriminator, enabling the generation of realistic images. One of the most prominent works is CycleGAN [14], which consists of two generators and two discriminators. These components are designed to translate images from one domain to another to achieve a close resemblance between the generated images and the real images from the target domain. The key innovation of CycleGAN lies in the use of a cycle-consistent loss, which enforces that an image translated to another domain and then back to the original domain retains its original structure. The cycle-consistency loss allows unsupervised training of the network (without paired images to serve as "ground-truth" labels), which is particularly important in medical image synthesis, where obtaining paired datasets can be challenging. By improving image translation quality and precision, CycleGAN has been applied to applications like MRI-to-CT translation to provide accurate electron density information for radiation therapy dose calculations [15].

6.2.1.2 Variational Autoencoders

Variational autoencoders (VAEs) are a type of generative model commonly used in unsupervised learning, capable of learning the latent space distribution of images and reconstructing high-quality images. This makes them highly relevant and readily applicable in medical image synthesis and reconstruction. UNIT [16] is an unsupervised image translation framework based on VAE with a shared latent space assumption, which allows images from different domains to be mapped to a common latent space. This facilitates cross-modal image translation, such as between MRI and CT images [17]. UNIT does not require paired datasets for training, making it particularly useful in scenarios where paired medical images are difficult to obtain.

6.2.1.3 Diffusion Models

Diffusion models are a class of probabilistic models used for image generation, where noise is iteratively added to corrupt and alter the image and then denoised in reverse to generate new data. These models have demonstrated excellent performance in image reconstruction and synthesis tasks. One foundational work is the denoising diffusion probabilistic model (DDPM) [13]. The training process of DDPM involves two stages: in the forward process, noise is gradually added to the data, creating a trajectory from the data distribution to a Gaussian distribution; in the reverse process, a neural network learns how to denoise, thereby generating realistic images from the noise. Building on the foundation of DDPM, Score-Based Stochastic Differential Equations (Score SDEs) [18] further advanced diffusion models by using stochastic differential equations to model the diffusion and denoising processes, providing a more flexible framework. Compared to DDPM, Score SDE is better suited for handling complex image generation tasks, especially in applications like compressed-sensing MRI [19] and sparse-view CT reconstruction [20]. By combining the diffusion process with stochastic differential equations that are based on the probability theory, Score SDE enhances the precision and stability of image generation while achieving more efficient image restoration during the reconstruction process. These developments have driven fast-emerging applications of diffusion models in the field of medical imaging. In the following sections, we will explore the specific applications of these models in various aspects of the simulation phase.

6.2.2 Image Reconstruction

Image reconstruction plays a critical role in the simulation phase of radiation therapy to provide 3D or 4D renderings of the human anatomy. AI enables the generation of high-quality images from low-quality or low-dose scans, as shown in Figure 6.2. AI can post-process images reconstructed by a conventional algorithm to enhance their quality (image-domain AI algorithms). It can also

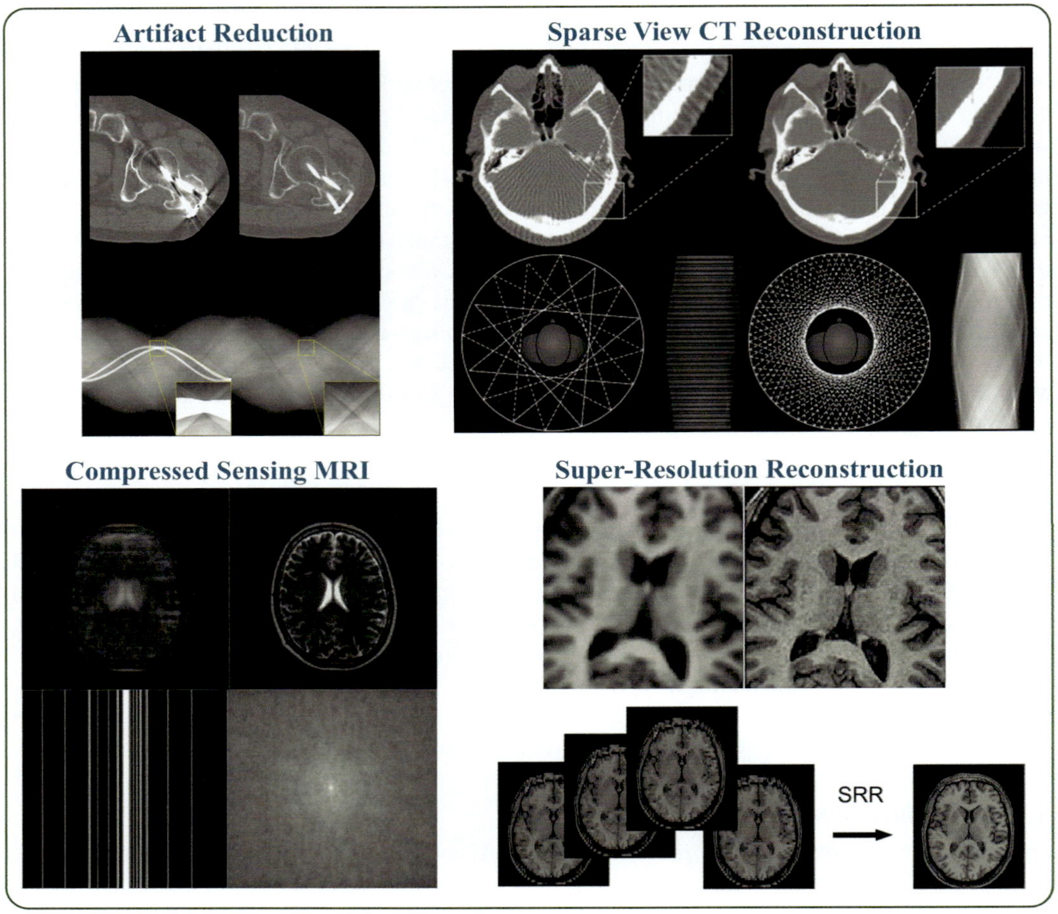

FIGURE 6.2 Illustration of specific applications in medical image reconstruction. **Top left**: AI-based metal artifact reduction on CT images; **Top right**: AI-based sinogram in-painting for sparse-view CT reconstruction; **Bottom left**: AI-based compressed-sensing MRI using sparsely sampled k-space data; **Bottom right**: AI-based MRI super-resolution reconstruction.

be directly integrated into the reconstruction workflow to convert raw signals into reconstructed images (signal-domain AI algorithms). Through deep learning networks, models can enhance the resolution and contrast of reconstructed images to optimize the visibility/delineation of tumors and normal tissues. The following outlines specific applications and relevant research in the field of image reconstruction.

6.2.2.1 Artifact Reduction

CT scans serve as a crucial source of anatomical information for delineating target areas and organs at risk (OARs), and the electron density information harbored in the CT pixel intensities is essential for radiation dose calculations. However, the presence of metal implants can affect CT image acquisition and introduce errors during CT image reconstruction, resulting in artifacts in the reconstructed images. These artifacts typically manifest as bright or dark streaks and are caused by factors such as beam hardening, photon starvation, edge effects, and scattering. For instance, dental implants, hip prostheses, and spinal metal screws frequently lead to pronounced metal artifacts. These artifacts not only impair the accuracy of organ and tumor contouring but introduce errors in

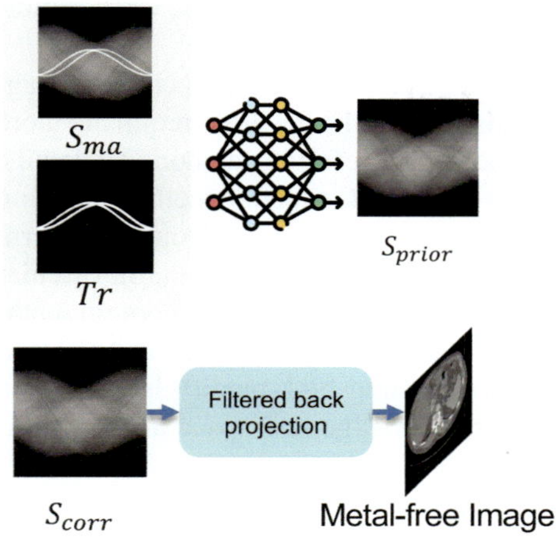

(a) CT metal artifact reduction framework that combines sinogram completion with prior information from the image domain.

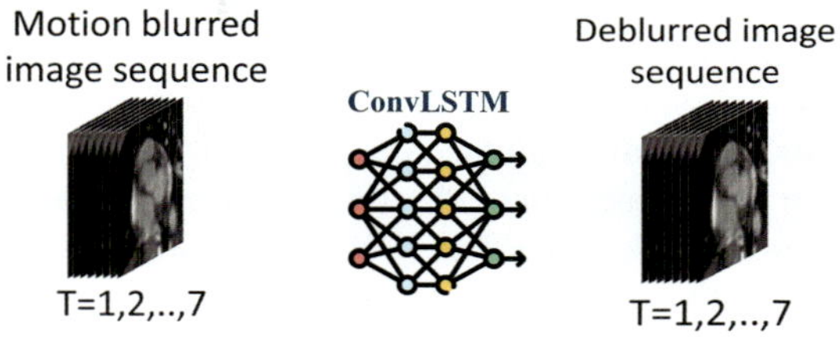

(b) MRI motion artifact reduction framework utilizing bi-directional convolutional long short-term memory (ConvLSTM) networks and multi-scale convolutions.

FIGURE 6.3 The schematic diagrams of different models for (a) CT metal artifact reduction and (b) MRI motion artifact reduction.

the derived electron densities, potentially leading to deviations in the radiation dose calculated for photon or particle beams and affecting the precision of treatments. To address this, many researchers have explored the use of AI techniques to reduce metal artifacts. These AI-driven approaches have significantly improved image quality and usability, facilitating more accurate contouring of tumors and normal tissues.

Early methods for metal artifact reduction primarily focused on independent processing in either the sinogram (signal) domain or the image domain. For example, Yu et al. proposed a framework that combines sinogram completion with prior information from the image domain [21]. As shown in Figure 6.3a, their approach leveraged two neural networks, SinoNet and PriorNet, to jointly recover metal-affected projection data, which was subsequently used to generate higher-quality CT images through filtered back projection (FBP). While this method demonstrated the potential of sinogram completion for reducing artifacts, the independent treatment of the sinogram and image domains limited its ability to fully eliminate the artifacts. Building on this, Wang et al. further advanced metal artifact reduction by proposing a dual-domain adaptive-scaling nonlocal network (DAN-Net) [22]. In their approach, adaptive scaling is first applied to the sinogram to preserve more tissue details. Then, a dual-domain network processes both the sinogram and the reconstructed CT image for further artifact removal. Residual sinogram learning and nonlocal modules were incorporated, significantly reducing the likelihood of secondary artifacts introduced from the neural network. This method's integrated approach to combine both sinogram and image domains markedly improved the overall image quality. As deep learning methods keep evolving, the focus shifted from purely reducing artifacts to enhancing model interpretability and accuracy. Wang et al. introduced a deep interpretable convolutional dictionary network (DICDNet) [23], which combined nonlocal characteristics of metal artifacts with a convolutional dictionary model and proximal gradient optimization techniques, resulting in a physically interpretable network architecture. The method effectively removed metal artifacts by improving the model's ability to identify and process these artifacts, demonstrating superior performance on both synthetic and clinical datasets. From the initial approaches focused on sinogram domain completion, to the introduction of dual-domain adaptive networks, and finally to physically interpretable models such as convolutional dictionary networks, these studies reflect the gradual evolution of metal artifact reduction techniques.

Each stage of development has contributed to enhanced artifact removal capabilities, while simultaneously improving the preservation of anatomical details in CT imaging.

Artifact reduction is not limited to metal artifacts in CT. In MRI, particularly in cardiac imaging, motion artifacts caused by patient movement present a distinct challenge, often requiring more sophisticated AI models to capture dynamic features over time while preserving anatomical details. To address motion artifacts in MRI, Lyu et al. proposed a motion artifact reduction method based on recurrent GANs [8]. As shown in Figure 6.3b, it employs bidirectional convolutional long short-term memory networks (ConvLSTM) and multi-scale convolutions to effectively capture cardiovascular dynamics, remove artifacts, and improve temporal resolution. Beyond purely image-domain methods, Cui et al. combined deep learning with k-space analysis to address motion artifacts by detecting phase encoding (PE) lines affected by motion and reconstructing high-quality images from unaffected k-space data [24]. Leveraging physics-based prior knowledge in k-space analysis, this innovative method improved the efficacy of motion artifact reduction in MRI.

Through these approaches, AI-driven artifact reduction techniques have advanced significantly, addressing lingering clinical challenges such as CT metal artifacts and MRI motion artifacts. These innovations support improved image quality, ultimately contributing to more precise tumor and organ contouring and enhanced accuracy in radiation therapy.

6.2.2.2 Super-Resolution Imaging

Super-resolution imaging leverages deep learning models to translate low-resolution medical images into high-resolution representations, improving the visibility of fine details and enabling more precise analysis and delineation of anatomical structures. This technique is particularly important in modalities such as MRI and CT, where clear visualization of anatomical structures and pathological features is critical for target localization and treatment planning. Medical images are often affected by noise, limited sensor resolution, and other hardware constraints, leading to reduced spatial resolution, which makes it challenging to discern minute details. Traditional image super-resolution techniques, such as interpolation, estimate new pixel values based on neighboring pixels but fail to recover high-frequency information. In contrast, deep learning-based super-resolution techniques employ advanced algorithms trained on large datasets to identify and restore missing high-frequency details through learned priors, producing images that closely match the original volumes. The AI-based approaches have demonstrated significant advantages over traditional methods, offering more detailed and accurate reconstructions. For example, Sánchez and Vilaplana proposed a 3D GAN-based model that utilizes 3D convolutions to leverage volumetric information for brain MRI super-resolution [25]. Although this method demonstrated promising results in outperforming classical interpolation techniques in 3D medical imaging, it did not fully exploit multi-contrast information, which could further enhance super-resolution performance. Lyu et al. addressed this limitation by proposing a multi-contrast MRI super-resolution framework [26]. Their approach integrated multi-contrast information into a high-level feature space rather than at the pixel level, resulting in images with higher structural similarity and peak signal-to-noise ratio compared to single-contrast methods. By employing both single-level non-progressive and two-level progressive networks, they demonstrated that the effective integration of multi-contrast information significantly improved image quality, particularly at higher up-sampling rates. Besides, Wu et al. introduced a novel brain MRI super-resolution method based on the DDPM [27]. This study incorporated a self-attention mechanism into DDPM to improve training speed and perceptual image quality. By leveraging DDPM's ability to generate fine details, the framework not only excelled in super-resolution for brain MRIs but showed potential applications in other anatomical regions, such as the spine and the knee sites. Beyond merely improving resolution, Chen et al. proposed a diagnosis-driven super-resolution framework that directly integrates super-resolution with diagnostic tasks [28]. Their multi-scale refined context network (MRC-Net) employed recursive temporal context distillation to reduce computational costs while enhancing super-resolution performance. Additionally, their diagnostic network introduced Sample Affinity Interaction (SAI) blocks to combine original images with super-resolution-enhanced images, effectively extracting and integrating discriminative features for diagnosis. This approach demonstrated that super-resolution techniques can be leveraged for image enhancement and to directly improve medical decision-making processes.

From the early adoption of GANs to the latest use of diffusion models, and the integration of multi-contrast information and multitask learning techniques, medical super-resolution imaging has undergone significant developments. These advancements have continually improved the resolution, structural fidelity, and treatment planning utility of medical images, laying a strong foundation for more precise and efficient cancer treatment.

6.2.2.3 Sparse-View and Low-Dose CT Reconstruction

For CT imaging, sparse-view and low-dose reconstruction are popular topics of research, primarily aimed at reducing radiation dose while maintaining image quality. Sparse-view CT reconstruction, for example, performs CT scanning by reducing the amount of projection data collected. Traditional CT scanning typically requires a large number of projection angles to generate high-quality reconstructions. However, a large number of projection angles will inevitably increase the imaging radiation dose. Sparse-view CT reconstruction reduces the sampling angles and compensates the information loss of under-sampling through advanced deep learning algorithms. For example, Yang et al. proposed an innovative Dual-Domain Diffusion Model (DDDM) specifically designed for sparse-view CT reconstruction [29], which is shown in Figure 6.4a. This model integrates both the sinogram and image domains and consists of a Sinogram Upgrading Module (SUM) and an Image

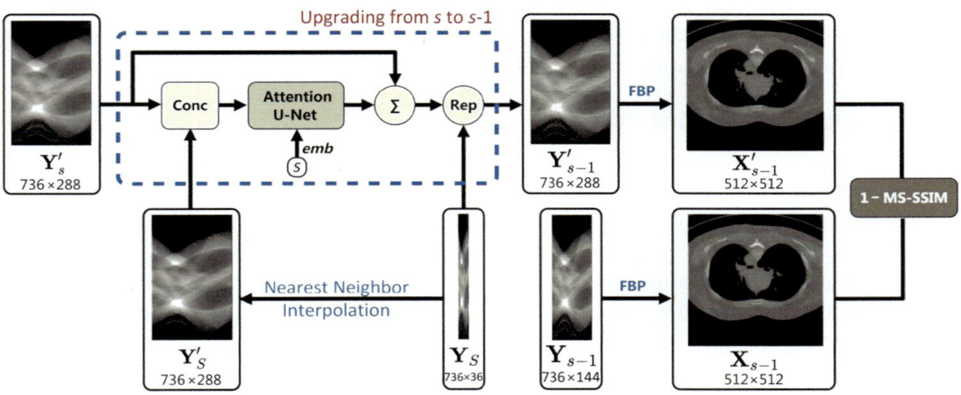

(a) Sinogram upgrading module for Sparse-view CT reconstruction.

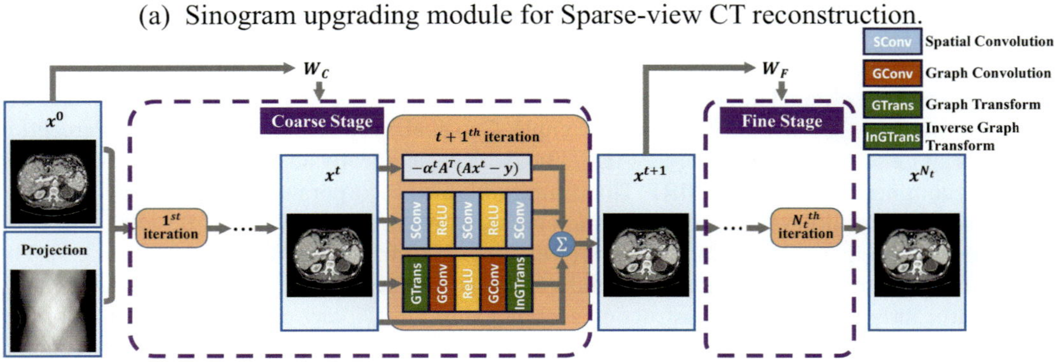

(b) Low-dose CT reconstruction framework utilizing graph convolution for non-local topological feature analysis and local pixel feature extraction.

FIGURE 6.4 The schematic diagrams of models for (a) sparse-view CT reconstruction (Reprint from Ref. [29]) and (b) low-dose CT reconstruction (Reprint from Ref. [30]).

Refining Module (IRM). The method demonstrates significant improvements over traditional deep learning models, not only excelling in classical similarity metrics but generalizing well to unseen anatomical sites.

In addition to reducing the number of projection angles, lowering the radiation intensities of the imaging source is another approach to reduce CT dose. Low-dose CT (LDCT) is also a prominent research area, as reduced photon counts in LDCT often lead to excessive noise and low signal-to-noise ratios (SNRs). Researchers have developed various AI-driven techniques to address the noise issues during the imaging process. For example, Xia et al. introduced a low-dose CT reconstruction network called MAGIC, which operates in both image and manifold spaces [31]. Leveraging the low-dimensional structure of medical image patches, the MAGIC model employs graph convolution to analyze nonlocal topological features and combines it with local pixel feature extraction in image space, achieving efficient noise suppression, as shown in Figure 6.4b. Experimental results show that MAGIC outperforms existing methods both quantitatively and qualitatively and demonstrates strong denoising performance even with limited labeled data. Additionally, Ding et al. proposed an adaptive hyperparameter deep learning approach for low-dose CT reconstruction. Their model is based on a half-quadratic splitting method and incorporates learnable image priors within a model-based iterative reconstruction (MBIR) framework, automatically adjusting hyperparameters to accommodate varying noise levels [32]. This method only needs to train a single universal model, which can generalize to data from different dose levels, showing robust and versatile performance.

In summary, many potent AI-driven CT reconstruction methods have been developed with specialized network structures and learning mechanisms to address specific imaging quality challenges. By combining domain-specific, physics-based prior knowledge with network-learned population priors, these methods effectively improved CT quality that is degraded by sparse-view and low-dose acquisitions, offering safer and more efficient imaging solutions for clinical applications.

6.2.2.4 Compressed-Sensing MRI

MRI is often limited by slow acquisition speeds, especially when high-resolution imaging is required. To address this limitation, researchers have developed various techniques to accelerate MRI scanning, with one of the most groundbreaking being compressed-sensing (CS)-MRI. CS-MRI allows for the reconstruction of high-quality images from under-sampled data, significantly reducing scanning time without compromising image quality. CS-MRI has proven particularly effective in scenarios that require rapid imaging, such as cardiac and pediatric MRI, where patient movements like breathing motion can negatively impact image quality. As the CS technology has matured, Siemens' MRI acceleration has received FDA approval and been successfully implemented in clinical practice, reducing the acquisition time for cardiac cine imaging from the traditional 4 minutes to just 16 seconds [33]. This advancement allows patients to breathe freely during scanning, eliminating the need to repeatedly hold their breath and greatly enhancing their overall clinical experience. Building on these clinical advancements, researchers continue to explore ways to further improve the performance of CS-MRI with AI. For example, Gao et al. proposed the Hierarchical Perception Adversarial Learning Framework (HP-ALF) [34], which specifically addresses the issue of aliasing artifacts commonly seen in CS-MRI. This framework also incorporates the advantages of adversarial learning, resulting in visually realistic and sharp reconstructed images. Besides, Sun et al. proposed a Deep Error Correction Network (DECN) to optimize CS-MRI reconstruction [35]. The DECN model incorporates a guidance module, an error correction module, and a data fidelity module, significantly improving reconstruction accuracy. For DECN, any existing CS-MRI algorithm can be used as a template module to guide the initial image reconstruction. Then, the error correction module employs a convolutional neural network (CNN) to correct structural errors in the template image, while the data fidelity module ensures image accuracy. Experimental results indicate that the DECN framework, with its error-correcting CNN, effectively compensates for structural errors in conventional inversion-based reconstruction, substantially enhancing the performance of existing CS-MRI methods.

Furthermore, Liu et al. investigated the clinical feasibility of AI-assisted compressed sensing (ACS) for MRI in patients with nasopharyngeal carcinoma (NPC) and compared its capabilities with those of parallel imaging (PI) [36]. In their study, 66 patients with pathologically confirmed NPC underwent MRI examinations of the nasopharynx and neck using both ACS and PI techniques on a 3.0-T MRI system. The ACS method was found to significantly reduce examination time while achieving superior image quality compared to PI ($p<0.0001$). Qualitative analyses further revealed that ACS provided better lesion detection, margin sharpness, and artifact reduction, as well as higher overall image quality. Inter-observer agreement for all qualitative metrics showed satisfactory-to-excellent consistency ($p<0.0001$). The results suggest that AI-ACS not only accelerates MRI scanning but enhances image quality, offering significant clinical benefits for patients with NPC by optimizing both imaging speed and diagnostic accuracy.

6.2.3 Image Synthesis

Medical image synthesis has become an important application of AI in the field of medical imaging. By converting data between different imaging modalities, image synthesis provides complementary anatomical/functional information, enhances image quality, and supports various radiation therapy tasks. This technology can generate images with improved contrast or simulate information from other imaging modalities, offering comprehensive guidance to the IGRT process. Image synthesis is not limited to commonly performed modality conversions, such as MRI-to-CT or CBCT-to-CT translations in Figure 6.5, but includes tasks like attenuation correction in PET/CT, and conversions between different MR contrast-weighted images.

Among these, MRI-to-CT and CBCT-to-CT image synthesis have become key applications of AI in the field of radiation therapy, as shown in Figure 6.5. The primary objective is to convert MRI or CBCT images into CT-equivalent images to provide accurate electron density information for

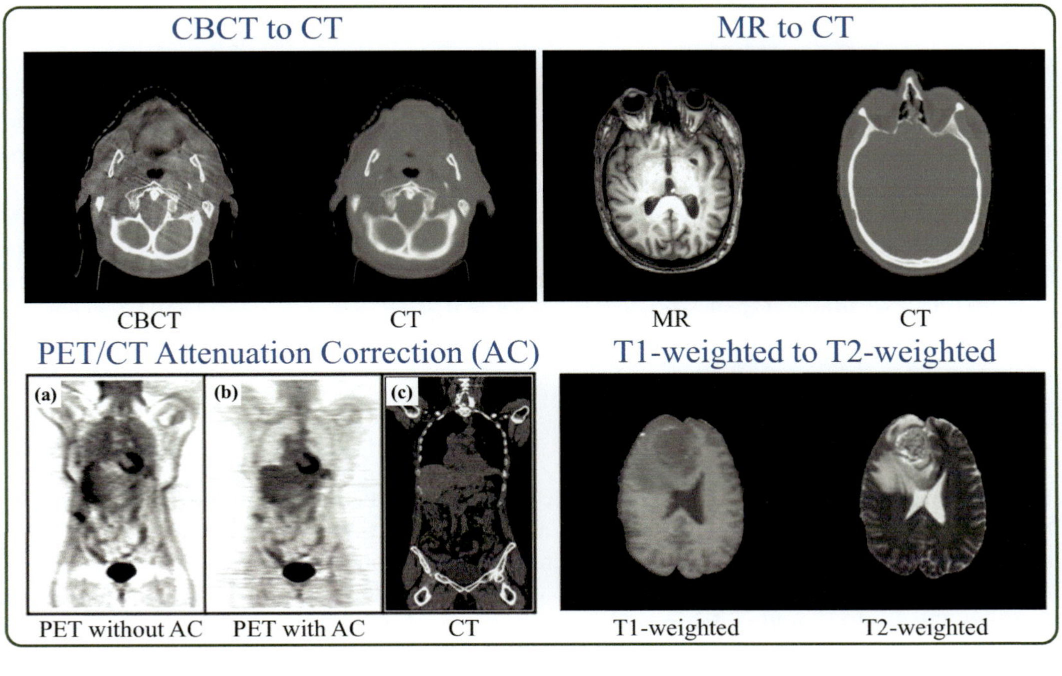

FIGURE 6.5 Example images for different image synthesis tasks. Examples from left to right: CBCT-to-CT synthesis; MRI-to-CT synthesis; CT synthesis from PET for attenuation correction; and the synthesis of T2-weighted MRI from T1-weighted acquisitions.

radiation dose calculation. While MRI offers significant advantages in soft-tissue contrast, it lacks the bone and electron density information provided by CT, making it less suitable for direct use in dose calculation. MRI-to-CT synthesis addresses this limitation by converting MRI data into complementary images that resemble CT for dose calculation and treatment planning. Similarly, due to degradations from amplified scatter and noise, CBCT images usually suffer from poor image contrast and inaccurate Hounsfield Unit (HU) values. CBCT-to-CT synthesis aims to improve the quality of CBCT to match that of the fan-beam CT, especially for adaptive radiation therapy (ART) scenarios that are heavily reliant on CBCT for tumor/organ segmentation and treatment planning. Liang et al. proposed a CycleGAN-based framework to generate CT images from CBCT [37], addressing the dose calculation errors in CBCT images caused by noise, artifacts, and inaccurate HU values. Li et al. introduced a Frequency-Guided Diffusion Model (FGDM) [38], which uses frequency-domain filters to guide the diffusion process, preserving the structural details of source domain (e.g., CBCT) images while generating high-quality images in the target domain (e.g., CT). Notably, it allows the model to be trained solely on target domain data without requiring paired source-target images. This zero-shot learning approach can directly translate images from one domain to another without prior exposure to source domain data during training. Furthermore, Li et al. introduced the Frequency-Decoupled Diffusion Model (FDDM) for MRI-to-CT conversion [39]. FDDM begins by extracting anatomical information from the MR image through an initial conversion module and then uses this information to guide a subsequent diffusion model that generates high-quality CT images. The model employs a dual-path reverse diffusion process to handle both low- and high-frequency information, striking a balance between image quality and anatomical accuracy.

In PET imaging, emitted positrons are attenuated by body tissues, causing inaccuracies in the detected signals. CT images, which provide high-resolution anatomical structure and tissue density information, allow for the calculation of attenuation coefficients for each tissue type. Therefore, attenuation correction (AC) using CT data can significantly improve the quantitative accuracy of PET images. Converting non-attenuation-corrected (NAC) PET images into attenuation-corrected (AC) PET images has critical importance in radiotherapy, as accurate attenuation correction enhances the activity localization precision of PET images, supporting accurate tumor localization and dose planning. For example, Hu et al. proposed a deep learning model based on the Wasserstein Generative Adversarial Network (WGAN) to generate synthetic attenuation-corrected PET (sAC PET) and synthetic CT (sCT) images from NAC PET images to reduce the imaging dose and address the misregistration/motion challenges between acquired PET-CT pairs [40].

Furthermore, synthesizing between multi-contrast MRIs of different sequences has shown substantial value. Kawahara and Nagata utilized a conditional GAN to perform conversions between T1- and T2-weighted MR images, providing an efficient solution for multi-contrast MRI applications [41]. This multimodal synthesis not only enhances the contrast properties of MRI data but also indirectly improves the generalizability of segmentation models trained on single-modality MR images.

6.2.4 Multimodal Image Registration

Multimodal image registration is a key practice in radiation therapy for improving the localization and contouring of anatomical structures and tumors. During the simulation stage of radiation therapy, multiple imaging modalities, such as CT, MRI, and PET, are often used, with each modality offering unique advantages in visualizing specific anatomical structures and physiological features. The goal of multimodal image registration is to align these different images accurately, providing a more comprehensive view of the tumor and surrounding tissues. In recent years, AI has significantly enhanced the efficiency and precision of multimodal image registration. AI-based registration algorithms can accurately correct spatial discrepancies between images from different modalities, aligning them within the same reference frame. This process not only improves the delineation of tumors and OARs but also integrates complementary information from different modalities to create a more complete image dataset to assist the development of more personalized treatment plans. For example, Balakrishnan et al. introduced the VoxelMorph framework [42], a fast learning-based method for deformable image registration, as shown in Figure 6.6a. Traditional image registration methods require iteratively optimizing an objective function for each pair of images, which can be time-consuming, especially for large datasets or complex deformation models. In contrast, VoxelMorph uses a CNN to map pairs of images and generate deformation fields in a "one-pass" fashion, making the registration process for new scans much faster. VoxelMorph offers two training strategies: unsupervised and semi-supervised. Even for the unsupervised setting, the model achieves accuracy comparable with state-of-the-art traditional methods while significantly speeding up computation. Following this, Chen et al. proposed the TransMorph model [43], which is based on a transformer architecture, as shown in Figure 6.6b. TransMorph addresses the limitations of CNNs in capturing long-range spatial relationships in images. Unlike convolutional networks, Transformers have a larger receptive field, allowing them to better understand spatial correspondences between moving and fixed images. TransMorph combines the strengths of both transformer and CNN architectures and includes variants such as diffeomorphic models for topology-preserving deformations and Bayesian models to estimate the registration uncertainty. However, VoxelMorph and TransMorph were not specifically optimized for multimodal registration, although they can be used for multimodal registration by using similarity loss functions robust to cross-modality intensity variations (normalized cross correlation, mutual information, etc.). Due to the substantial differences in image information between modalities (e.g., MRI and CT), deep learning registration algorithms alone may struggle to capture these differences effectively. As a result, many studies

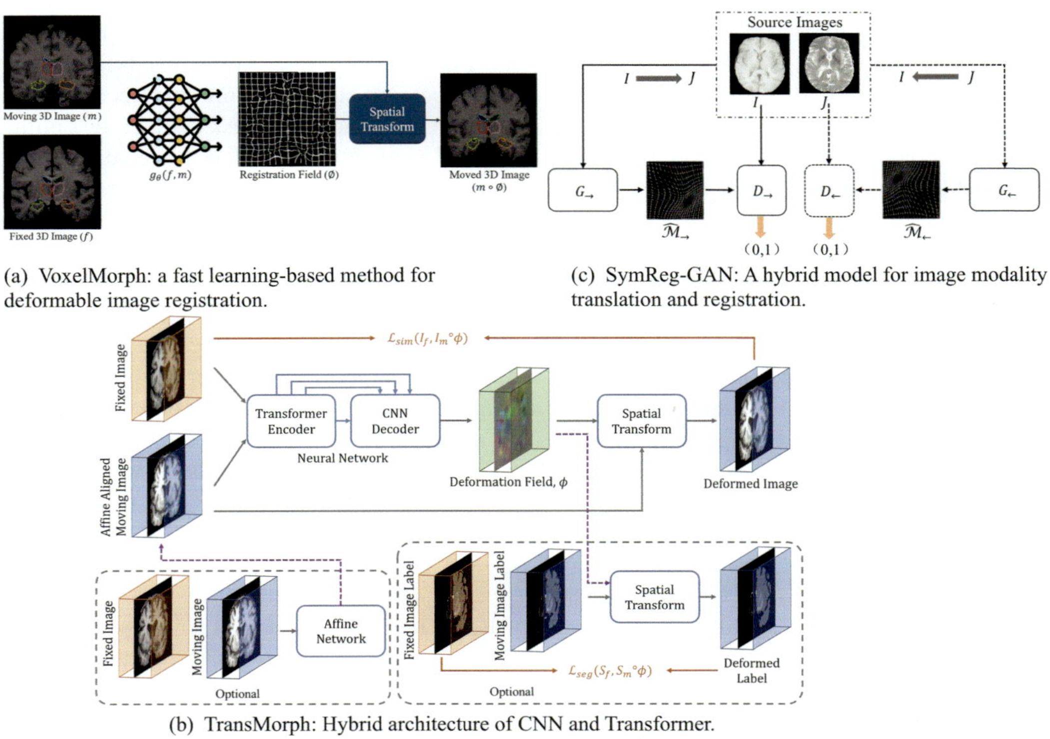

(a) VoxelMorph: a fast learning-based method for deformable image registration.

(c) SymReg-GAN: A hybrid model for image modality translation and registration.

(b) TransMorph: Hybrid architecture of CNN and Transformer.

FIGURE 6.6 The schematic diagrams of architectures for various image registration models. (a) VoxelMorph, (b) TransMorph (Reprint from Ref. [43]), and (c) SymReg-GAN (Reprint from Ref. [44]).

have combined modality translation/synthesis with registration to achieve better alignment across different modalities. Zheng et al. introduced SymReg-GAN (Figure 6.6c), a symmetric image registration method based on GANs [44]. SymReg-GAN incorporates bidirectional spatial transformations, encouraging registered images to return to their original state after an inverse transformation, thereby reducing biases introduced by traditional unidirectional registration. It also employs a conditional GAN framework to harmonize images from different modalities for multimodal registration. By adopting a semi-supervised strategy, the model can learn effectively from both labeled and unlabeled data.

As shown in Figure 6.6, from VoxelMorph's CNN-based structure to TransMorph's Transformer architecture and SymReg-GAN's symmetric GAN framework, these methods improve the efficiency and accuracy of unimodal or multimodal image registration through various mechanisms. AI-assisted multimodal image registration allows us to obtain more complete anatomical/functional information, offering more reliable support for tumor localization and radiation therapy planning.

6.2.5 Automatic Segmentation and Contouring

In recent years, with the advancement of deep learning technology, automatic segmentation and contouring have become increasingly prevalent and important in radiation therapy. Automatic segmentation significantly improves the efficiency of identifying tumor targets and OARs, and reduces the variability caused by subjective manual contouring. Numerous automatic segmentation models are available, each showing strengths and weaknesses depending on specific applications and datasets. To better understand the performance of these models in medical image segmentation, several key studies are introduced below. Ronneberger et al. introduced the famous U-Net architecture [45], one of the pioneering works in medical image segmentation. The network consists of a contracting path and a symmetric expanding path, allowing it to capture contextual information while performing precise localized segmentation. Building on U-Net, many variants have since been developed, with nnU-Net being one of the most notable [46]. nnU-Net is a self-configuring segmentation method that automatically adjusts pre-processing steps, network architecture selection, training strategy, and post-processing steps for different segmentation tasks, achieving optimal results without manual intervention. Beyond U-Net-based segmentation models, Ma et al. proposed MedSAM [47], a foundational model aimed at achieving universal medical image segmentation. Trained with a large dataset of paired medical images and masks that cover 10 imaging modalities and more than 30 cancer types, MedSAM has demonstrated robustness and high accuracy across a wide range of tasks. Another noteworthy contribution is TotalSegmentator [48], a model capable of automatically and robustly segmenting 104 anatomical structures in CT images, including 27 organs, 59 bones, 10 muscles, and 8 vessels. Tested on a large dataset of clinical data, the model achieved a Dice similarity coefficient of 0.943, significantly outperforming other publicly available segmentation models. These studies highlight the immense potential of automatic segmentation technology in radiation therapy. By efficiently and accurately identifying and segmenting tumor and normal tissue regions, these models are especially beneficial in time-sensitive scenarios like adaptive radiotherapy.

6.3 AI FOR RT DELIVERY

In addition to treatment simulation, the advent of IGRT marked a paradigm shift by integrating imaging technologies directly into the treatment delivery process. Traditionally, radiation therapy relied on surface markers on patients to guide daily radiation delivery. However, the complex anatomy and the dynamic nature of tumor positions often necessitated large safety margins, which, although facilitating tumor coverage, inadvertently increased radiation exposure to surrounding healthy tissues [49]. Real-time imaging within treatment sessions enables clinicians to account for anatomical changes, organ motion, and patient positioning variations. Intra-treatment imaging techniques such as CBCT, ultrasound, and MRI are now commonly employed to verify and adjust the treatment setup/plans, ensuring precise dose delivery to the tumor while minimizing damage to adjacent healthy tissues.

In recent years, AI has emerged as a transformative tool for imaging guidance during radiotherapy delivery [49]. For example, AI can improve the efficiency and accuracy of cross-domain image registration, making it possible to quickly register treatment planning images with limited imaging signals captured during beam delivery (for instance, a single X-ray projection), which enables real-time tumor tracking to guide and optimize motion management techniques. This development allows machines and clinicians to respond dynamically to changes in tumor position and patient anatomy, delivering radiation doses that are more accurate and tailored to individual patient needs. Machine learning models can also predict tumor motion based on historical and real-time data, allowing the system to function with minimum latency to maximize the treatment precision [50]. Additionally, deep learning models facilitate accurate dose verification during [51] and post-treatment [52], enabling delivery quality checks and adaptive dose adjustments when necessary.

6.3.1 AI for Imaging Guidance during RT Delivery

The integration of imaging systems, such as CBCT and MRI, into linear accelerators has been a pivotal advancement in IGRT, enabling on-board (patient on the treatment couch) and real-time visualization of patient anatomy and treatment delivery. These imaging guidance techniques allow for accurate on-board patient positioning and real-time inference throughout the radiotherapy session. CBCT, for example, provides 3D imaging that helps verify patient setup and adjust for anatomical changes, such as tumor shrinkage or organ motion, which may occur throughout the treatment course [53]. Recently, the integration of MRI into medical linear accelerator (LINAC) systems has introduced new possibilities for IGRT by offering superior soft-tissue contrast without additional ionizing radiation exposure [54]. This is particularly beneficial for tumors in areas where clear visualization of soft tissues is critical.

Compared with pre-treatment imaging during simulation, intra-treatment imaging usually has a much stricter demand on acquisition efficiency, due to the treatment time constraint, and the frequency and variability of patient motion (e.g., breathing and peristalsis). Traditional imaging methods often experience a trade-off between image quality and acquisition speed, which can hinder on-board imaging, real-time monitoring, and treatment adaptation strategies. The application of AI in on-board and real-time imaging has opened new avenues for improving the efficiency and quality of image acquisition processes in radiotherapy. Recent advances in AI-based reconstruction algorithms for limited-angle CBCT and motion-resolved 4D-CBCT/MRI enable faster imaging while preserving high image quality. AI-based methods are being developed for real-time tumor/anatomy monitoring and motion tracking using extremely limited on-board imaging samples, as well as for motion prediction to offset the latencies of imaging and treatment adaptation techniques.

6.3.1.1 Limited-Angle On-Board CBCT Reconstruction

Compared with sparse-view CBCT, limited-angle CBCT acquires projections from a limited scan angle (not necessarily sparse), which is usually a more challenging reconstruction problem due to the complete omission of a large angle span. Limited-angle acquisitions allow faster imaging (accounting for the gantry rotation speed limit of on-board CBCT systems) and are usually the only CBCT option in clinics due to mechanical blockage/constraints caused by ancillary systems or patient size. As radiotherapy treatments usually involve radiation beams delivered sparsely or continuously along an arc trajectory, limited-angle CBCTs can be acquired throughout the treatment delivery with continuous limited-angle gantry sweeping to monitor the patients' anatomy and reconstruct the delivered dose. However, reconstruction using traditional algorithms such as

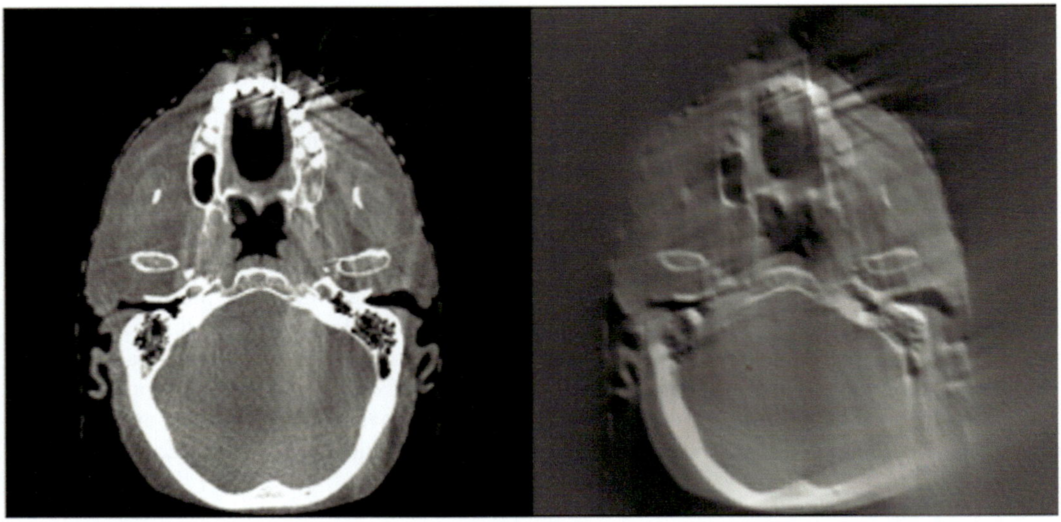

FIGURE 6.7 Illustrations of limited-angle CBCT reconstruction with the Feldkamp-Davis-Kress (FDK) algorithm. On the left is the full-angle image. On the right is the limited-angle reconstruction with a scan angle $[0°,120°]$.

filtered back-projection-based Feldkamp-Davis-Kress (FDK) algorithm [55] would yield severe limited-angle artifacts, as shown in Figure 6.7. MBIR methods have improved upon FDK by incorporating regularization techniques to enforce image priors, such as image smoothness or image gradient sparsity [56], but they remain computationally expensive and are less effective when projection data is highly limited. Deformation-driven (deformation vector field-based) methods address these challenges by leveraging prior information, such as pre-treatment CT or CBCT, and modeling the current anatomy as a deformation of the prior volume. For example, Ren et al. proposed a method that uses a deformation vector field (DVF) to morph a prior CT/CBCT into new 3D images representing new patient anatomy, based on limited-angle projections [57]. Nevertheless, such methods face challenges from dependency on accurate priors and high computational demands, limiting the robustness and efficiency of clinical applications. Their accuracy is also potentially degraded under large anatomical changes between prior/new imaging.

Recently, this field has seen a significant shift toward deep learning-based approaches, which leverage data-driven priors to better handle the missing information from limited-angle scanning. DL-based models are trained to infer missing data from the limited-angle acquisitions and imaging priors, resulting in reconstructed images that retain essential anatomical details. One notable example is the use of GANs for sinogram in-painting. Li et al. [58] proposed a GAN-based approach for limited-angle reconstruction using a patch-GAN architecture to in-paint missing sinogram data. The generator learns to map limited-angle sinograms to full-angle sinograms by minimizing an adversarial loss alongside a mean absolute error (MAE) loss for better data consistency. The in-painted full-angle sinogram is then used with traditional methods like filtered back-projection or simultaneous algebraic reconstruction technique with total variation regularization (SART-TV), significantly reducing artifacts and improving image quality even for narrow scan angles like 60°. Hu et al. [59] developed the Structure-Enhanced Attention Network (SEA-Net) for limited-angle CBCT reconstruction. SEA-Net employs a dual-network design comprising an Image Restoration Network (IR-Net) to reduce artifacts and a Structure Enhancement Network (SE-Net) to recover high-frequency details. The architecture incorporates residual dense attention blocks for advanced feature extraction and a spatial attention module to focus on artifact-prone regions, significantly improving

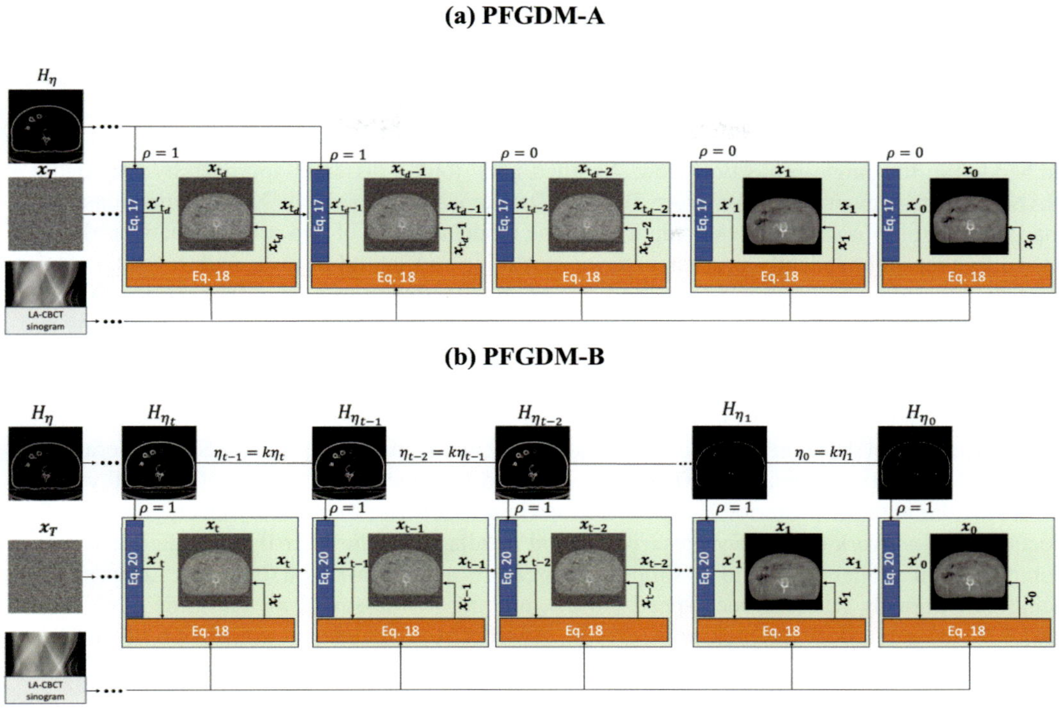

FIGURE 6.8 Workflow diagrams of PFGDM (Reprint from Ref. [61]).

reconstruction quality. Additionally, diffusion models are also employed in limited-angle image reconstruction. Liu et al. [60] introduced DOLCE, a diffusion probabilistic model designed specifically for limited-angle reconstruction. This model integrates a conditional diffusion process with data-consistency updates, iteratively refining the image reconstruction based on the limited-angle sinogram. The unique strength of DOLCE lies in its ability to quantify reconstruction uncertainty, a crucial feature in clinical settings where error estimation benefits informed decision-making. It outperformed state-of-the-art models like diffusion posterior sampling (DPS), achieving a higher peak signal-to-noise ratio (PSNR) and generating consistent results across diverse datasets, including both medical images and industrial CT scans. Building on diffusion-based methods, Xie et al. proposed a Prior Frequency-Guided Diffusion Model (PFGDM) specifically tailored for limited-angle CBCT (LA-CBCT) reconstruction. Their method utilizes a conditional diffusion model, where high-frequency anatomical details extracted from prior CT scans serve as a strong regularization prior, enhancing structural preservation during reconstruction. As shown in Figure 6.8, PFGDM was designed with two variants: PFGDM-A, which phases out the prior information after a preset iteration step to accommodate anatomical differences between the prior CT and to-be-reconstructed CBCT, and PFGDM-B, which continuously introduces the prior with an adaptive threshold to gradually reduce its influence. The approach outperformed existing LA-CBCT reconstruction techniques, demonstrating robust performance across various scan angles and anatomical sites, including scenarios with extremely limited scan angles [61].

A growing focus has now been formed on extremely limited-angle reconstruction, with several notable advancements in single-projection CBCT reconstruction methods. One of the pioneering works in this area is by Shen et al. [62], who introduced a deep learning model for single-projection CBCT reconstruction, using a hierarchical network architecture comprising three main components: a representation network, a transformation module, and a generation network. The representation network extracts 2D features from the input projection image, while the transformation module reshapes these 2D features into a 3D tensor, effectively learning the mapping between 2D projections and 3D anatomical structures. The generation network then uses these transformed features to predict the volumetric CBCT image. The training was performed with synthetic digitally reconstructed radiograph (DRR)–CBCT pairs generated from augmented 4D-CT datasets, allowing the model to integrate patient-specific prior information and decode hidden anatomical details embedded in the single-projection view. Another study took a different approach by employing a GAN-based framework to reconstruct 3D CBCT volumes from biplanar X-ray projections rather than relying solely on a single-view input [63]. The model consists of two parallel encoder–decoder networks that independently process anterior–posterior and lateral X-rays, with a feature fusion module integrating information from both views. It effectively uses skip connections to bridge 2D and 3D feature maps, addressing the dimensionality mismatch. Additionally, the training process involves a combination of mean squared error (MSE) loss and adversarial loss, along with a CycleGAN-based style transfer to align synthetic DRRs with real X-ray images, improving the quality of the reconstructed 3D CBCT images. In a recent advancement, Loÿen et al. used a lighter, CNN-based model designed for real-time radiotherapy applications [64]. Unlike Shen's hierarchical approach, this patient-specific network is streamlined to directly reconstruct 3D CBCT volumes from singular anterior-posterior X-ray projections in a voxel-wise manner. By leveraging skip connections, the network effectively preserves spatial details and reduces artifacts while maintaining computational efficiency. Due to its simpler architecture and optimization for speed, Loÿen's model achieves extremely fast inference speed (50 μs), making it well-suited for real-time clinical scenarios where rapid decision-making is crucial. Another study employed a diffusion-based model for single-projection CBCT reconstruction. X-CBCT-DDPM [65] employs a dual-model diffusion framework consisting of a Projection-DDPM and a CBCT-DDPM to reconstruct 3D CBCT volumes from a single X-ray projection. The Projection-DDPM first generates synthetic full-view X-ray projections, which are processed through a Geometric Transformation Module (GTM) using the FDK algorithm for initial volumetric reconstruction. This preliminary CBCT volume then serves as a guiding prior for the CBCT-DDPM, which iteratively denoises the volume using a 3D Attention V-net, progressively refining the image by transforming Gaussian noise into anatomically accurate details. A recently proposed deep learning-based framework [66] utilized two orthogonal kV X-ray projections to quickly reconstruct 3D volumetric images for image-guided proton FLASH radiotherapy. It comprises four modules: projection acquisition, deep learning-based image reconstruction (InverseNet3D), image quality assessment, and treatment evaluation using water equivalent thickness (WET) to detect anatomical changes. Tested on 30 lung cancer patients, it demonstrated robust image quality and real-time performance, demonstrating future potential for clinical usage. In response to the growing interest in multimodal imaging models, the Advanced Surface Imaging (A-SI) framework, a diffusion model-based approach, was developed for real-time volumetric image reconstruction from single-angle X-ray projections in surface-guided radiotherapy (SGRT) [67]. It combines high-frequency optical surface imaging (OSI) with low-frequency single-angle X-ray projections to generate Optical Surface-Derived CBCT (OSD-CBCT). By integrating surface imaging with sparse X-ray projections, the method reduces radiation exposure while maintaining high image quality and anatomical accuracy. By training a hierarchical neural network with patient-specific data, 3D CBCT images can be reconstructed from a single or few 2D X-ray projections with an average inference time of 0.5 seconds per CBCT [62].

Limited-angle CBCT reconstruction has made significant progress, evolving from traditional iterative methods to advanced deep learning approaches that leverage data-driven priors. These modern techniques, including GAN-based and diffusion-based models, have demonstrated promising results in handling incomplete projection data and reducing artifacts. Despite these advancements, challenges remain, particularly in maintaining reconstruction accuracy across diverse anatomical sites and under extremely limited scan angles. Future work may focus on integrating multimodal data and improving robustness to variations in patient anatomy, which could further enhance clinical utility and patient outcomes.

6.3.1.2 Motion-Resolved 4D-CBCT/MRI and Dynamic CBCT/MRI Reconstruction

Patient motion remains a significant challenge in radiotherapy. To address this, 4D-CBCT and 4D-MRI techniques have been developed to capture patient motion patterns to define the target better and improve on-board patient setup. Sonke et al. [68] pioneered the use of 4D-CBCT to enhance frameless stereotactic body radiotherapy (SBRT), developing respiratory-correlated imaging to significantly reduce geometric uncertainties and achieve high precision in lung target definition and treatment. Nielsen et al. [69] conducted a comprehensive analysis involving a large cohort of peripheral lung SBRT patients, utilizing 4D-CBCT to measure and track tumor motion across multiple treatment fractions. Their study revealed that while initial tumor motion estimates from planning 4D-CT scans were relatively accurate, significant variations occurred in subsequent fractions, emphasizing the need for frequent motion assessments using on-board 4D-CBCT. Despite advancements in 4D-CBCT for patient motion monitoring, the traditional 4D-CBCT techniques face significant limitations [70]. Under the assumption of periodic motion, 4D-CBCT uses retrospective phase sorting to bin cone-beam projections into semi-static phase bins. The phase-binned projections were subsequently reconstructed into corresponding 3D CBCT volumes, each representing a motion state along a nominal motion curve. The phase-binning process substantially reduces the number of projections available in each bin for CBCT reconstruction. Consequently, 4D-CBCT either suffers from under-sampling artifacts and limited image quality, or has to acquire more projections to ensure sufficient sampling in each phase bin, which leads to prolonged scan time and increased imaging dose. To improve the image quality of 4D-CBCT without incurring additional scan time/dose, recent 4D-CBCT reconstructions have turned to AI-driven methods. By integrating U-Net-based CNNs into a simultaneous motion estimation and image reconstruction (SMEIR) [71] framework, Huang et al. addressed the challenge of accurately estimating lung DVFs for motion-compensated 4D-CBCT reconstruction [72], where traditional intensity-driven 2D-3D deformation techniques fall short due to insufficient intensity variations. The 2D-3D lung DVFs were initially estimated using an SMEIR algorithm and then fine-tuned by a U-Net-based CNN, which leveraged prior motion information and anatomical features to enhance DVF accuracy. Such a method allowed precise motion estimation and enabled the reconstruction of high-quality 4D-CBCT images using only 80 projections per phase. In another study, Zhang et al. utilized a CNN to reduce streaking artifacts in initial phase-correlated Feldkamp-Davis-Kress (PCF) reconstructions for 4D-CBCT, enabling the generation of high-quality motion models directly from on-board 4D-CBCT images [73]. By integrating these CNN-enhanced images into motion-compensated reconstruction, the framework effectively resolves inter-phase respiratory motion while maintaining phase-specific details. Building on this foundation, their subsequent work further evolved by integrating deep learning-based groupwise registration into the motion-compensated reconstruction framework, achieving near real-time phase-resolved 4D-CBCT reconstruction [74]. Figure 6.9

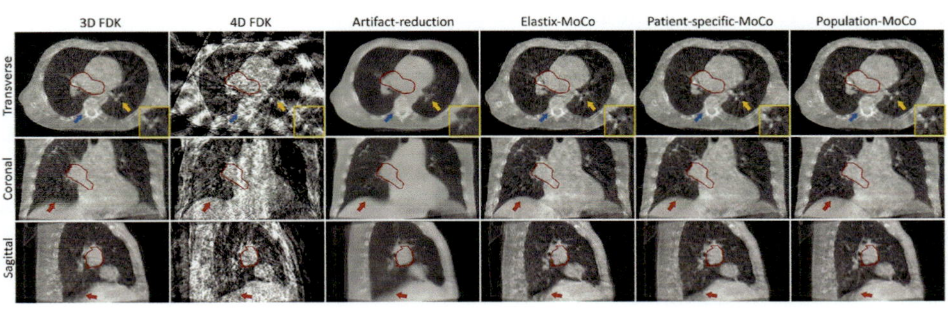

FIGURE 6.9 Example reconstruction results for a real patient scan using different reconstruction methods, including those with deep learning-based groupwise registration (Patient-specific-MoCo and Population-MoCo) [74]. Tumor regions are indicated by red contours. The display range is [−0.002, 0.028] mm^{-1} (Reprint from Ref. [74]).

shows the reconstruction results of one 4D-CBCT phase by different methods for a real patient scan with motion.

In addition to the under-sampling and image artifact challenge, the periodic motion assumption inherent in motion phase sorting of 4D-CBCT restricts its ability to accurately capture irregularities such as baseline shifts, drifts, and variations in breathing amplitude or frequency. The temporal resolution of 4D-CBCT is also constrained by the number of respiratory bins, leading to intra-bin motion artifacts. To address such challenges, AI-based techniques that can reconstruct dynamic CBCT volumes (a CBCT for each X-ray projection) and build comprehensive motion models to describe motion without phase-binning were developed. AI-based dynamic CBCT reconstruction not only overcomes the challenges of temporal resolution limits but enables the capture of complex and irregular motion patterns, paving the way for more precise and efficient motion management in radiation therapy. Zhang et al. proposed the STINR framework [75] that uses implicit neural representations (INRs) to decouple the dynamic CBCT reconstruction into solving separate spatial and temporal components, where multilayer perceptrons (MLPs) are employed to model the static reference volume and time-varying motion DVFs independently. By deforming the optimized static reference volume with time-varying DVFs, the dynamic CBCT sets can be solved. By integrating prior knowledge through PCA-based motion models, STINR reduces the complexity of reconstructing dynamic CBCTs from limited projection data and optimizes the reconstruction directly from patient-specific projections without pre-training, making it robust to irregular or non-periodic motions. To alleviate the dependency on well-defined prior motion models, PMF-STINR was subsequently proposed [76], which employs a one-shot learning approach that does not rely on prior anatomical or motion models for dynamic CBCT reconstruction. Similar to STINR, PMF-STINR decouples the dynamic CBCTs into spatial and temporal components using INRs. Additionally, a data-driven B-spline-based motion model learns motion basis components (MBCs) directly from cone-beam projections, bypassing the need for prior motion modeling. PMF-STINR has been validated on digital and physical phantom studies, as well as real patient datasets, demonstrating robust performance in accurately reconstructing dynamic CBCTs and capturing complex motion patterns without requiring pre-acquired motion/anatomical models.

Similar to 4D-CBCT, 4D-MRI enables dynamic visualization of anatomical and motion information with superior soft-tissue visibility [77,78], which is especially beneficial for motion-impacted abdominal sites with limited X-ray contrast. However, significant challenges remain for 4D-MRI, including elongated acquisition and reconstruction time, under-sampling artifacts after motion binning, and low spatial resolution. With the recent advancements in deep learning, multiple AI-driven 4D-MRI studies have been proposed to account for those challenges. Dracula [79], a 3D U-Net dCNN [45,80] model, significantly accelerated the reconstruction of heavily under-sampled 4D MRI data by reducing processing time from 9 to 12 hours (MoCo-HDTV) or 10 minutes (GRASP) to just 28 seconds. The model was trained and evaluated on data from 67 subjects, achieving high structural similarity (SSIM=0.97) with minor artifacts. Despite slight blurring, the images were clinically acceptable for delineating tumors and OARs, enabling real-time clinical applications. Murray et al. proposed Movienet [81] for 4D-MRI reconstruction, which employs a modified U-Net architecture to operate directly in the image domain, bypassing the computationally expensive k-space data-consistency checks typical of iterative CS approaches like GRASP. It exploits space–time–coil correlations while enforcing motion preservation, which is achieved by sorting respiratory motion states linearly from expiration to inspiration during training. This strategy eliminates the need for explicit motion constraints, reducing reconstruction times to less than 1 second. To address the spatial-resolution limitations of 4D-MRI, Park et al. proposed an Autoencoder-Inspired Convolutional Network Super-Resolution (ACNS) [82] method that utilizes nonlinear mapping to recover missing spatial information by learning the relationship between low-resolution (LR) and high-resolution (HR) MRI features, achieving real-time resolution enhancement of 4D imaging in MRI-guided radiation therapy.

However, similar to 4D-CBCT, 4D-MRI's reliance on retrospective sorting into "motion bins" [83] assumes regular and reproducible motion, often not aligning with clinical reality [84]. Irregular motion patterns can lead to degraded image quality, such as blurriness and ghosting, and the averaged motion curves fail to capture clinically significant irregularities. This limitation poses challenges in determining appropriate radiotherapy margins and accurately accumulating delivered radiation doses. Therefore, reconstructing dynamic MRI is highly desirable in clinics. Biswas et al. introduced a deep learning-based solution for dynamic MRI reconstruction, MoDL-SToRM [85], that combines deep-learned CNN priors with SToRM regularization, which leverages nonlocal redundancies in the data to capture respiratory and cardiac motion patterns. By formulating reconstruction as an optimization problem and unrolling it into a deep network, MoDL-SToRM achieves high-quality reconstructions with a fivefold reduction in scan time compared to conventional SToRM. This model-based approach applies patient-specific information, resulting in reconstructions that effectively minimize noise and artifacts even under high under-sampling ratios. In comparison, an unsupervised deep-learning-based method, time-dependent deep image prior (TD-DIP), uses a generative CNN with a mapping network and a time-varying latent manifold to capture temporal dependencies without requiring pre-trained data or patient-specific priors [86]. Evaluated on cardiac cine and fetal MRI, it demonstrated superior motion fidelity and higher SSIM scores than baseline methods, such as GRASP, without needing heartbeat markers or gating. While MoDL-SToRM's strength lies in integrating patient-specific motion information through SToRM priors, TD-DIP's unsupervised approach bypasses the need for explicit prior information, instead relying on the temporal consistency within the acquired data. Currently, most of the dynamic MRI studies are limited to 2D cine imaging. A recent work, STINR-MR [83], employs spatial and temporal INRs to reconstruct 3D cine-MRI from highly under-sampled k-space data (Figure 6.10). Similar to STINR for dynamic CBCT reconstruction, it uses a joint approach that combines image reconstruction and intra-scan deformable registration, where the spatial INR models the reference 3D MR image, and the temporal INR captures intra-scan dynamic motion through DVFs. A PCA-based motion model is incorporated to regularize the solution, enabling efficient and accurate reconstruction of high-resolution 3D cine-MRI with a temporal resolution of less than 100 ms. Compared with STINR, the PCA motion model in STINR-MR can either be derived from prior 4D-MRI scans or directly from the dynamic MR scan. With the help of AI, the motion-resolved 4D-CBCT/MRI and dynamic CBCT/MRI are seeing improved image quality and more accurate motion models, allowing precise characterization of patient-specific motion patterns to guide more accurate radiotherapy planning, on-board adaptation, and treatment delivery.

6.3.1.3 Real-Time X-Ray-Based Imaging for Treatment Monitoring

Techniques like 4D-CBCT and dynamic CBCT serve as valuable tools to capture patient-specific motion patterns and require a scan time of 1 minute or longer. However, the relatively long scan time prohibits 4D-CBCT and dynamic CBCT from real-time, instantaneous motion tracking and monitoring. Traditionally, 2D planar imaging using X-rays has been the primary method for capturing real-time intra-treatment anatomy to guide radiotherapy interventions, largely due to its rapid imaging speed and well-established clinical workflows. However, a major drawback of X-ray imaging is its limited soft-tissue contrast, which makes it difficult to accurately localize tumors and monitor motion, especially for sites including the liver and pancreas. To address this issue, advanced X-ray-guided radiotherapy systems like CyberKnife, Radixact, and VERO use implanted radio-opaque fiducial markers as reference points to track target motion [89]. CyberKnife, for instance, employs the Synchrony™ Respiratory Tracking System, using implanted gold fiducials that are tracked with orthogonal X-rays to build a correlation model between the movement of internal markers and external surface surrogates on the patient. This allows for real-time beam adjustments to account for surrogate-indicated target motion. Similarly, Radixact updates a motion correlation model periodically using X-ray imaging, enabling dynamic multi-leaf collimator (MLC) adjustments to maintain alignment with the moving target. However, these markers offer only point-based

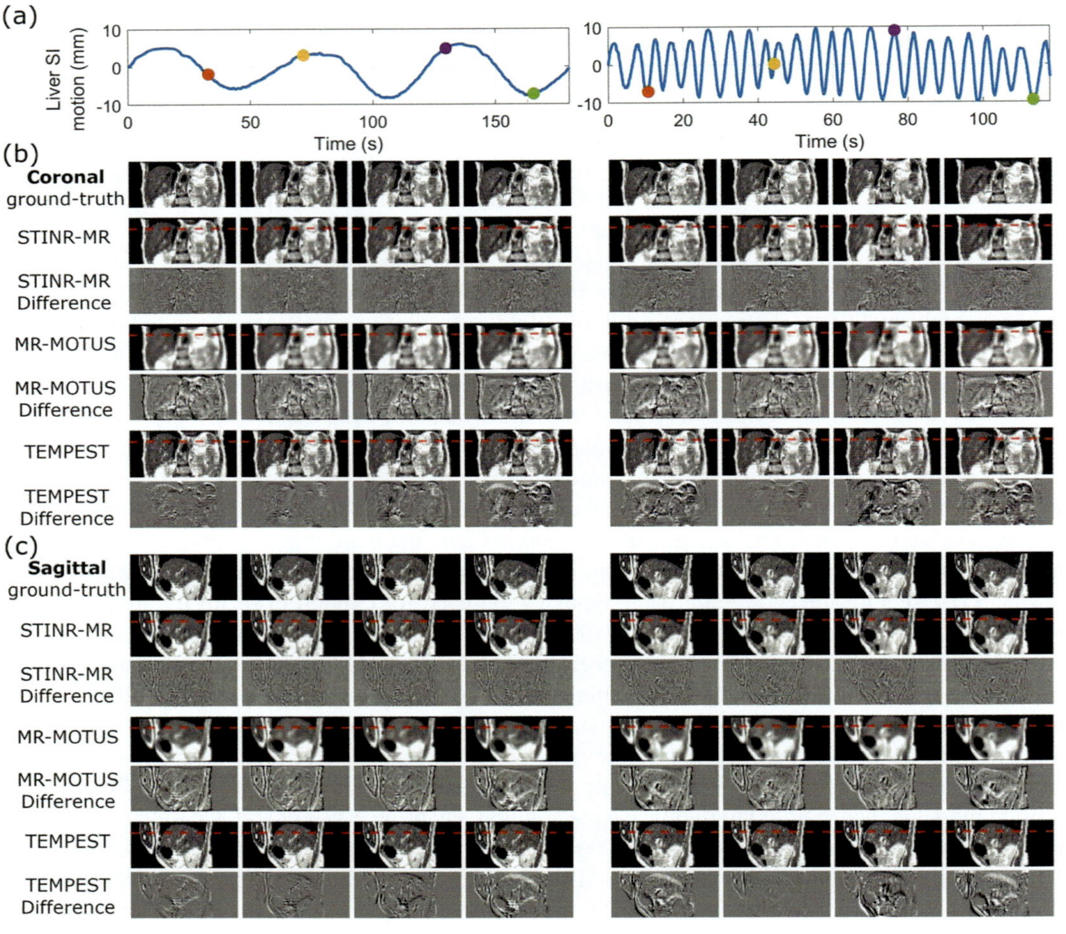

FIGURE 6.10 Comparison of reconstructed dynamic cine-MR images using STINR-MR [83] (offline PCA), MR-MOTUS [87], and TEMPEST [88] methods, alongside the "ground-truth" images, in the (b) coronal and (c) sagittal views for both slow (left column) and irregular (right column) breathing scenarios from the patient simulation study. MR-MOTUS and TEMPEST are two available methods for comparison. Corresponding difference images are also provided for each method. The top panels (a) display the liver motion trajectories in the SI direction as solved by STINR-MR, with the selected motion states marked by dots for visual comparison (Reprint from Ref. [83]).

localization and may shift over time, potentially compromising their reliability. In recent years, AI-based techniques have emerged as a promising alternative, offering non-invasive solutions for normal tissue and tumor tracking from X-ray images without the need for fiducial markers. Even in cases where the anatomy is difficult for the human eyes to discern, these techniques have demonstrated the ability to accurately identify and track tumors [42]. Broadly, there are two types of X-ray-based, real-time imaging approaches: those that directly localize the tumor/target on X-ray projections and those that infer 3D motion/images from these projections for volumetric anatomy tracking.

The first approach focuses on directly identifying the tumor or target from X-ray projection data. Zhao et al. trained a deep learning model on over 800 annotated kV X-ray projection images to directly localize the prostate targets [90]. The model accurately identifies the prostate target location from anterior-posterior (AP) and lateral images, achieving deviations of 0.7–2.21 mm in the AP direction and 1.23–2.20 mm laterally compared to human annotations. The method also performs consistently with fiducial marker-based and CBCT-based localizations and shows potential for real-time tracking within 200 ms per image. Building on this foundation, Zhao et al. further developed a patient-specific approach for pancreatic tumor localization using synthetic training data derived from planning CT (pCT) images [91]. This evolution involved the generation of DRRs incorporating deformation, rotation, and translation to simulate inter- and intra-fractional anatomical variations for model training. The updated method achieved comparable accuracy to fiducial-based approaches, with mean absolute differences under 2.6 mm and concordance correlation coefficients above 93%, while maintaining a real-time processing speed of 100–200 ms. These advancements demonstrate the progress of deep learning methods in personalized, markerless tumor localization solutions that are non-invasive, cost-effective, and clinically feasible for IGRT applications. Another notable study introduced a convolutional recurrent neural network (CRNN) to localize lung tumors in real time from continuously acquired X-ray projections [92]. The CRNN combines convolutional neural networks to extract spatial features from X-ray projections with recurrent neural networks (RNNs) to model temporal motion patterns. A delta image approach was used to highlight tumor motion between consecutive projections, while frequent recalibrations based on rigid registrations with planning 4D-CT templates ensured robustness. The CRNN achieved a 3D localization error of 1.3 ± 1.4 mm with a low latency of 20 ms. Fu et al. first introduced the concept of target decomposition to enhance target contrast in kV projection images, presenting a significant advancement over traditional approaches [93]. The proposed target decomposition method distinguishes tissues based on their spatial locations relative to the tumor, rather than relying on differences in attenuation coefficients as in dual-energy imaging. They implemented this concept using a patient-specific conditional GAN model, trained on paired DRRs and decomposed target images (DTIs) generated from lung 4DCT volumes. The method then produces synthetic DTIs (sDTIs) from real-time kV projection images acquired during treatment to significantly enhance tumor contrast. Tumor tracking was performed via template matching using sDTIs and pre-generated tumor templates. Validated on nine patients with implanted Calypso beacons, the method achieved an average absolute mean error of 0.8 ± 0.7 mm in the superior-inferior (SI) direction and 0.9 ± 0.8 mm in the in-plane left-right direction, demonstrating sub-voxel accuracy and robust tracking performance. These results highlight the method's clinical potential, particularly its suitability for real-time markerless tumor tracking with a total latency of approximately 70 ms. However, while the above-mentioned approaches offer rapid and accurate tumor localization, they are usually limited to estimating motion in 2D planes and do not provide volumetric information about anatomical changes/deformation during treatment.

The key idea of the second approach is to generate 3D images from singular 2D X-ray projections for subsequent 3D tumor localization or extrapolate 3D deformable motion from singular 2D X-ray projections for DVF-driven tumor localization. For the former reconstruction-driven approaches, as mentioned in Section 2.1.1, limited-angle CBCT reconstruction has evolved toward extreme scenarios using one or two X-ray projections for instantaneous volumetric imaging. Based on the real-time volumetric image, tumors can be further localized through segmentation. Leveraging multitask learning (MTL), the RT-SRTS method achieves real-time (70 ms), simultaneous CBCT reconstruction and tumor segmentation from a single X-ray projection with CNN trained on patient-specific data [94]. While mapping 2D X-ray projections to 3D volumes has shown promising advancements, such as improved accuracy and real-time performance, these methods can face challenges related to the lack of reconstruction robustness and missed anatomical details. Additionally, these approaches often require post-processing steps, such as segmentation, and do not directly yield DVFs for capturing detailed motion dynamics. To address these limitations, DVF-driven methods have emerged as an alternative approach for resolving 3D motion directly from singular X-ray projections. Instead of directly mapping 2D images to 3D volumes, Voxelmap [95] introduces a patient-specific deep learning framework that maps 2D images to 3D DVFs, enabling 3D motion estimation and volumetric imaging during lung cancer radiotherapy. Leveraging the nonlinear mathematics of manifolds, the model learns patient-specific respiratory motion patterns from standard clinical 4D-CT and 2D X-ray imaging workflows. The architecture combines an encoding arm to extract latent features from 2D image pairs, a decoding arm to reconstruct 3D DVFs, and optional integration layers to encourage diffeomorphic transformations. Tested on data from two lung cancer patients, Voxelmap achieved submillimeter accuracy in estimating thoracoabdominal motion (e.g., 0.1 ± 0.5 mm along the left-right axis) and volumetric imaging with high fidelity. The model demonstrated real-time performance with an inference time of 50 ms, enabling seamless integration into clinical workflows. Similarly, Foote et al. proposed a real-time 2D-3D deformable registration framework leveraging deep learning for lung radiotherapy targeting [96]. The method begins by creating a patient-specific low-rank motion subspace from respiratory-correlated CT (4D-RCCT) data, capturing principal components of lung deformations during breathing. DRRs are generated using these deformations to simulate 2D fluoroscopic images, which are then used to train a DenseNet model. The trained neural network approximates the inverse mapping of the complex deformation-projection relationship, predicting the deformation state of the anatomy from live 2D X-ray images. The framework achieves real-time performance with inference throughput exceeding 1,000 images per second and demonstrates a maximum deformation error below 2 mm, significantly reducing registration error compared to optimization-based approaches. Wei et al. [97] proposed a CNN-based method to achieve real-time three-dimensional tumor localization from single X-ray projections. In their framework, a CNN regression model was trained to map singular X-ray projections to motion parameters derived from a PCA-based motion model. The method incorporated intensity correction to minimize discrepancies between DRRs and real X-ray projections, along with a data augmentation technique that added realistic noise patterns to improve model robustness. During treatment, the CNN model estimated tumor position within submillimeter precision while avoiding the computational overhead of traditional iterative approaches. After that, Zhang et al. introduced 2D3D-RegNet [98], an unsupervised, end-to-end deep learning framework for 2D-3D deformable image registration, targeting real-time DVF-driven CBCT estimation. The method employs a U-Net-based architecture with differentiable forward-projection layers for 2D-3D mapping and DVF inversion modules for inverse-consistent registration. It aligns prior high-quality CT/CBCT images with limited X-ray projections to estimate new on-board CBCTs. In experiments, 2D3D-RegNet demonstrated substantial improvements in accuracy and efficiency over traditional iterative 2D-3D registration methods, solving DVFs within seconds as opposed to hours. Another deep learning-based volumetric tumor tracking method uses a Swin Transformer network to align 2D cone-beam X-ray projections with 3D planning CT images through hybrid data augmentation, style correction using a GAN for realistic image adaptation, and efficient encoding–decoding processes, enabling fast and accurate DVF-driven tumor localization with 1.5 mm RMSE in under 51 ms [99]. Figure 6.11 shows the tumor registration visualization of their work. However, most of the DVF-driven methods for single X-ray real-time volumetric target tracking are focused on the anatomical site of the lung, which has favorable X-ray contrast for relatively easier deformable registration and mapping. For low X-ray contrast sites like the liver, respiration-induced motion is as significant and similarly requires real-time tumor motion tracking and monitoring. Figure 6.12 shows a series of works that are proposed to volumetrically localize moving liver tumors with a single X-ray projection. The MeshRegNet-Bio method [100] combines a graph neural network (GNN) with biomechanical modeling to achieve real-time liver tumor localization from a single on-board X-ray projection, as shown in Figure 6.12a. It predicts liver surface deformation from a single X-ray projection using a patient-specific GNN, which is followed by biomechanical modeling to solve intra-liver motion for volumetric tumor tracking. The biomechanical modeling step helps to infer physically and physiologically plausible volumetric liver motion from hyper-elastic liver tissue models, without relying on the limited X-ray imaging intensity contrast to solve DVFs. To further improve the accuracy of real-time liver and liver tumor motion tracking, shown in Figure 6.12b, the Surf-X-Bio framework [101] was proposed for real-time 3D liver tumor localization by combining OSI and a single X-ray projection as input to offer complementary information. In addition, it also

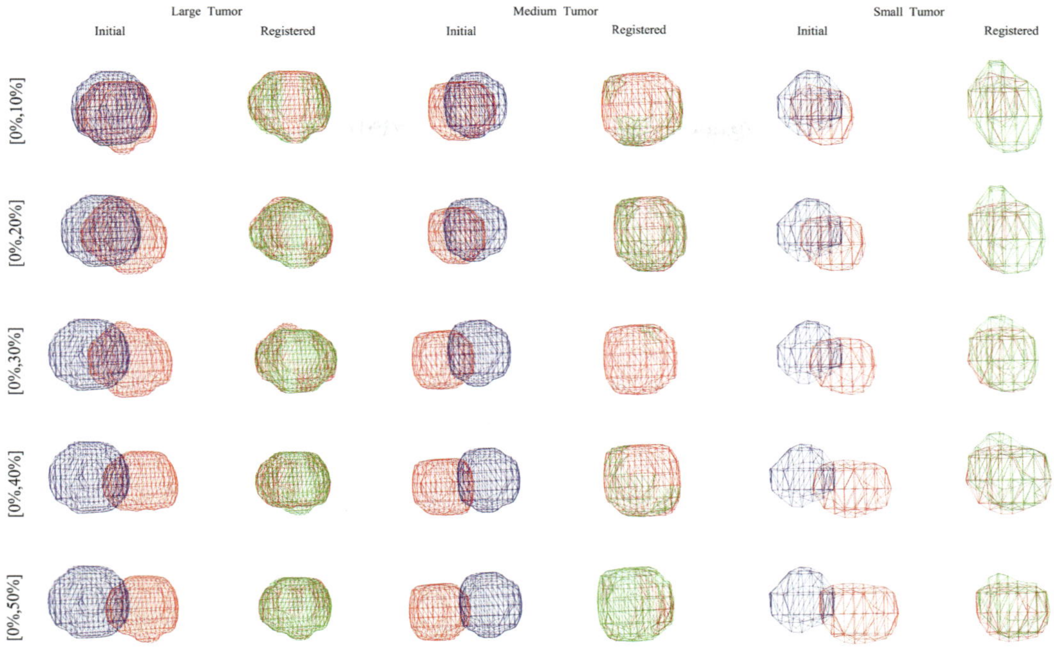

FIGURE 6.11 Tumor registration/localization results of a deep learning-driven, single X-ray projection-based volumetric tumor tracking method using a Swin Transformer network [99]. From left to right, the alignment results for three tumor types—large, medium, and small—are shown. The first, third, and fifth columns depict unaligned images, while the second, fourth, and sixth columns show aligned images. In each image, the red tumor represents the "ground truth," the blue tumor corresponds to the prior planning CT (moving tumor), and the green tumor illustrates the moved tumor after model inference (Reprint from Ref. [99]).

develops a deep learning-driven biomechanical model to substantially accelerate the biomechanical modeling process from minutes to less than 1 second. This framework demonstrates robustness in cases with large motion and when parts of the liver boundary are not captured by the limited field of view of the X-ray. Both MeshRegNet-Bio and Surf-X-Bio, however, used angle-specific projections to train angle-specific models. Thus, different models are needed for different projection angles. To overcome this issue, the X360 method [102] was further proposed to estimate volumetric liver motion in real-time from a single, arbitrarily angled X-ray projection, as shown in Figure 6.12c. It combines deep learning-based feature extraction with sequential rigid and deformable registration modules. The model utilizes a geometry-aware feature pooling layer to incorporate angle-specific projection information, enabling angle-agnostic inference of liver boundary motion. This geometry-aware pooling mechanism bridges the pixel-based X-ray feature maps and graph-based liver surface nodes by projecting 3D nodes onto 2D feature maps with physics-driven, angle-aware projecting layers, to extract the most relevant features for the subsequent registration models. By leveraging a combination of population-based and patient-specific deep learning models, these techniques enable accurate volumetric liver and liver tumor motion tracking based on a single X-ray projection (or with additional surface imaging), offering great potential for X-ray-based motion monitoring and treatment adaptation/intervention for traditionally challenging, low-contrast sites like the liver. Figure 6.13 shows the visualization of real-time liver tumor localization results of MeshRegNet-Bio.

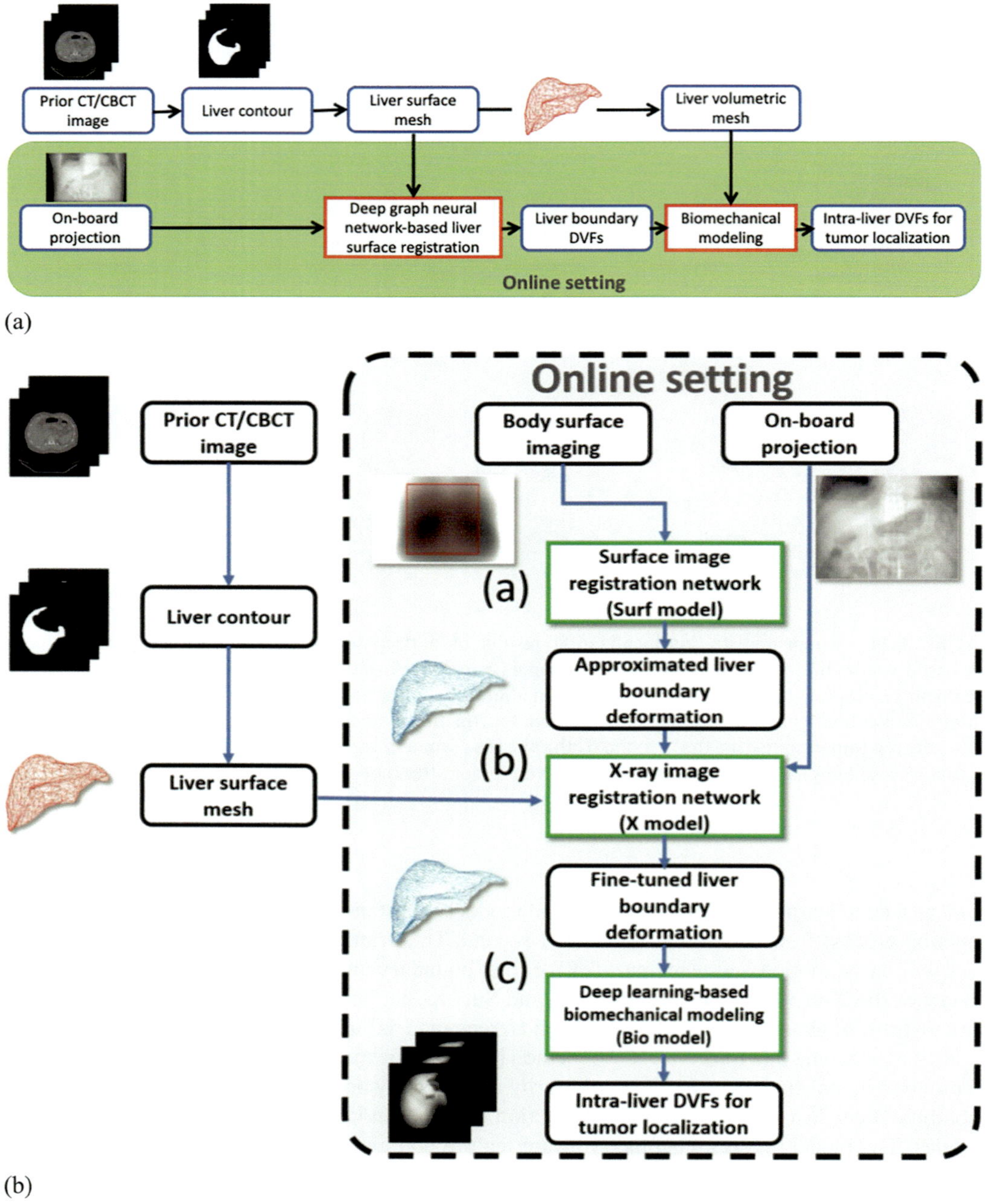

FIGURE 6.12 A series of single X-ray projection-based liver and liver tumor deformable motion estimation methods.

(*Continued*)

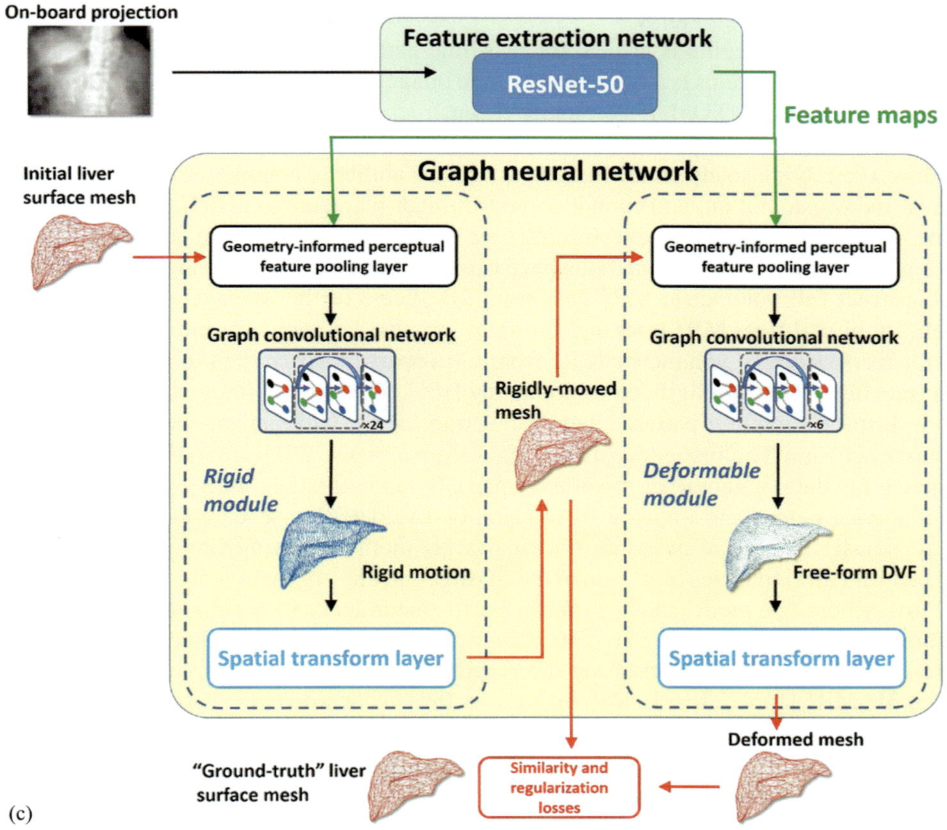

FIGURE 6.12 ***(Continued)*** A series of single X-ray projection-based liver and liver tumor deformable motion estimation methods.

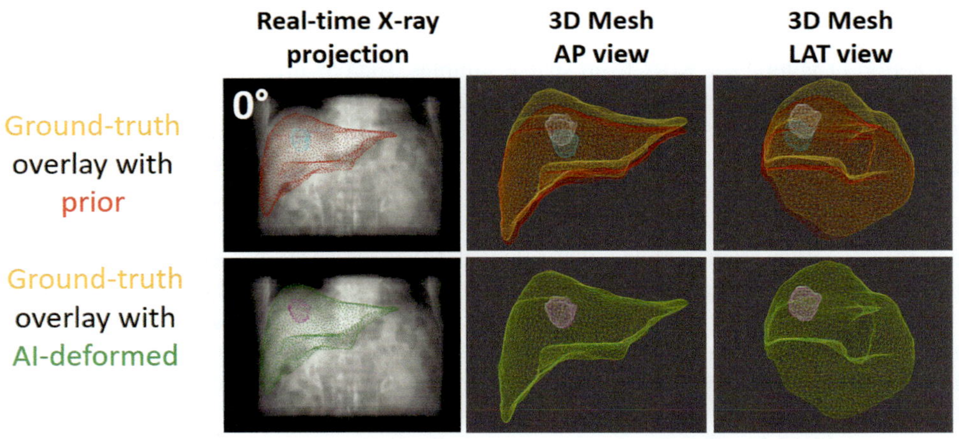

FIGURE 6.13 Visualization of deep learning-based real-time liver imaging via MeshRegNet-Bio, by capturing the instantaneous motion of the liver as 3D deformable meshes from a single X-ray projection. The columns show the prior non-motion-resolved (upper) and deformed (lower) liver volumetric meshes projected onto the single X-ray projection at 0° (column 1), or onto the "ground-truth" meshes from two different views (column 2: anterior-posterior view; column 3: lateral view). The prior non-motion-resolved meshes were shown in red (liver) and cyan (tumor), the deformed ones in green (liver) and magenta (tumor), and the ground-truth ones in yellow (liver) and white (tumor).

6.3.1.4 Real-Time MR Imaging for Treatment Monitoring

In MRgRT, fast MR imaging is critical for real-time patient monitoring. Similar to X-ray-based imaging, MR-guided systems typically acquire cine images limited to 2D planes. Waddington et al. used motion-encoded AUTOMAP to rapidly reconstruct 2D radial MRI data, offering real-time performance suitable for adaptive radiotherapy, where speed is crucial for managing tumor motion [103]. However, relying solely on 2D imaging limits the ability to comprehensively track complex, 3D tumor and organ motion, and cannot correct through-plane motion [104], which is critical for ensuring accurate dose delivery and minimizing radiation exposure to surrounding healthy tissues. To address this, AI-driven methods have been developed to estimate 3D deformable motion and reconstruct full volumetric MRI data from 2D slices, further enhancing the precision and applicability of real-time MRI tracking. Liu et al. proposed a geometry-informed deep learning model for reconstructing volumetric MRI from ultra-sparse k-space data to enable real-time 3D motion tracking during MRI-guided radiotherapy [105]. The method integrates geometric priors, including k-space sampling patterns and spatial transforms, with patient-specific priors learned by a neural network. The model consists of three components: a 2D generation network to complete sparse 2D data, a geometry module to map 2D representations into volumetric space, and a 3D refinement network to improve image quality. Evaluated on seven abdominal patients, the model demonstrated high accuracy in tracking target motion, with median gross tumor volume (GTV) centroid discrepancies of <1 mm in the SI direction and approximately 1 mm in other directions. Furthermore, the model showed robustness to anatomical and positional changes over time. Instead of directly reconstructing 3D-MR images, Wei et al. used an unsupervised multi-branch CNN to estimate the DVF representing the respiratory motion from coronal cine-MRI and the reference 3D-MRI [106]. The 3D-MR image was then reconstructed by applying the estimated DVF to deform the reference 3D-MRI. The method was validated on data from eight liver cancer patients, achieving high Dice similarity coefficients (DSCs >96.1%) for liver contour estimation and minimal blood vessel localization errors (<2.6 mm) across imaging planes. Reconstruction was completed within 100 ms, meeting real-time requirements for tumor tracking radiotherapy. Liu et al. proposed a prior-augmented implicit neural representation (NeRP) learning framework [107] that utilizes two 3D MRI scans (at in-hale and ex-hale states) as priors to enable real-time 3D MRI estimation for motion monitoring. NeRP models the relationship between voxel coordinates and intensities using a neural network, enabling efficient interpolation and extrapolation of motion states. This method augments sparse priors to create a range of motion phases, which regularize the reconstruction of volumetric MRI from sparse samples, such as orthogonal 2D cine-MRI slices. Evaluated on seven hepatocellular carcinoma patients, the method achieved high reconstruction fidelity (PSNR: 38.02 dB, SSIM: 0.98) and sub-voxel accuracy in 3D motion tracking, as demonstrated by GTV motion analysis. In addition to 2D-to-3D MRI mapping, researchers have also explored 3D-to-3D data mapping to convert highly under-sampled 3D MRIs to high-quality MRIs for IGRT. Terpstra et al. introduced TEMPEST [88], a deep learning framework for real-time 3D motion estimation from highly under-sampled MRI, which allows subsequent DVF-driven 3D-to-3D mapping. Their approach uses a multi-resolution CNN trained on respiratory-resolved 4D MRI, where "ground-truth" DVFs are derived from an optical flow algorithm applied to CS reconstructions. Once trained, TEMPEST infers 3D DVFs for 3D-to-3D mapping in under 200 ms, meeting the stringent sub-500 ms latency requirement for MRI-guided radiotherapy. They validated TEMPEST on digital (XCAT) and physical (QUASAR) phantoms, CT data, and volunteer MR scans on an MR-LINAC, consistently showing <2 mm mean motion errors at typical acceleration factors, with resilience to artifacts and cross-modality generalizability. Shao et al. proposed KS-RegNet, an unsupervised k-space-driven network for real-time MRI motion estimation [108]. It utilizes a U-Net architecture combined with k-space data fidelity loss, leveraging a fully sampled prior image and highly under-sampled real-time k-space data to predict DVFs. Evaluated on cardiac cine and abdominal 4D-MRI datasets, KS-RegNet outperformed traditional methods like

Elastix, achieving higher DICE scores (up to 0.894) and lower center-of-mass errors (1.01 mm), while maintaining a low latency (600 ms). Its robust performance with severe under-sampling facilitates accurate, real-time 3D motion tracking, enhancing MR-guided radiotherapy by enabling dynamic tumor localization and adaptive treatment plans.

Looking forward, the development of fast and robust volumetric MR imaging and motion-tracking techniques is essential for intra-treatment motion monitoring and real-time plan adaptation for MRgRT. A more advanced k-space acquisition strategy, preferably in 3D, will enable more efficient volumetric data sampling to derive accurate motion representations and promote advanced delivery strategies like beam gating and MLC tracking. In addition to respiratory motion, slower motion like peristalsis or faster motion like cardiac beating may also be potentially addressed with MRgRT thanks to its superior soft-tissue contrast and the development of AI-driven imaging and motion-tracking strategies.

6.3.1.5 AI for Motion Prediction

Rapid and real-time motion prediction is essential to prevent additional latency in adaptive radiotherapy, making AI, with its short inference time, an ideal solution. An early study by Teo et al. [109] employed an MLP model for real-time tumor motion prediction. The approach utilized a sliding temporal window to extract input features from patient respiratory data. The model was optimized with historical offline patient tumor motion trajectories. Following this, long short-term memory (LSTM) networks, which are designed to capture long-term dependencies in sequential data, have proven effective for predicting respiratory motion based on historical patterns [110]. Wang et al. [111] proposed a novel approach utilizing a deep bidirectional long short-term memory (Bi-LSTM) network for respiratory motion prediction in real-time tumor tracking. The study leveraged a seven-layer Bi-LSTM model trained on respiratory motion data from over 100 lung cancer patients. The Bi-LSTM architecture effectively captured long-term dependencies in the data, and it was particularly effective in scenarios with longer latency (e.g., 400 ms), achieving superior accuracy compared to traditional models like ARIMA [112] and ADMLP-NN [113]. Following this study, Lin et al. [114] explored a different LSTM-based approach, focusing on optimizing hyperparameters to further enhance prediction accuracy. Their model demonstrated superior accuracy in predicting respiratory motion, outperforming conventional artificial neural network (ANN) models [115]. Importantly, this study demonstrated the critical role of hyperparameter tuning in LSTM models, which influenced subsequent research to adopt similar rigorous optimization strategies for enhanced predictive performance.

The performance of LSTMs is further enhanced when applied to MRI data, as MRI offers superior soft-tissue contrast compared to X-rays, enabling more precise tumor localization, especially in challenging cases involving irregular breathing. This improved accuracy in visualizing the tumor and surrounding tissues provides high-quality input data for LSTMs, leading to more reliable motion predictions. In a study by Lombardo et al. [116], the authors implemented both offline and online LSTM models for predicting tumor centroid positions using 4 Hz cine-MRI data from MR-LINAC treatments. The offline LSTM was trained on a dataset comprising over 13 hours of motion data, while the online version incorporated a re-optimization scheme to adapt to recent respiratory patterns in real time. The online LSTM achieved better accuracy, reducing the RMSE significantly compared to baseline linear regression models, particularly for longer prediction horizons (e.g., 500 ms). Based on this work, they further evaluated the performance of LSTM-based models for real-time tumor contour prediction in MR-guided radiotherapy (MRgRT) [117]. They compared a standard LSTM model (LSTM-shift), a convolutional LSTM (ConvLSTM), and a convolutional LSTM with spatial transformer layers (ConvLSTM-STL). The LSTM-shift model, optimized in both offline and online modes, was designed to predict future centroid positions and align the last observed contour. The study found that the online LSTM-shift outperformed the more complex ConvLSTM models, achieving a Hausdorff distance of 1.2 mm and demonstrating robustness across varying patient respiratory patterns. Overall, these AI-based approaches offer an efficient solution for motion prediction, significantly enhancing the precision of real-time adaptive radiotherapy. Future directions may focus on integrating multimodal data and refining algorithms to handle more complex and irregular motion patterns, ultimately enhancing the robustness and clinical applicability of AI-driven real-time tumor localization.

6.3.2 Post-Treatment Follow-Up

6.3.2.1 Image Standardization and Harmonization

After the full radiotherapy course concludes, patients will return to the clinic for scheduled follow-ups and receive periodical imaging. The follow-up imaging helps monitor the tumor response and the side effects, with potential drug interventions or follow-up treatments available if warranted. Quantitative models, especially AI-based models, can be derived based on these follow-up images to enable treatment response and side effects predictions before their actual manifestation to allow earlier, and usually more effective, interventions. The follow-up images can also be combined with pre-treatment and during-treatment images to further enhance a model's predictive power. However, to develop such models, the variability in imaging acquisition protocols across clinical sites remains a significant challenge, as the follow-up images may not be consistently acquired using the same machine/protocol. And even larger differences can exist between pre-treatment, during-treatment, and post-treatment images. Differences in factors including image slice thickness, CT tube current, MR sequence parameters, and image reconstruction kernels can lead to diverse image appearances. This variability increases inter- and intra-observer discrepancies when these images are interpreted by clinicians. Similarly, they can significantly impact the reproducibility of predictive imaging biomarkers and resulting AI models, potentially compromising the accuracy of clinical assessments.

Achieving uniform imaging protocols across diverse healthcare settings is a complex task, as each institution may have different operational practices. Furthermore, even if protocol unification were possible, inherent differences among scanner manufacturers introduce additional variabilities. To address these challenges, AI-based approaches have been developed to standardize and harmonize imaging datasets through post-processing, helping to minimize inter-scan variability and mitigate its effects on downstream applications. Figure 6.14 shows two categories of harmonization. One effective approach involves the use of generative AI models, such as GANs, to normalize images acquired from different platforms and protocols. By converting images to a consistent

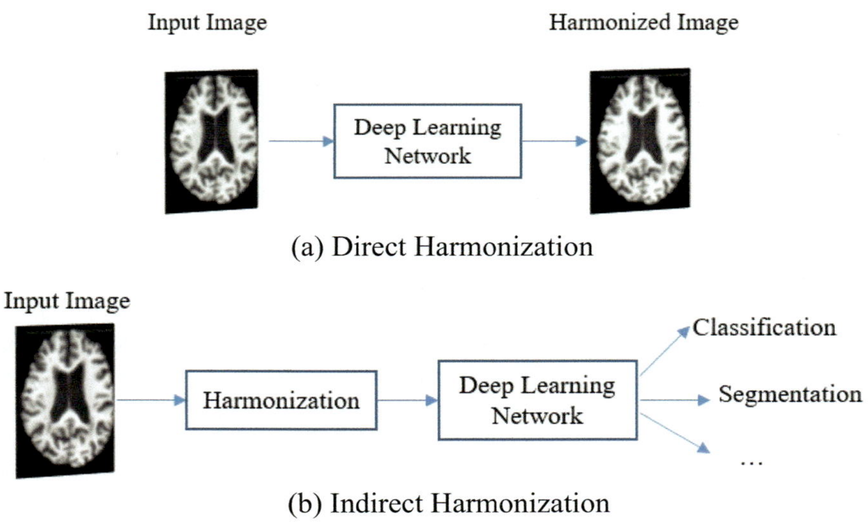

FIGURE 6.14 Classification of harmonization based on network outputs (Reprint from Ref. [118]).

standard, these models can improve the uniformity of datasets, enhancing the performance of subsequent tasks like automated contouring, extraction of imaging biomarkers, and prediction of treatment outcomes [119]. For example, GANs have been used to transform images from various scanner types or settings into a unified representation, effectively reducing discrepancies that arise from differences in acquisition parameters [120]. This harmonization process not only supports more accurate quantitative analysis but also enhances the reliability of AI models trained on these images by providing more consistent input data.

These advancements highlight the potential of AI to streamline clinical workflows by reducing the need for rigid acquisition standardization across institutions. By leveraging deep learning models, healthcare providers can address the variability introduced by different imaging protocols and equipment manufacturers, paving the way for more consistent and reproducible imaging data that can be utilized across various clinical and research settings.

6.3.2.2 Side Effects Detection

Accurate and early identification of treatment-related side effects is crucial for adopting early interventions and improving overall treatment outcomes. Side effects, such as radiation pneumonitis, mucositis, and skin toxicity, can vary in severity and impact patient quality of life, necessitating timely and precise monitoring throughout and after the course of treatment. Recent studies have explored the application of AI for detecting and predicting these side effects, leveraging imaging and clinical data to enable more personalized patient care.

Traditional methods of side effects assessment rely on manual evaluation, which can be subjective and prone to variability among clinicians. In recent years, AI, particularly DL and machine learning (ML) techniques, has been employed to analyze radiological images and detect subtle, early changes indicative of side effects. For example, AI algorithms have been developed to identify radiation-induced lung damage, such as pneumonitis and fibrosis, by analyzing CT scans taken during and after thoracic radiotherapy [121]. CNNs have been particularly effective in detecting these changes by learning patterns associated with tissue damage, allowing for the early identification of complications before they become symptomatic [122]. Similarly, in head-and-neck radiotherapy, AI models have been used to detect early signs of mucositis and xerostomia by analyzing MRI or CT images. These models often rely on texture analysis and radiomic features to distinguish between normal and affected tissues. Recent studies have constructed prediction models using textural features extracted from various imaging modalities, including CT, MRI, and PET, to identify early changes indicative of side effects. For instance, CNNs trained on T2-weighted (T2W) MRI or diffusion-weighted imaging (DWI) data have been used to predict the onset of mucositis with promising accuracy, helping clinicians intervene earlier and adjust treatment plans accordingly [123,124].

While imaging-based models have shown promise, detecting side effects accurately often requires more than just image data. A recent study utilized radiomics and dosiomics features from CT images, along with clinical factors like age and body mass index (BMI), to train ML models that could predict the likelihood of patients developing moderate to severe radiation dermatitis. The study found that integrating these data types significantly enhanced the model's predictive performance, achieving an area under the curve (AUC) of 0.83, which outperformed models based solely on traditional clinical or dosimetric parameters [125].

Another key challenge in side effects detection is the need for accurate and consistent segmentation of affected regions. Traditional methods often involve manual contouring, which is labor-intensive and subject to inter-observer variability. Recent advancements in AI have enabled the automation of this process, improving consistency and efficiency. Auto-segmentation models, such as U-Net and its variants, facilitate the analysis of how radiation affects near-tumor tissues. A recent work developed a DL-based tool, DeepTOP, which integrates automated tumor segmentation and clinical outcome prediction using MRI data [126]. The approach employed a U-Net with a codec structure for segmentation and a three-layer CNN for prediction, enhanced by a weight distribution algorithm to improve accuracy. DeepTOP was trained and validated using 1,889 MRI slices from 99 patients in a multicenter clinical trial, achieving a Dice coefficient of 0.79 and slice-specific sensitivity of 0.98 for segmentation. For outcome prediction, it demonstrated an accuracy of 0.789, with specificity and sensitivity of 0.725 and 0.812, respectively.

Despite the progress, several challenges remain in the application of AI for side effects detection. One major issue is the need for large, diverse datasets to train robust models that generalize well across different patient populations and clinical settings. The lack of external validation in many studies means that the reported models may not perform consistently across various institutions. Looking ahead, integrating large language models (LLMs) could enhance side effects detection by leveraging their ability to process and correlate multimodal data, such as imaging, clinical records, and patient-reported outcomes. LLMs can interpret text-based data alongside imaging features, potentially leading to more accurate, holistic assessments of patient side effects and supporting more personalized adaptive radiotherapy strategies.

REFERENCES

1. Chandarana, H., et al., Emerging role of MRI in radiation therapy. *Journal of Magnetic Resonance Imaging*, 2018. 48(6): pp. 1468–1478.
2. MacManus, M., et al., Use of PET and PET/CT for radiation therapy planning: IAEA expert report 2006–2007. *Radiotherapy and Oncology*, 2009. 91(1): pp. 85–94.
3. Metcalfe, P., et al., The potential for an enhanced role for MRI in radiation-therapy treatment planning. *Technology in Cancer Research & Treatment*, 2013. 12(5): pp. 429–446.
4. Kry, S.F., et al., AAPM TG 158: measurement and calculation of doses outside the treated volume from external-beam radiation therapy. *Medical Physics*, 2017. 44(10): pp. e391–e429.
5. Specht, L. and A.K. Berthelsen. PET/CT in radiation therapy planning. In *Seminars in Nuclear Medicine*. 2018 Jan. **48**(1): pp. 67–75.
6. Speirs, C.K., et al., PET-based radiation therapy planning. *PET Clinics*, 2015. 10(1): pp. 27–44.
7. Gjesteby, L., et al., Metal artifact reduction in CT: where are we after four decades? *IEEE Access*, 2016. 4: pp. 5826–5849.
8. Lyu, Q., et al., Cine cardiac MRI motion artifact reduction using a recurrent neural network. *IEEE Transactions on Medical Imaging*, 2021. 40(8): pp. 2170–2181.
9. Obuchowicz, R., M. Strzelecki, and A. Piórkowski, Clinical applications of artificial intelligence in medical imaging and image processing—a review. *Cancers (Basel)*, 2024. **16**(10): p. 1870.
10. Dayarathna, S., et al., Deep learning based synthesis of MRI, CT and PET: review and analysis. *Medical Image Analysis*, 2023. **92**: p. 103046.
11. Goodfellow, I., et al., Generative adversarial nets. In *Proceedings of the 28th International Conference on Neural Information Processing Systems - Volume 2*, Montreal, Canada 2014. Vol. 27, pp. 2672–2680.
12. Kingma, D.P., Auto-encoding variational bayes. arXiv preprint arXiv:1312.6114, 2013.
13. Ho, J., A. Jain, and P. Abbeel, Denoising diffusion probabilistic models. *Advances in Neural Information Processing Systems*, 2020. 33: pp. 6840–6851.
14. Zhu, J.-Y., et al., Unpaired image-to-image translation using cycle-consistent adversarial networks. In *2017 IEEE International Conference on Computer Vision (ICCV)*, Venice, Italy, 2017.
15. Liu, Y., et al., CT synthesis from MRI using multi-cycle GAN for head-and-neck radiation therapy. *Computerized Medical Imaging and Graphics*, 2021. 91: p. 101953.
16. Liu, M.-Y., T. Breuel, and J. Kautz, Unsupervised image-to-image translation networks. In *Proceedings of the 31st International Conference on Neural Information Processing Systems*, Long Beach, California, USA, 2017. Vol. 30, pp. 700–708.
17. Paavilainen, P., S.U. Akram, and J. Kannala. Bridging the gap between paired and unpaired medical image translation. In Engelhardt, S., et al. *Deep Generative Models, and Data Augmentation, Labelling, and Imperfections. DGM4MICCAI DALI 2021*, Strasbourg, France.
18. Song, Y., et al., Score-based generative modeling through stochastic differential equations. In 9th International Conference on Learning Representations, {ICLR} 2021, Virtual Event, Austria, May 3-7, 2021, OpenReview.net. https://dblp.org/rec/conf/iclr/0011SKKEP21.bib}, bibsource={dblp computer science bibliography, https://dblp.org .
19. Chung, H. and J.C. Ye, Score-based diffusion models for accelerated MRI. *Medical Image Analysis*, 2022. 80: p. 102479.

20. Song, Y., et al., Solving inverse problems in medical imaging with score-based generative models. arXiv preprint arXiv:2111.08005, 2021.
21. Yu, L., et al., Deep sinogram completion with image prior for metal artifact reduction in CT images. *IEEE Transactions on Medical Imaging*, 2020. 40(1): pp. 228–238.
22. Wang, T., et al., DAN-Net: dual-domain adaptive-scaling non-local network for CT metal artifact reduction. *Physics in Medicine & Biology*, 2021. 66(15): p. 155009.
23. Wang, H., et al., DICDNet: deep interpretable convolutional dictionary network for metal artifact reduction in CT images. *IEEE Transactions on Medical Imaging*, 2021. 41(4): pp. 869–880.
24. Cui, L., et al., Motion artifact reduction for magnetic resonance imaging with deep learning and k-space analysis. *PloS One*, 2023. 18(1): p. e0278668.
25. Sánchez, I. and V. Vilaplana, Brain MRI super-resolution using 3D generative adversarial networks. arXiv preprint arXiv:1812.11440, 2018.
26. Lyu, Q., et al., Multi-contrast super-resolution MRI through a progressive network. *IEEE Transactions on Medical Imaging*, 2020. 39(9): pp. 2738–2749.
27. Wu, Z., et al., Super-resolution of brain MRI images based on denoising diffusion probabilistic model. *Biomedical Signal Processing and Control*, 2023. 85: p. 104901.
28. Chen, Z., et al., Super-resolution enhanced medical image diagnosis with sample affinity interaction. *IEEE Transactions on Medical Imaging*, 2021. 40(5): pp. 1377–1389.
29. Yang, C., et al., A dual-domain diffusion model for sparse-view CT reconstruction. *IEEE Signal Processing Letters*, 2024. **31**: pp. 1279–1283.
30. Xia, W., et al., MAGIC: manifold and graph integrative convolutional network for low-dose CT reconstruction. arXiv preprint arXiv:2008.00406, 2020.
31. Xia, W., et al., MAGIC: manifold and graph integrative convolutional network for low-dose CT reconstruction. *IEEE Transactions on Medical Imaging*, 2021. 40(12): pp. 3459–3472.
32. Ding, Q., et al., Deep learning with adaptive hyper-parameters for low-dose CT image reconstruction. *IEEE Transactions on Computational Imaging*, 2021. 7: pp. 648–660.
33. Ye, J.C., Compressed sensing MRI: a review from signal processing perspective. *BMC Biomedical Engineering*, 2019. 1(1): p. 8.
34. Gao, Z., et al., Hierarchical perception adversarial learning framework for compressed sensing MRI. *IEEE Transactions on Medical Imaging*, 2023. 42(6): pp. 1859–1874.
35. Sun, L., et al., A deep error correction network for compressed sensing MRI. *BMC Biomedical Engineering*, 2020. 2: pp. 1–12.
36. Liu, H., et al., AI-assisted compressed sensing and parallel imaging sequences for MRI of patients with nasopharyngeal carcinoma: comparison of their capabilities in terms of examination time and image quality. *European Radiology*, 2023. 33(11): pp. 7686–7696.
37. Liang, X., et al., Generating synthesized computed tomography (CT) from cone-beam computed tomography (CBCT) using CycleGAN for adaptive radiation therapy. *Physics in Medicine & Biology*, 2019. 64(12): p. 125002.
38. Li, Y., et al., Zero-shot medical image translation via frequency-guided diffusion models. *IEEE Transactions on Medical Imaging*, 2023. **43**: pp. 980–993.
39. Li, Y., et al., FDDM: unsupervised medical image translation with a frequency-decoupled diffusion model. arXiv preprint arXiv:2311.12070, 2023.
40. Hu, Z., et al., Obtaining PET/CT images from non-attenuation corrected PET images in a single PET system using Wasserstein generative adversarial networks. *Physics in Medicine & Biology*, 2020. 65(21): p. 215010.
41. Kawahara, D. and Y. Nagata, T1-weighted and T2-weighted MRI image synthesis with convolutional generative adversarial networks. reports of practical. *Oncology and Radiotherapy*, 2021. 26(1): pp. 35–42.
42. Balakrishnan, G., et al., Voxelmorph: a learning framework for deformable medical image registration. *IEEE Transactions on Medical Imaging*, 2019. 38(8): pp. 1788–1800.
43. Chen, J., et al., Transmorph: transformer for unsupervised medical image registration. *Medical Image Analysis*, 2022. 82: p. 102615.
44. Zheng, Y., et al., SymReg-GAN: symmetric image registration with generative adversarial networks. *IEEE Transactions on Pattern Analysis and Machine Intelligence*, 2021. 44(9): pp. 5631–5646.
45. Ronneberger, O., P. Fischer, and T. Brox. U-net: convolutional networks for biomedical image segmentation. In *Medical Image Computing and Computer-Assisted Intervention–MICCAI 2015: 18th International Conference,* Munich, Germany, October 5–9, 2015, *proceedings, part III* 18. 2015. Springer.

46. Isensee, F., et al., nnU-Net: a self-configuring method for deep learning-based biomedical image segmentation. *Nature Methods*, 2021. 18(2): pp. 203–211.
47. Ma, J., et al., Segment anything in medical images. *Nature Communications*, 2024. 15(1): p. 654.
48. Wasserthal, J., et al., TotalSegmentator: robust segmentation of 104 anatomic structures in CT images. *Radiology: Artificial Intelligence*, 2023. **5**(5): e230024. doi: 10.1148/ryai.230024. PMID: 37795137; PMCID: PMC10546353.
49. Zhao, W., et al., Artificial intelligence in image-guided radiotherapy: a review of treatment target localization. *Quantitative Imaging in Medicine and Surgery*, 2021. 11(12): pp. 4881–4894.
50. Kawamura, M., et al., Revolutionizing radiation therapy: the role of AI in clinical practice. *Journal of Radiation Research*, 2023. 65(1): pp. 1–9.
51. Yan, S., et al., Quality assurance for online adaptive radiotherapy: a secondary dose verification model with geometry-encoded U-Net. Machine Learning*: Science and Technology*, 2024. 5(4): p. 045013.
52. Yang, X., et al., Real-time onboard volumetric imaging for tumor tracking during treatment and post-treatment dose verification. *International Journal of Radiation Oncology, Biology, Physics*, 2024. 120(2): pp. S193–S194.
53. Letourneau, D., et al., Cone-beam-CT guided radiation therapy: technical implementation. *Radiotherapy and Oncology*, 2005. 75(3): pp. 279–286.
54. Kerkmeijer, L.G., et al., The MRI-linear accelerator consortium: evidence-based clinical introduction of an innovation in radiation oncology connecting researchers, methodology, data collection, quality assurance, and technical development. *Frontiers in Oncology*, 2016. 6: p. 215.
55. Feldkamp, L.A., L.C. Davis, and J.W. Kress, Practical cone-beam algorithm. *Journal of the Optical Society of America A*, 1984. 1(6): pp. 612–619.
56. Zhang, H., et al., Regularization strategies in statistical image reconstruction of low-dose x-ray CT: a review. *Medical Physics*, 2018. 45(10): pp. e886–e907.
57. Ren, L., et al., A novel digital tomosynthesis (DTS) reconstruction method using a deformation field map. *Medical Physics*, 2008. 35(7): pp. 3110–3115.
58. Li, Z., et al., A sinogram inpainting method based on generative adversarial network for limited-angle computed tomography. In *Proc. SPIE 11072, 15th International Meeting on Fully Three-Dimensional Image Reconstruction in Radiology and Nuclear Medicine*, 1107220, Philadelphia, PA, USA, 2019.
59. Hu, D., et al., SEA-Net: Structure-Enhanced Attention Network for Limited-Angle CBCT Reconstruction of Clinical Projection Data. *IEEE Transactions on Instrumentation and Measurement*, 2023. **72**: p. 4507613.
60. Liu, J., et al., DOLCE: a model-based probabilistic diffusion framework for limited-angle ct reconstruction. In *2023 IEEE/CVF International Conference on Computer Vision (ICCV)*, Paris, France, 2023, pp. 10464-10474. Doi: 10.1109/ICCV51070.2023.00963.
61. Xie, J., et al., Prior frequency guided diffusion model for limited angle (LA)-CBCT reconstruction. *Physics in Medicine & Biology*, 2024. 69(13): p. 135008.
62. Shen, L., W. Zhao, and L. Xing, Patient-specific reconstruction of volumetric computed tomography images from a single projection view via deep learning. *Nature Biomedical Engineering*, 2019. 3(11): pp. 880–888.
63. Ying, X., et al., X2CT-GAN: reconstructing CT from biplanar X-rays with generative adversarial networks. In *2019 IEEE/CVF Conference on Computer Vision and Pattern Recognition (CVPR)*, Long Beach, CA, USA, 2019, pp. 10611–10620.
64. Loÿen, E., D. Dasnoy-Sumell, and B. Macq, Patient-specific three-dimensional image reconstruction from a single X-ray projection using a convolutional neural network for on-line radiotherapy applications. *Physics and Imaging in Radiation Oncology*, 2023. 26: p. 100444.
65. Pan, S., et al., Patient-specific 3D volumetric CBCT image reconstruction with single x-ray projection using denoising diffusion probabilistic model. In *Proc. SPIE 12931, Medical Imaging 2024: Imaging Informatics for Healthcare, Research, and Applications*, 129310P (2 April 2024) San Diego, California, United States.
66. Chang, C.W., et al., Deep learning-based fast volumetric image generation for image-guided proton FLASH radiotherapy. *Research Square*, 2023. doi: 10.21203/rs.3.rs-3112632/v1. Update in: IEEE Trans Radiat Plasma Med Sci. 2024 Nov;8(8):973–983. doi: 10.1109/trpms.2024.3439585. PMID: 37546731; PMCID: PMC10402267
67. Pan, S., et al., Patient-specific CBCT synthesis for real-time tumor tracking in surface-guided radiotherapy. arXiv:2410.23582v2, 2024.

68. Sonke, J.J., et al., Frameless stereotactic body radiotherapy for lung cancer using four-dimensional cone beam CT guidance. *International Journal of Radiation Oncology, Biology, Physics*, 2009. 74(2): pp. 567–574.
69. Nielsen, T.B., et al., Tumour motion analysis from planning to end of treatment course for a large cohort of peripheral lung SBRT targets. *Acta Oncologica*, 2021. 60(11): pp. 1407–1412.
70. Zhang, Y., et al., A review on 4D cone-beam CT (4D-CBCT) in radiation therapy: Technical advances and clinical applications. *Medical Physics*, 2024. 51(8): pp. 5164–5180.
71. Wang, J. and X. Gu, Simultaneous motion estimation and image reconstruction (SMEIR) for 4D cone-beam CT. *Medical Physics*, 2013. 40(10): p. 101912.
72. Huang, X., et al., U-net-based deformation vector field estimation for motion-compensated 4D-CBCT reconstruction. *Medical Physics*, 2020. 47(7): pp. 3000–3012.
73. Zhang, Z., et al., Deep learning-based motion compensation for four-dimensional cone-beam computed tomography (4D-CBCT) reconstruction. *Medical Physics*, 2023. 50(2): pp. 808–820.
74. Zhang, Z., et al., Fast motion-compensated reconstruction for 4D-CBCT using deep learning-based groupwise registration. *Biomedical Physics & Engineering Express*, 2025. 11(1): p. 015030.
75. Zhang, Y., et al., Dynamic cone-beam CT reconstruction using spatial and temporal implicit neural representation learning (STINR). *Physics in Medicine & Biology*, 2023. 68(4): p. 045005.
76. Shao, H.-C., et al., Dynamic CBCT imaging using prior model-free spatiotemporal implicit neural representation (PMF-STINR). *Physics in Medicine & Biology*, 2024. 69(11): p. 115030.
77. Stemkens, B., E.S. Paulson, and R.H.N. Tijssen, Nuts and bolts of 4D-MRI for radiotherapy. *Physics in Medicine & Biology*, 2018. 63(21): p. 21TR01.
78. Curtis, A.D. and H.-L.M. Cheng, Primer and historical review on rapid cardiac CINE MRI. *Journal of Magnetic Resonance Imaging*, 2022. 55(2): pp. 373–388.
79. Freedman, J.N., et al., Rapid 4D-MRI reconstruction using a deep radial convolutional neural network: Dracula. *Radiotherapy and Oncology*, 2021. 159: pp. 209–217.
80. Çiçek, Ö., et al., 3D U-Net: learning dense volumetric segmentation from sparse annotation. In *Medical Image Computing and Computer-Assisted Intervention—MICCAI 2016*. 19th International Conference, Athens, Greece, October 17-21, 2016. Cham: Springer International Publishing.
81. Murray, V., et al., Movienet: deep space–time-coil reconstruction network without k-space data consistency for fast motion-resolved 4D MRI. *Magnetic Resonance in Medicine*, 2024. 91(2): pp. 600–614.
82. Park, S., et al., Autoencoder-inspired convolutional network-based super-resolution method in MRI. *IEEE Journal of Translational Engineering in Health and Medicine*, 2021. 9: p. 1800113.
83. Shao, H.-C., et al., 3D cine-magnetic resonance imaging using spatial and temporal implicit neural representation learning (STINR-MR). *Physics in Medicine & Biology*, 2024. 69(9): p. 095007.
84. Yasue, K., et al., Quantitative analysis of the intra-beam respiratory motion with baseline drift for respiratory-gating lung stereotactic body radiation therapy. *Journal of Radiation Research*, 2022. 63(1): pp. 137–147.
85. Biswas, S., H.K. Aggarwal, and M. Jacob, Dynamic MRI using model-based deep learning and SToRM priors: MoDL-SToRM. *Magnetic Resonance in Medicine*, 2019. 82(1): pp. 485–494.
86. Yoo, J., et al., Time-dependent deep image prior for dynamic MRI. *IEEE Transactions on Medical Imaging*, 2021. 40(12): pp. 3337–3348.
87. Huttinga, N.R.F., et al., Nonrigid 3D motion estimation at high temporal resolution from prospectively undersampled k-space data using low-rank MR-MOTUS. *Magnetic Resonance in Medicine*, 2021. 85(4): pp. 2309–2326.
88. Terpstra, M.L., et al., Real-time 3D motion estimation from undersampled MRI using multi-resolution neural networks. *Medical Physics*, 2021. 48(11): pp. 6597–6613.
89. Wilcox, S., et al., Respiration-induced organ motion compensation: a review. *Annals of Biomedical Engineering*, 2024. **53**: pp. 271–283.
90. Zhao, W., et al., Visualizing the invisible in prostate radiation therapy: markerless prostate target localization via a deep learning model and monoscopic Kv projection x-ray image. *International Journal of Radiation Oncology, Biology, Physics*, 2018. 102(3): pp. S128–S129.
91. Zhao, W., et al., Markerless pancreatic tumor target localization enabled by deep learning. *International Journal of Radiation Oncology, Biology, Physics*, 2019. 105(2): pp. 432–439.
92. Wang, C., et al., Technical Note: 3D localization of lung tumors on cone beam CT projections via a convolutional recurrent neural network. *Medical Physics*, 2020. 47(3): pp. 1161–1166.
93. Fu, Y., et al., Deep learning-based target decomposition for markerless lung tumor tracking in radiotherapy. *Medical Physics*, 2024. 51(6): pp. 4271–4282.

94. Zhu, M., et al., RT-SRTS: angle-agnostic real-time simultaneous 3D reconstruction and tumor segmentation from single X-ray projection. *Computers in Biology and Medicine*, 2024. 173: p. 108390.
95. Hindley, N., C.-C. Shieh, and P. Keall, A patient-specific deep learning framework for 3D motion estimation and volumetric imaging during lung cancer radiotherapy. *Physics in Medicine & Biology*, 2023. 68(14): p. 14NT01.
96. Foote, M., et al., Real-time 2D-3D deformable registration with deep learning and application to lung radiotherapy targeting. In *26th International Conference, IPMI 2019*, Hong Kong, China, June 2–7, 2019. pp. 265–276.
97. Wei, R., et al., Convolutional Neural Network (CNN) based three dimensional tumor localization using single x-ray projection. *IEEE Access*, 2019. 7: pp. 37026–37038.
98. Zhang, Y., An unsupervised 2D-3D deformable registration network (2D3D-RegNet) for cone-beam CT estimation. *Physics in Medicine & Biology*, 2021. **66**(7): p. 074001.
99. Dai, J., et al., Volumetric tumor tracking from a single cone-beam X-ray projection image enabled by deep learning. *Medical Image Analysis*, 2024. 91: p. 102998.
100. Shao, H.-C., et al., Real-time liver tumor localization via a single x-ray projection using deep graph neural network-assisted biomechanical modeling. *Physics in Medicine & Biology*, 2022. 67(11): p. 115009.
101. Shao, H.-C., et al., Real-time liver tumor localization via combined surface imaging and a single x-ray projection. *Physics in Medicine & Biology*, 2023. 68(6): p. 065002.
102. Shao, H.-C., et al., Real-time liver motion estimation via deep learning-based angle-agnostic X-ray imaging. *Medical Physics*, 2023. 50(11): pp. 6649–6662.
103. Waddington, D.E.J., et al., Real-time radial reconstruction with domain transform manifold learning for MRI-guided radiotherapy. *Medical Physics*, 2023. 50(4): pp. 1962–1974.
104. Spieker, V., et al., Deep learning for retrospective motion correction in MRI: a comprehensive review. *IEEE Transactions on Medical Imaging*, 2024. 43(2): pp. 846–859.
105. Liu, L., et al., Real time volumetric MRI for 3D motion tracking via geometry-informed deep learning. *Medical Physics*, 2022. 49(9): pp. 6110–6119.
106. Wei, R., et al., Real-time 3D MRI reconstruction from cine-MRI using unsupervised network in MRI-guided radiotherapy for liver cancer. *Medical Physics*, 2023. 50(6): pp. 3584–3596.
107. Liu, L., et al., Volumetric MRI with sparse sampling for MR-guided 3D motion tracking via sparse prior-augmented implicit neural representation learning. *Medical Physics*, 2024. 51(4): pp. 2526–2537.
108. Shao, H.-C., et al., Real-time MRI motion estimation through an unsupervised k-space-driven deformable registration network (KS-RegNet). *Physics in Medicine & Biology*, 2022. 67(13): p. 135012.
109. Teo, T.P., et al., Feasibility of predicting tumor motion using online data acquired during treatment and a generalized neural network optimized with offline patient tumor trajectories. *Medical Physics*, 2018. 45(2): pp. 830–845.
110. Lombardo, E., et al., *Evaluation of real-time tumor contour prediction using LSTM networks for MR-guided radiotherapy*. Radiotherapy and Oncology, 2023. 182: p. 109555.
111. Wang, R., et al., A feasibility of respiration prediction based on deep Bi-LSTM for real-time tumor tracking. *IEEE Access*, 2018. 6: pp. 51262–51268.
112. Khashei, M. and M. Bijari, A novel hybridization of artificial neural networks and ARIMA models for time series forecasting. *Applied Soft Computing*, 2011. 11(2): pp. 2664–2675.
113. Sun, W., et al., Respiratory signal prediction based on adaptive boosting and multilayer perceptron neural network. *International Journal of Radiation Oncology Biology Physics*, 2016. 96(2): p. E702.
114. Lin, H., et al., Towards real-time respiratory motion prediction based on long short-term memory neural networks. *Physics in Medicine & Biology*, 2019. 64(8): p. 085010.
115. Yun, J., et al., An artificial neural network (ANN)-based lung-tumor motion predictor for intrafractional MR tumor tracking. *Medical Physics*, 2012. 39(7): pp. 4423–4433.
116. Lombardo, E., et al., Offline and online LSTM networks for respiratory motion prediction in MR-guided radiotherapy. *Physics in Medicine & Biology*, 2022. **67**(9): p. 095006.
117. Romaguera, L.V., et al., Prediction of in-plane organ deformation during free-breathing radiotherapy via discriminative spatial transformer networks. *Medical Image Analysis*, 2020. 64: p. 101754.
118. Abbasi, S., et al., Deep learning for the harmonization of structural MRI scans: a survey. *BioMedical Engineering OnLine*, 2024. 23(1): p. 90.
119. Zuo, L., et al., An overview of disentangled representation learning for MR image harmonization. In S. Kevin Zhou and Hayit Greenspan and Dinggang Shen (eds), *Deep Learning for Medical Image Analysis* (Second Edition), 2024: pp. 135–152. https://www.sciencedirect.com/science/article/pii/B9780323851244000143. https://doi.org/10.1016/B978-0-32-385124-4.00014-3

120. Bashyam, V.M., et al., Deep generative medical image harmonization for improving cross-site generalization in deep learning predictors. *Journal of Magnetic Resonance Imaging*, 2022. 55(3): pp. 908–916.
121. Wang, L., et al., Computed tomography-based delta-radiomics analysis for discriminating radiation pneumonitis in patients with esophageal cancer after radiation therapy. *International Journal of Radiation Oncology* Biology* Physics*, 2021. 111(2): pp. 443–455.
122. Giordano, F.M., et al., Radiation-induced pneumonitis in the era of the COVID-19 pandemic: artificial intelligence for differential diagnosis. *Cancers (Basel)*, 2021. **13**(8): p. 1960.
123. Shin, J., et al., MRI radiomics model predicts pathologic complete response of rectal cancer following chemoradiotherapy. *Radiology*, 2022. 303(2): pp. 351–358.
124. Shaish, H., et al., Radiomics of MRI for pretreatment prediction of pathologic complete response, tumor regression grade, and neoadjuvant rectal score in patients with locally advanced rectal cancer undergoing neoadjuvant chemoradiation: an international multicenter study. *European Radiology*, 2020. 30(11): pp. 6263–6273.
125. Lee, T.F., et al., Utilizing radiomics and dosiomics with AI for precision prediction of radiation dermatitis in breast cancer patients. *BMC Cancer*, 2024. 24(1): p. 965.
126. Li, L., et al., Accurate tumor segmentation and treatment outcome prediction with DeepTOP. *Radiotherapy and Oncology*, 2023. 183: p. 109550.

7 Adaptive Radiation Therapy

Yao Zhao, Xinru Chen, Dong Joo Rhee, and Jinzhong Yang

7.1 INTRODUCTION

7.1.1 Overview of Adaptive Radiation Therapy (ART)

Adaptive radiation therapy (ART) has been evidenced as a promising technique for improving the quality of treatment delivery by accounting for anatomical variations such as changes in tumor volume, normal tissue deformation, weight loss, and variations in patient position from day to day [1–3]. ART involves modifications to the original treatment plan based on repeated daily imaging of the patient during a course of treatment. By adapting the original treatment plan, ART aims to increase the effectiveness of radiotherapy and reduce toxicity to surrounding healthy tissues.

Historical progress in ART has been facilitated by advancements in imaging technologies and treatment planning systems (TPS). The development from two-dimensional (2D) to three-dimensional conformal radiation therapy (3D-CRT) improved tumor targeting through better imaging. Advances such as intensity-modulated radiation therapy (IMRT) and volumetric modulated arc therapy (VMAT) further enhanced dose distribution, allowing highly conformal dose delivery while sparing organs at risks (OARs). The integration of image-guided radiation therapy (IGRT) represented a substantial leap forward, providing real-time imaging during treatment delivery and facilitating adjustments based on daily anatomical variations [4]. ART builds upon these technologies, enabling treatment plans to be modified based on daily imaging. Early implementations of ART involved periodic replanning, but this process was time-consuming and required significant manual effort. Recent developments in artificial intelligence (AI) have addressed these limitations by automating and streamlining the ART workflow, making it more practical and efficient for routine clinical use [5–7].

7.1.2 Workflow of ART

The ART workflow typically starts with initial imaging—commonly a simulation computed tomography (CT) or magnetic resonance imaging (MRI) scan—used for treatment planning. Clinicians then perform target and OAR delineation, after which the dose distribution is optimized and calculated within a dedicated TPS. Once the plan is approved, the patient begins the course of therapy. During each treatment fraction, intra- and inter-fractional variations in patient anatomy may be detected via daily imaging, which can include cone-beam computed tomography (CBCT) on conventional Linacs, CT-on-rails, or MRI for MR-Linac platforms. If clinically significant variations are observed, an updated treatment plan can be generated to accommodate changes in tumor volume, OAR positions, or tissue heterogeneities. Depending on the clinical scenario, there are various levels of ART [8–10]:

- **Offline adaptation** occurs over multiple fractions, where observed changes drive a replanning process for subsequent sessions.
- **Online adaptation** occurs immediately prior to or even during treatment, in which the plan is re-optimized in near real time to reflect daily anatomical variations.

DOI: 10.1201/9781003480365-8

- **Real-time adaptation** is an emerging approach where frequent or continuous imaging guidance (e.g., MRI) allows for on-the-fly adjustments of beam positioning and dose distributions within a single treatment fraction.

Regardless of the level of adaptation, plan verification remains a critical component of the workflow. Updated plans must undergo rigorous quality assurance (QA) procedures to ensure compliance with patient- and machine-specific safety criteria. Finally, dose delivery is performed, often followed by post-delivery verification to confirm that the planned dose aligns with the delivered dose.

CT-based ART workflows typically involve daily CBCT imaging on conventional linear accelerators. CBCT provides information on patient anatomy but may suffer from reduced soft-tissue contrast and imaging artifacts (e.g., scatter, truncation) relative to simulation CT. The images are then registered to the planning CT, and the radiation oncologist or medical physicist evaluates whether target/OAR displacement needs plan adaptation. Various vendors now offer integrated solutions (e.g., Ethos) that enable online plan re-optimization and automated contour modification [11,12].

MRgART workflows leverage high-contrast MRI to delineate soft-tissue structures, enabling more precise identification of the target and OARs. Unlike CT, MRI inherently lacks electron density information, which poses challenges for dose calculation and necessitates synthetic CT (sCT) generation or hybrid MR-CT protocols. Clinical platforms (e.g., Elekta Unity) integrate an MRI scanner with a linear accelerator to enable online adaptation based on high-quality soft-tissue imaging. The detailed anatomical visualization in MRgART can enhance confidence in target localization and margin reduction. However, integrating MRI into radiotherapy introduces additional complexities, such as magnetic field-induced dose perturbations and longer treatment times associated with online plan re-optimization [13,14].

7.1.3 Technological Foundations

The successful implementation of ART relies on robust imaging capabilities, advanced TPS, and efficient workflows that can accommodate rapid re-optimization.

CT-based imaging remains the backbone of current ART implementations [15]. It provides quantitative electron density information essential for dose calculation. Onboard CBCT systems afford daily imaging, with suboptimal soft-tissue contrast compared to simulation CT. Nevertheless, iterative reconstruction algorithms and novel artifact-reduction techniques continue to enhance CBCT quality. MRI is increasingly adopted in ART due to superior soft-tissue contrast and the ability to perform real-time or near real-time imaging without ionizing radiation. High-field MRI-Linacs and low-field MRI-Linacs enable clinicians to visualize tumor and organ motion concurrently with beam delivery [16–18]. Advances in fast imaging sequences (e.g., radial acquisition, compressed sensing) and motion management techniques help mitigate geometric distortion and respiratory motion artifacts, thereby improving the accuracy of MR-based ART. The integration of novel sequences, such as T2-weighted or cine MRI, provides real-time anatomical information, enabling gating or real-time plan adaptation.

TPS for ART must incorporate robust, time-efficient algorithms for re-optimization and dose recalculation. Monte Carlo-based and advanced convolution/superposition approaches can accurately account for heterogeneities, magnetic field effects, and varying tissue densities [19]. Online adaptive TPS platforms typically involve automated steps for contour propagation, dose projection, and plan optimization, all within an expedited workflow to minimize patient on-couch time. In CT-based ART (e.g., Ethos), embedded algorithms utilize machine learning models to guide plan re-optimization by referencing databases of historically validated plans [20]. In MR-guided ART (MRgART), commercial solutions (e.g., Monaco-based online planning for Elekta Unity [16]) incorporate real-time magnetic field corrections and refined optimization objectives. Emerging solutions aim to reduce adaptation time from tens of minutes to just a few minutes, thereby maximizing clinical feasibility.

7.1.4 Role of AI in ART

Nowadays, AI offers powerful tools to address the growing complexity and time demands of ART. Within ART, AI could contribute to several key domain:

- Enhancing ART through Improved Imaging and Contour Delineation: AI-driven methods can enhance the quality of daily imaging by suppressing noise, reducing artifacts, and extracting anatomical features that facilitate more accurate target delineation [21]. Accurate delineation of tumor volumes and OARs is critical for ART, especially in the presence of anatomical changes. AI-driven imaging technologies significantly improve this process through advanced segmentation and registration methods. Convolutional neural networks (CNNs) have proven highly effective in automating the segmentation of tumors and OARs from imaging modalities such as CT and MRI [6,13].
- Facilitating Automated Treatment Planning: Advanced machine learning (ML) models can reduce the time-intensive nature of plan generation by leveraging prior knowledge (e.g., through knowledge-based planning (KPB)) [22,23]. AI also aids in dose prediction and optimization, allowing for the iterative adjustment of treatment parameters to achieve desired dose distribution. This automation enhances consistency and plan quality while significantly reducing the time and resources required for manual planning [24].
- Enabling Real-Time Adaptation: Emerging AI systems now aim to continuously monitor anatomical changes during treatment delivery and predict the need for on-the-fly plan modifications. AI might have the potential to integrate real-time imaging data with predictive models to anticipate anatomical changes and adjust treatment plans accordingly [6].

In addition to these technical contributions, AI-driven predictive analytics offer the potential to model both tumor response and treatment-related toxicities throughout treatment. By integrating clinical, imaging, and dosimetric data, AI models can predict tumor response and identify patients at higher risk for radiation-induced toxicities. These insights enable clinicians to determine when and how to adapt treatment plans, ensuring a more personalized treatment. Taken together, these advancements enhance ART by improving precision, consistency, and adaptability, while alleviating the workload for clinicians.

This chapter explores the use of AI in both CT-based and MR-guided ART, highlighting the current state-of-the-art technologies, clinical implementation workflows, and emerging innovations.

7.2 CT-BASED ART AND AI APPLICATIONS

7.2.1 CT Imaging in ART

CT imaging serves as the primary modality for planning and daily guidance in many ART workflows. By providing daily anatomical information with electron density data, CT-based techniques enable accurate dose calculations, tumor delineation, and OARs segmentation [15].

CBCT has been widely used on conventional Linac for daily patient imaging. By comparing daily CBCT images to the planning CT, clinicians can detect variations in target and OARs, thus prompting plan adaptation if deviations exceed clinically acceptable thresholds. However, CBCT imaging is susceptible to artifacts and image quality degradation due to scattered radiation, detector limitations, and truncated field of view. These artifacts can introduce uncertainties in target localization and limit the reliability of quantitative analyses such as Hounsfield unit (HU) measurements for dose recalculation [25]. Frequent QA checks are required to maintain geometric fidelity and HU accuracy, as recommended by the American Association of Physicists in Medicine (AAPM) Task Group reports (e.g., AAPM TG-179, TG-142) [26,27]. Despite these challenges, recent advances in reconstruction algorithms, scatter correction methods, and hardware design continue to enhance CBCT-based ART workflows, facilitating real-time decision-making and more precise daily adaptation.

7.2.2 AI-Driven Image Analysis and Processing for CT-Based ART

7.2.2.1 Automated Segmentation and Contouring

While CBCT-based ART enables the recalculation of radiation dose on updated patient anatomy prior to irradiation, accurate and efficient segmentation of targets and OARs remains a key challenge in ART workflow. Manual OAR delineation constitutes a significant portion of the time required for ART replanning, whereas auto-contouring could substantially improve ART workflow efficiency [28]. Recently, the advances in AI-driven tools have greatly increased the clinical acceptance of automatically delineated contours for daily dose optimization and treatment planning.

AI-driven auto-segmentation approaches are predominantly based on fully convolutional networks, particularly UNet [29] and ResNet [30] variants. Among these, the UNet architecture is most widely applied, featuring an encoder–decoder structure that forms a characteristic Ushaped architecture. The nnU-Net framework, which is fully self-configuring, is frequently used as a baseline and adapted for specific clinical needs [31]. Performance evaluation of auto-segmentation models typically involves both qualitative assessment and quantitative metrics. These quantitative metrics can be broadly categorized into volume-based and distance-based measures, which assess contour agreement with reference delineations [32]. In CBCT-based ART, conventional auto-contouring methods primarily rely on propagating planning CT contours to daily CBCT images via deformable image registration (DIR). However, DIR-based contours may be less robust, particularly in cases of significant anatomical deformation or weight loss [33]. Numerous studies have shown that deep learning-based auto-segmentation achieves higher accuracy than traditional approaches. Feasibility studies using auto-segmentation in ART have been explored in various cancer types [11,34–39]. Those clinical evaluations indicate that deep learning-based auto-contouring achieves performance comparable to manual segmentation while reducing inter-observer variability and expediting the ART workflow. Notably, some commercial ART systems still employ DIR-based auto-contouring methods [40]. Given the higher accuracy and computational efficiency of deep learning models, they are expected to further streamline the ART workflow. Nevertheless, before integrating AI-based segmentation tools into clinical practice, it is crucial to consider potential limitations related to dataset variability. Differences in image quality, acquisition parameters, and institutional protocols can affect model performance. To mitigate these challenges, a patient-specific segmentation workflow has been proposed [41]. This approach utilizes planning CT images and daily images from the initial treatment fractions to refine the segmentation model, thereby improving segmentation accuracy for subsequent fractions. Such adaptive strategies can enhance the reliability of AI-driven segmentation in ART.

7.2.2.2 Image Registration and Alignment

Image registration is an important step in CT-based ART workflow, ensuring that the daily CBCT image is accurately aligned with the reference planning CT. Inaccurate registration may lead to poor contour propagation from CT to CBCT, suboptimal dose distributions, inadequate target coverage, and/or elevated normal tissue toxicity. Recently, advances in AI have substantially augmented registration workflows, enabling more efficient and robust alignment across different imaging sessions [42,43].

Conventional registration methods typically employ intensity-based or feature-based algorithms. Intensity-based algorithms (e.g., mutual information, cross-correlation) leverage pixel or voxel values to identify optimal spatial transforms, whereas feature-based approaches utilize predefined landmarks, contours, or anatomical structures to guide alignment [44,45]. Although these traditional methods can yield acceptable performance for rigid or small deformations, they often struggle with significant anatomical changes, organ deformation, or artifacts in CBCT images. Moreover, the computational burden of deformable registration can be considerable, limiting real-time or online adaptation. To address these limitations, deep learning-based registration algorithms have been proposed, which learn complex spatial transformations from training data rather than iteratively searching parameter space [42,43]. Such approaches typically employ CNNs to predict dense deformation vector fields (DVFs) that align daily CBCT with the planning CT. These methods generally fall into three general categories based on the availability of ground-truth deformation information:

- Supervised Approaches: Models are trained on pairs of images with known ground-truth DVFs (often derived from high-quality deformable registrations, synthetic phantoms, or manually annotated landmarks) [42,46]. While supervised methods can achieve impressive accuracy, their performance is heavily dependent on the reliability of the ground-truth DVFs. In clinical practice, the complexity and variability of anatomical deformations may not always be fully captured by these ground-truth datasets, potentially limiting the accuracy of supervised models.
- Weakly Supervised Approaches: Weakly supervised models mitigate the dependency on extensive ground-truth DVFs by using partial guidance (e.g., sparse landmark correspondences or structural delineations) [47]. These approaches can be more robust against inter-patient variability, particularly if they incorporate additional constraints (e.g., segmentations of OARs) during training and prediction.
- Unsupervised Approaches: Unsupervised registration methods eliminate the need for ground-truth DVFs by utilizing similarity metrics (e.g., cross-correlation, mutual information) as loss functions to train the models. These models are trained to deform images by maximizing similarity metrics, offering greater flexibility when ground-truth DVFs are unavailable. Notably, the VoxelMorph framework, introduced by Balakrishnan et al. [48], exemplifies an unsupervised learning approach that employs a spatial transformer network (STN) [49] to generate deformed images during the training process, thereby enhancing registration accuracy without reliance on annotated data.

Many studies have demonstrated that AI-enhanced registration leads to reduced alignment errors and decreased inter- and intra-observer variability in CT-based ART, particularly for anatomical sites prone to large deformations (e.g., abdomen) [50]. For example, Liang et al. [51] introduced a deep unsupervised learning framework for automated prostate contour propagation from planning to CBCT images in ART. Their regional deformable model, enhanced with narrow-band mapping, was trained on 180 CBCT volumes and validated on independent datasets, demonstrating superior performance. Similarly, Hu et al. [52] designed the dual attention module to deal with large intensity differences between CT and CBCT images. When evaluated on the lung dataset, their method achieved a dice similarity coefficient (DSC) of 89.74% and a Structural Similarity Index (SSIM) of 86.34%, outperforming traditional methods. Cao et al. [53] further advanced the application of unsupervised model for CT-to-CBCT image registration by introducing the edge-guided attention module and the cross-domain attention module. Their results demonstrated a substantial decrease in registration errors, especially in regions with high anatomical complexity and motion. In addition, transformer-based architectures such as Swin–VoxelMorph [54] and TransMorph [55] have made significant contributions to the field of DIR. Swin–VoxelMorph integrates Swin Transformer [56] modules with the traditional [48] framework, enhancing the model's ability to capture both local and global anatomical features. Similarly, TransMorph incorporates transformer-based modules to improve contextual understanding, enabling more accurate deformation predictions [55]. Beyond direct CT-to-CBCT registration, methods for generating sCT from CBCT have been developed. These approaches utilize generative adversarial networks (GANs) [57] and other deep learning architectures to synthesize high-quality CT images that closely resemble planning CT scans. By transforming CBCT images into sCT, the contrast and anatomical visualization can be enhanced, thereby facilitating more accurate image registration. Liang et al. [58] demonstrated that GAN-based CT synthesis from CBCT reduced image artifacts and improved the alignment precision between CBCT and planning CT, leading to more accurate contour propagation.

In clinical practice, the integration of AI-based registration can significantly streamline adaptive workflows by reducing the time required for manual contour adjustments and iterative optimization. This efficiency is especially critical in settings utilizing online ART, where rapid and accurate registration is essential. Furthermore, by ensuring more precise alignment of anatomical structures, AI-based registration has the potential to improve dosimetric accuracy, resulting in enhanced target coverage and greater sparing of critical structures throughout the treatment course. Current research is focused on incorporating AI-driven registration into comprehensive ART platforms that include auto-segmentation, dose recalculation, and plan re-optimization.

7.2.2.3 Artifact Reduction and Image Enhancement

CBCT imaging is inherently prone to artifacts, many of which are also present in conventional CT but are exacerbated by the cone-beam geometry and lower radiation dose used for safety considerations. Scatter artifacts arise due to photon scattering within the patient, leading to reduced contrast and streaking artifacts. Beam hardening artifacts occur when lower-energy photons are preferentially absorbed by high-density structures, resulting in cupping artifacts or dark streaks around metallic implants and bones. Metal artifacts are primarily caused by the presence of implants or other high-Z materials, which lead to excessive photon attenuation and scattered radiation reaching the detector, producing severe streaking and dark-band artifacts. Motion artifacts result from patient movement or respiratory motion during image acquisition, manifesting as blurring, ghosting, or double-edge effects. Additionally, the cone-beam geometry and dose reduction strategies introduce lower spatial resolution and additional streaking artifacts, further degrading CBCT image quality.

Traditional artifact correction approaches, such as iterative filtering [59] and Monte Carlo-based modeling [60], have been explored to mitigate these issues. However, their application is often limited by significant computational complexity and extended processing times, making them less feasible for real-time clinical use [61]. In recent years, deep learning-based models have demonstrated superior efficiency in addressing CBCT artifacts. Studies have shown that CNNs can effectively perform denoising and artifact reduction in both the volume and projection domains [62–64]. Furthermore, specialized deep learning models have been developed to enable small field-of-view (FOV) acquisitions while maintaining high image quality, thereby reducing scan time and facilitating rapid CBCT acquisition [65–67]. AI-driven approaches have also shown promise in reducing metal artifacts [68–70] and mitigating motion-induced blurring [71–73], thereby enhancing the overall usability of CBCT images in ART.

In the current ART workflow, dose calculation is typically performed either on deformed planning CT images or directly on CBCT following appropriate corrections. Improving CBCT quality to approximate that of CT—a process referred to as sCT generation—is preferable to DIR of planning CT due to the uncertainties associated with DIR-based methods [61]. Deep learning models, including CNNs and GANs [57], have demonstrated strong potential for generating high-fidelity sCT images from CBCT. The GAN framework, originally developed for image style transfer, employs a generator to synthesize images and a discriminator to differentiate real from synthetic images, utilizing adversarial training to enhance output quality. More advanced architectures, such as cycle-consistent GAN (CycleGAN) [74], incorporate cycle consistency constraints, eliminating the need for perfectly aligned voxel-wise image pairs. These AI-driven approaches have been successfully applied to generate high-quality sCT images across various anatomical sites, improving the accuracy of dose calculations and facilitating more precise ART adaptation [75–80].

7.2.3 AI in Treatment Planning for CT-Based ART

With the advent of onboard CBCT integrated into linear accelerators, CT-based ART has emerged as a promising approach to enhancing precision in radiotherapy. ART can be performed in two primary settings: offline and online workflows. While offline ART has demonstrated significant success and led to improved patient outcomes in various clinical scenarios, online adaptive therapy has historically faced considerable challenges. The primary obstacle involves the lengthy time required to generate an adaptive treatment plan while the patient remains immobilized on the treatment table, which is often impractical in a clinical setting.

Recent advances in computational algorithms have begun to address these limitations, enabling the automation of key processes such as contouring and treatment planning. These innovations have greatly reduced the time required for plan adaptation, bringing the concept of online ART closer to routine clinical feasibility. For example, the Varian Ethos system (Varian Medical Systems, Palo Alto, CA, USA) supports streamlined online adaptive workflows, significantly cutting re-optimization and contour review time to under 20 minutes [81].

The rapid progress in AI technologies has further revolutionized adaptive treatment planning. AI-driven algorithms for automated contouring, including DIR techniques and deep learning models, improve both the speed and accuracy of these processes [15,82]. For instance, the Ethos system employs intelligent prioritization of optimization goals and conflict resolution strategies, facilitating efficient plan adaptation while ensuring adherence to clinical objectives [83]. Emerging strategies also incorporate ML models to predict dose distributions and automatically generate dose–volume histograms (DVHs) tailored to individual patient anatomies. These approaches minimize reliance on manual intervention, improving workflow efficiency and consistency [84]. Moreover, comparative studies of commercial systems have shown that CBCT-based ART platforms yield clinical outcomes comparable to MRI-guided systems like Unity (Elekta AB, Stockholm, Sweden) and MRIdian (ViewRay Inc., Denver, CO, USA), with the advantage of lower implementation costs and broader accessibility [85,86].

7.2.3.1 Automated Treatment Planning

Automated treatment planning has evolved considerably, transitioning from traditional knowledge-based planning (KBP) to advanced AI-driven techniques. KBP, one of the earliest approaches, leverages historical treatment data to develop predictive models for generating treatment plans. These models ensure consistency in plan quality and reduce variability, providing a strong starting point for optimization. Several commercial systems, such as Varian's RapidPlan, incorporate patient-specific geometry and historical dose distributions into the planning process, effectively streamlining treatment workflows [22,23].

Within the context of ART, KBP remains a foundational tool. It facilitates rapid adjustments to treatment plans as patient anatomy changes during therapy. Strategies such as adding extra planning structures and iteratively refining model parameters have demonstrated the potential for fully automated workflows, minimizing manual intervention [22,23]. More recently, AI-driven methods have advanced the field by automating complex aspects of dose distribution planning. Among these, reinforcement learning (RL) and its subset, deep reinforcement learning (DRL), have shown considerable promise. These approaches optimize planning by modeling iterative decision-making within predefined constraints. For instance, deep Q-networks (DQN) have been successfully applied to treatment scenarios, learning optimal beam configurations to maximize target coverage while sparing OARs [87–89]. An example of a DRL application is the Virtual Treatment Planner Network (VTPN), which mimics human planner behavior by dynamically adjusting treatment planning parameters (TPPs). These systems analyze DVHs and iteratively refine plans to achieve high-quality results [87]. Another innovative approach, the Functional automatic treatment PlannIng Network (FatPIN), integrates functional characteristics of DVHs to enhance learning efficiency and adaptability, allowing it to generalize across varied patient anatomies and clinical scenarios [90].

While these developments significantly reduce planning time and variability, challenges remain. These challenges include improving training data quality, enhancing the interpretability of AI-driven decisions, and addressing the computational complexity of DRL frameworks [7,89]. Future research may benefit from hybrid models that merge the robustness of KBP with the adaptability of AI-based methods to further refine automated planning for ART.

7.2.3.2 Predictive Modeling for Treatment Adaptation

An emerging frontier in ART is predictive modeling to guide treatment adaptation. AI models that predict tumor response to radiation are pivotal for identifying the need for plan adjustments during therapy. These models rely on longitudinal imaging data, tumor biology, and various patient-specific factors to project changes in tumor volume, position, or other features. For instance, CNNs are widely used to extract spatial features from medical images, enabling the assessment of tumor morphology and predicting responses to therapy. Furthermore, recurrent neural networks (RNNs) complement CNNs by analyzing temporal sequences, such as imaging data from multiple treatment sessions, to evaluate tumor progression. Moreover, advanced models like attention mechanisms and transformers are increasingly integrated to focus on critical data features, thereby improving predictive accuracy [91]. Additionally, ensemble approaches that combine imaging data with clinical parameters, such as patient demographics and molecular biomarkers, enhance the robustness of predictions and guide personalized treatment decisions.

Radiomics-based predictive models further enhance ART by extracting high-dimensional imaging features and correlating them with treatment outcomes. For instance, radiomic analyses have identified early biomarkers, which are crucial for guiding dose escalation or de-escalation strategies [7,91,92]. These approaches also leverage "dosiomics," the analysis of dose distribution patterns, to refine predictions of normal tissue complications, including radiation dermatitis and xerostomia [92,93].

Predictive analytics also support clinical decision-making by estimating likely treatment outcomes and toxicity risks. AI algorithms that predict whether adaptive interventions will benefit specific patients can optimize resource use and treatment prioritization. Studies indicate that incorporating predictive models into ART workflows can improve tumor control rates and reduce treatment-related complications [92]. Moreover, multi-institutional datasets and harmonized imaging protocols are vital for enhancing model generalizability and encouraging widespread clinical adoption [91–93].

7.2.4 Real-Time Monitoring and Dose Adjustment in CT-Based ART

While CT-based ART relies on daily CBCT imaging to address inter-fractional changes, emerging AI-driven methodologies are expanding their capabilities to manage intrafractional motion, such as respiratory dynamics, gastrointestinal peristalsis, and transient patient shifts. These real-time or near real-time monitoring strategies aim to mitigate dosimetric uncertainties that arise from unaccounted anatomical motion, thereby preserving target coverage and minimizing dose to OARs. Though inherently constrained by the limited temporal resolution of CBCT compared to MRI-guided systems, recent advances in AI-enhanced imaging, predictive modeling, and markerless tracking are bridging this gap, aiming to facilitate real-time adaptation even in CT-based workflows.

7.2.4.1 Intra-Fraction Imaging and Motion Management

CT-based systems employ periodic kV/MV planar imaging or rapid CBCT acquisitions to monitor anatomical motion during treatment. These modalities are augmented by AI to improve tracking accuracy and reduce latency:

- Internal Fiducial Tracking: Radiopaque markers (e.g., gold seeds) implanted near tumors are tracked using kV/MV projections. Deep learning algorithms, such as CNNs, have been developed to enhance marker detection in low-contrast or artifact-prone images. For example, Liang et al. [94] demonstrated that a fully convolutional network (FCN)-based model achieved 98.6% and 95.6% fiducial identification precision and recall in orthogonal X-ray images from CyberKnife. The mean (±SD) centroid error between the predicted fiducial markers and the ground truth was 0.25 ± 0.47 pixels on the test data. However, fiducial placement is invasive, prompting interest in markerless tracking.

- Accelerated CBCT Imaging: Accelerated gantry rotation systems, such as the Halcyon 2.0, are capable of acquiring volumetric CBCT images in under 15 seconds. To mitigate motion artifacts and enhance image quality, artificial intelligence-driven reconstruction algorithms—specifically those combining compressed sensing with GANs—have been developed. AI-based reconstructions can reduce motion artifacts and shorten the time needed for image acquisition, thereby moving closer to real-time volumetric imaging. A feasibility study by Lu et al. [95] conducted a feasibility study demonstrating that a geometry-guided deep learning technique can rapidly and accurately reconstruct CBCT images from sparsely sampled data. While compressed sensing techniques have successfully reduced the number of required projections to achieve low-dose CBCT, the resulting image sparsity remains insufficient for real-time volumetric imaging demands. Consequently, recent efforts have focused on generating volumetric images from single X-ray projections using either two-dimensional–three-dimensional (2D–3D) registration techniques or ML approaches, often integrating a lung motion model as prior knowledge. Yang et al. [96] proposed TransNet, a GAN-based model designed to learn patient-specific 2D–3D transformations and generate volumetric images from a single projection. This approach holds the potential to enable real-time CBCT imaging during the delivery of lung stereotactic body radiation therapy (SBRT), thereby facilitating accurate and active motion management.

Beyond advancements in intra-fraction imaging, AI has been explored for tumor motion prediction during CT-based ART. Unlike reactive motion management strategies, AI enables proactive anticipation of tumor trajectories, facilitating real-time adjustments to beam delivery and dose distribution [97]. A common strategy involves viewing tumor motion as a temporal sequence problem. By capturing the dependencies between consecutive breathing cycles, RNNs—or their variants like Long Short-Term Memory (LSTM) networks—can learn to forecast short-term fluctuations in tumor position [98,99]. These models typically rely on historical intrafractional signals, including real-time kV/MV projection data or external surrogate signals (e.g., respiratory belts, surface markers), and then predict future tumor locations. For instance, Wang et al. [100] reported that an LSTM-based architecture could predict respiratory motion and internal liver motion 0.6 mm of ground truth, enabling beam gating with minimal latency. Besides simple point-based motion prediction, more advanced CNN-based frameworks focus on learning anatomical deformations directly from imaging data. These methods often incorporate patient-specific models derived from 4D CT scans or historical CBCT datasets. By continuously updating the learned deformation fields, the network anticipates how tumor and OAR geometries will evolve over the course of a breathing cycle. Edmunds et al. [101] proposed the use of Mask Region CNN (Mask R-CNN) to automate diaphragm segmentation in CBCT images for real-time lung tumor tracking. Trained on 3,499 raw CBCT projections from ten lung cancer patients, the model achieved robust diaphragm localization with a mean tracking error of 4.4 mm, requiring no manual intervention.

7.2.4.2 Dynamic Dose Adjustment via AI-Driven Automation

Dynamic dose adjustment in CT-based ART represents a critical frontier in minimizing geometric uncertainties and optimizing therapeutic outcomes. Once intrafractional anatomical shifts or deformations are detected, AI-driven systems enable rapid re-optimization of beam parameters to align dose delivery with real-time target and OAR configurations [102].

A primary challenge in real-time adaptation is the computational burden of accurate dose calculation. Traditional dose calculation methods, such as Monte Carlo simulations or convolution/superposition algorithms, are computationally intensive and impractical for real-time adaptation. In response, deep learning approaches have emerged as an effective tool, enabling rapid dose prediction while preserving dosimetric fidelity. DL-based dose calculation frameworks typically employ

CNNs to learn the complex relationship between patient anatomy, beam configuration, and resultant dose distribution [103,104]. The initial application of deep learning models was to boost the accuracy of pencil beam dose calculation to approach the accurate dose distribution calculated using the Monte-Carlo (MC) simulation [105]. Based on that, Fan et al. [106] developed a 3D deep residual U-Net to predict dose distributions directly from CT and fluence map inputs. The model first converts 2D fluence maps into 3D volumes using a ray traversal algorithm, which projects beamlet intensities along divergent ray lines to approximate 3D energy deposition. However, this approach faced challenges when applied to VMAT, where the MLC operates in dynamic mode, leading to more complex dose distributions. Additionally, projecting fluence maps onto 3D volumes introduced divergence effects, potentially omitting certain voxels and compromising dose accuracy. To overcome these limitations, Liang et al. [107] incorporated additional parameters such as projected fluence maps, CT images, radiological depth, and source-to-voxel distance into their models. Utilizing a dataset of 44 head and neck VMAT plans, their network achieved an average gamma pass rate of 98.75% under the criteria of 2% dose difference and 3 mm distance-to-agreement, demonstrating high fidelity to treatment planning system-calculated dose distributions.

Following the calculation of updated dose distributions, re-optimizing beam parameters is the next critical step. Traditional optimization algorithms often rely on iterative processes that can be time-intensive. Emerging AI methodologies address these limitations through data-driven automation, enabling sub-minute re-optimization with clinical-grade precision. KBP, widely adopted for initial treatment plan generation, has been extended to ART by leveraging historical plan libraries and ML models [22,23]. By training ML models on institutional repositories of high-quality plans, KBP systems predict optimal beam parameters (e.g., fluence maps, MLC sequences) that align with current anatomical geometries. In addition, RL has emerged as a transformative approach for autonomous beam parameter selection. RL agents, trained to maximize reward functions tied to dosimetric objectives (e.g., target coverage, OAR sparing), iteratively refine beam angles and MLC segments [87,90]. A detailed discussion of these methods is presented in Section 7.2.3.1.

7.2.5 Clinical Implementation (Ethos)

The Ethos platform (Varian Medical Systems), a leading commercial solution for CT-based online ART, was introduced in 2020 [12]. This platform integrates deep learning technologies to facilitate real-time anatomical segmentation, dose re-optimization, and QA. By streamlining online ART workflows, Ethos effectively addresses both inter- and intrafractional anatomical variations. A hallmark of the Ethos system is its ability to combine CBCT imaging with AI-driven automation, enabling on-table treatment adaptation within a time frame of 15–25 minutes per fraction [108]. This streamlined workflow encompasses several critical steps, including automated segmentation of anatomical structures, clinician review and optional editing of the auto-generated contours, plan re-optimization, dose calculation, and a comprehensive QA check [109,110]. The entire workflow is structured into three key stages:

7.2.5.1 High-quality CBCT Imaging

Obtaining high-quality images rapidly is essential for accurate auto-segmentation and efficient on-table adaptation within the limited treatment time available. Ethos employs the Halcyon 2.0 system, which utilizes iterative reconstruction techniques to produce high-quality CBCT images. These images are deemed acceptable for ART applications, supporting precise and reliable adaptation. Building on this capability, the integration of the new HyperSight imaging system introduces novel features, including an extended FOV of up to 70 cm and advanced reconstruction techniques that significantly enhance image quality [111]. HyperSight offers imaging acquisition in under 6 seconds, which is approximately ten times faster than [61] conventional linear-accelerator-based imaging systems [112]. This rapid imaging capability facilitates single-breath-hold scans, a critical feature for effective motion management in the treatment of thoracic and abdominal tumors.

Moreover, HyperSight enables dose calculations directly on the acquired CBCT images, eliminating the need for additional imaging registration.

7.2.5.2 Deep Learning Auto-Segmentation

Following the acquisition of daily CBCT images, the Ethos platform employs CNNs to automatically contour 70+ anatomical structures (targets and OARs) in real time. The auto-segmentation model has been trained on a diverse dataset collected from multiple clinical centers, ensuring its robustness and reliability across varied patient populations. The supervised learning framework used for neural network training utilized hundreds of images paired with ground-truth contours to optimize the model's performance. While clinicians retain the ability to revise these auto-generated contours, the high accuracy of the automated segmentation often minimizes the need for manual adjustments, significantly reducing the time required for contouring. For instance, in breast cancer, AI-generated contours for the critical structures achieved an average DSC exceeding 0.9, demonstrating high fidelity to expert-delineated contours. Additionally, the repeatability of the AI-based segmentation has been rigorously evaluated, with DSC values nearing 1 and mean Hausdorff 95% distances consistently below 0.15 mm [108]. These metrics highlight the precision and consistency of the auto-segmentation process, reinforcing its value in ART clinical workflows.

7.2.5.3 Treatment Planning Workflow

The Intelligent Optimization Engine (IOE) and RapidPlan are integral components of the Varian Ethos platform, a cutting-edge ART system. The automated treatment planning workflow in Ethos differs significantly from the conventional planning processes. The primary distinction lies in the automated optimization performed by the IOE, a core element of the Ethos TPS. The IOE automates and streamlines the generation of radiotherapy plans by translating a ranked and ordered list of clinical goals—representing the physician's intent—into optimization objectives [12,83]. This process incorporates additional heuristics and optimization structures that are managed internally by the system, beyond the user's direct control. Careful consideration of the ranked clinical goals is essential, as they are also used in generating online adaptive treatment plans that account for dosimetric trade-offs associated with daily anatomical variations. The IOE-driven optimization process facilitates intuitive decision-making by clinicians, enabling effective comparisons between scheduled and adapted plans based on dosimetric outcomes [113].

RapidPlan, a KBP tool, complements the IOE by utilizing ML algorithms trained on a database of prior clinical plans. It predicts achievable DVHs for new patients to guide plan optimization within the Ethos environment. However, the effectiveness of RapidPlan in this context depends on the construction and quality of the RapidPlan model. By offering institution-specific planning protocols, RapidPlan reduces inter-planner variability and enhances overall planning consistency. To ensure the quality of online ART treatments, the Ethos treatment unit integrates Mobius 3D-Adapt as an independent plan QA tool. In a retrospective study conducted by Zhao et al. [114], patient-specific QA for 16 adaptive plan sessions demonstrated a gamma passing rate of 99% (± 0.7%), highlighting the reliability of the system in delivering accurate and adaptive treatment plans.

Clinical implementations of Ethos have been reported across multiple disease sites, demonstrating the potential of AI-driven CT-based ART to improve both treatment precision and workflow efficiency. Several institutions have employed Ethos for daily adaptive prostate radiotherapy, a setting where bladder and rectal filling can shift the target substantially. Moazzezi et al. [39] reported that 96% of fractions for prostate treatments required edits to the auto-segmented contours. For the majority of patients, Ethos's online adaptive workflow improved CTV D98% coverage and reduced normal tissue doses, particularly in cases where the anatomy of the day might have led to dose metrics exceeding clinical thresholds. These improvements were achieved without requiring manual edits, demonstrating the efficiency and clinical utility of the Ethos platform. In head and neck cancer treatment, the Ethos system addresses the challenges posed by complex anatomy and dynamic changes in patient weight or tumor shrinkage. Case series have demonstrated that

Ethos-based adaptive treatments maintain robust tumor coverage while sparing critical structures such as the salivary glands and spinal cord. The AI contouring tools allow for precise adjustments in regions prone to significant anatomical variations, ensuring that dose prescriptions remain accurate throughout the course of treatment. Nasser et al. [115] evaluated the utility of online adaptation with the Ethos CBCT-guided system for head and neck cancer patients, reporting that online-adapted plans optimized dose distribution to the updated daily anatomy, maintained target coverage and homogeneity, and improved sparing of OARs in a time-efficient manner.

The successful implementation of the Ethos system necessitates a multidisciplinary team comprising radiation oncologists, medical physicists, dosimetrists, and radiation therapists, all proficient in AI-driven workflows. Comprehensive training protocols and well-defined standard operating procedures (SOPs) are essential to ensure that staff can efficiently manage daily adaptive tasks while accurately identifying potential errors. While the Varian Ethos system represents a significant advancement in ART, several limitations need attention. Current studies highlight challenges in AI-driven auto-segmentation accuracy for anatomically complex regions, such as overlapping structures (e.g., prostate–bladder interface) or post-surgical seromas in breast cancer, where manual corrections remain necessary [20,39,108]. Furthermore, the system's dependency on high-quality CBCT imaging introduces challenges in low-contrast regions (e.g., soft-tissue boundaries in head and neck cases), where segmentation errors may propagate into suboptimal dose distributions. To address these limitations, ongoing research focuses on two key strategies. First, federated learning frameworks aim to enhance the generalizability of AI models by training on multi-institutional datasets. Second, hybrid AI-human workflows are being developed to integrate clinician feedback, enabling real-time error correction and improving the robustness of adaptive planning. These initiatives hold promise for further refining the Ethos system and expanding its clinical utility.

7.3 MR-GUIDED ART AND AI APPLICATIONS

7.3.1 Overview of MR-Linac Technology

MRgART represents an advanced approach in radiation oncology, leveraging onboard MRI to refine and personalize radiation delivery based on anatomical and physiological changes throughout the treatment course. The integration of high-resolution MRI with radiation therapy offers several advantages over CT-based approaches, particularly in terms of superior soft-tissue contrast, real-time motion tracking, and precise treatment adaptation.

One of the primary limitations of CBCT-guided radiation therapy is its inadequate soft-tissue resolution, which can compromise the accurate delineation of target volumes and OARs. In contrast, onboard MRI in MR-guided radiotherapy systems enables superior soft-tissue visualization, thereby facilitating more precise tumor contouring. This is particularly beneficial for tumors in anatomically complex regions, such as the pancreas, prostate, and abdominal oligometastases, where improved tissue differentiation can enhance treatment accuracy and safety. Another key advantage of MRgART is its ability to acquire imaging data during radiation delivery. Unlike CBCT, which captures images before treatment and is susceptible to motion artifacts, MRI can continuously monitor anatomical structures during beam delivery without the need for implanted fiducials or external motion management devices. This real-time visualization capability enables more precise motion management through gated radiation delivery, where the beam is activated only when the target remains within a predefined boundary. This approach mitigates the need for large Planning Target Volume (PTV) expansions, thereby improving tumor targeting while minimizing radiation exposure to surrounding healthy tissues. The integration of MR-guided motion management strategies, such as deep inspiration or deep expiration breath-hold techniques, further refines treatment precision and reduces normal tissue toxicity.

Three MR-Linac systems are currently available or under development for MRgART: the ViewRay MRIdian, MagnetTx Aurora-RT, and Elekta Unity [13,17,116,117]. These systems integrate MRI with linear accelerators to enable real-time imaging and adaptive replanning, though their clinical adoption and technological maturity vary significantly. The MagnetTx Aurora-RT is a low-field (0.5 T) MR-Linac system designed with an open-bore, in-line geometry to mitigate the electron return effect. It received both Food and Drug Administration (FDA) and Conformité Européenne (CE) approvals, and began treatment in 2023 [118]. However, published clinical data on the Aurora-RT remain limited. Its open-bore design could offer ergonomic benefits for patient positioning and may simplify integration of additional hardware for motion management or treatment delivery. The ViewRay MRIdian system was one of the first low-field MRI-guided RT platforms to receive FDA clearance [119]. It combines a 0.35 T MRI scanner with a radiation delivery unit. Early versions employed three cobalt-60 sources mounted on a ring gantry to deliver radiation at a dose rate of 550 cGy/min. Later upgrades replaced the cobalt sources with a 6-MV flattening filter-free (FFF) linear accelerator capable of delivering at least 600 MU/min at a 90-cm isocenter. The low-field MRI environment of the MRIdian system reduces certain magnetic field effects—such as the electron return effect—and allows for continual soft-tissue imaging during beam delivery. A landmark innovation in this domain is the Elekta Unity MR-Linac (Elekta AB, Stockholm, Sweden), the first clinically deployed high-field (1.5 T) hybrid system integrating a 7-MV FFF linear accelerator with a Philips MRI scanner [16]. Approved for clinical use in 2018 (CE mark and FDA), the Unity system features a 70-cm bore diameter and a unique design where the radiation beam is perpendicular to the magnetic field orientation. Recent advancements, such as Elekta's Comprehensive Motion Management (CMM) system (released in 2023), have expanded motion management capabilities to include beam gating and multi-level respiratory tracking, addressing limitations of earlier versions restricted to tumor motion monitoring.

The online adapt-to-shape workflow of MRgART using the Elekta Unity system has been reported with a median treatment duration of 46 minutes (range: 31–85 minutes) for head and neck cancer [10]. This prolonged workflow underscores the need for AI-driven automation to enhance efficiency, streamline segmentation, and facilitate real-time treatment adaptation. While the integration of AI into CT-based ART has been extensively reviewed in Section 7.2, MRgART presents a distinct set of technical and clinical challenges that necessitate specialized AI solutions. The following sections will focus on AI applications specifically designed for MRgART, highlighting strategies that leverage MRI's strengths while addressing its inherent limitations, such as the absence of electron density information. AI methodologies that are conceptually similar to those already discussed in Section 7.2 will not be reiterated here but will instead be examined in the context of their adaptation to MRI-based workflows.

7.3.2 AI-Driven Applications for MRgART

7.3.2.1 Automated Segmentation and Contouring

Automated segmentation for MRgART builds upon many of the AI-driven techniques developed for CT-based auto-segmentation (see Section 7.2.2.1) while addressing the unique challenges and advantages of MRI-based workflows. The primary advantage of MRI over CT in segmentation is its superior soft-tissue contrast, which allows for more precise delineation of target volumes and OARs. This is particularly evident in prostate cancer, where T2-weighted MRI provides enhanced tumor conspicuity, reducing inter-observer variability and improving segmentation consistency compared to CT-based delineations.

Given the time-sensitive nature of online MRgART, automated segmentation solutions are critical for reducing physician workload and enhancing workflow efficiency [120]. Since the CNNs for MRI-based segmentation in 2017 [121], deep learning-based methods have consistently outperformed atlas-based and handcrafted segmentation methods. Similar to CT-based ART, significant advancements in MRgART have been achieved through deep learning models, mainly those based on the U-Net architecture, which has demonstrated superior accuracy in segmenting both tumors and normal tissues. A major challenge in MRgART is the need for rapid and accurate segmentation under strict time constraints while the patient remains on the treatment couch [120,122]. Furthermore, as fractionated treatment generates an increasing volume of imaging data with expert-delineated contours, there is a growing interest in developing patient-specific auto-segmentation models that incorporate prior knowledge from initial treatment planning to improve segmentation accuracy for subsequent fractions. Two main approaches have been proposed for patient-specific segmentation in MRgART:

Fine-Tuning a Baseline Model (BM): A cohort-based BM is first trained on a large dataset of patients with similar anatomical and pathological characteristics. This BM is then fine-tuned using a given patient's planning MRI and corresponding expert contours, allowing the model to adapt to patient-specific anatomical features. Moreover, imaging data and expert contours from previous fractions can be incorporated into an iterative fine-tuning process, progressively refining segmentation accuracy over the course of treatment [123–125].

Training a Patient-Specific Model from Scratch: Instead of relying on a pre-trained cohort-based BM, a unique model is trained exclusively on an individual patient's data. This model may be progressively updated throughout the treatment course, incorporating new fraction imaging and expert segmentations in a continuous learning process [126].

Both approaches have demonstrated improved performance over generalized segmentation models, yet each presents distinct trade-offs [122]. Patient-specific models can more effectively account for intra-patient anatomical variations, leading to improved segmentation accuracy within an individual treatment course. However, these models require continuous training, increasing computational demands, and may exhibit reduced performance in cases of substantial anatomical changes over time. Conversely, cohort-based models offer greater generalizability across patients but may lack the precision required for real-time adaptation during fractionated treatments.

Beyond anatomical imaging, MRI facilitates the integration of functional sequences, such as diffusion-weighted imaging (DWI) and dynamic contrast-enhanced (DCE) MRI, which provide complementary biological information. The incorporation of multiparametric MRI (mpMRI) data into segmentation workflows has been shown to enhance tissue differentiation, improving the identification of tumor subregions with distinct biological properties. By capturing both structural and physiological characteristics, mpMRI can refine auto-segmentation models, reducing reliance on manual contouring and mitigating inter-observer variability. Recent studies have explored the application of deep learning-based auto-segmentation using mpMRI data in the context of MRgART. Wahid et al. [127] investigated the use of mpMRI-based deep learning models for automatic segmentation of oropharyngeal cancer primary gross tumor volumes (GTVp), incorporating anatomical (T1-weighted, T2-weighted MRI) and functional imaging parameters (apparent diffusion coefficient [ADC], volume transfer constant [Ktrans], and extracellular extravascular volume fraction [Ve]). Their study demonstrated that multiparametric input channels improved segmentation accuracy, with the T2+T1 model outperforming other configurations in key evaluation metrics, including DSC, sensitivity, and surface distance measures. Notably, their best-performing model (T2+T1) produced segmentations that were indistinguishable from ground-truth delineations in a Turing test conducted with three expert radiation oncologists ($p > 0.05$). These findings highlight the potential of auto-segmentation leveraging mpMRI to enhance accuracy, robustness, and clinical consistency in MRgART.

7.3.2.2 Image Registration and Alignment

Robust DIR is a critical component of MRgART, as it enables the accurate spatial mapping of daily MR images to the reference CT image [10,128]. Accurate registration is important for the propagation of target and OAR contours, accurate dose recalculation, and reliable dose accumulation over successive treatment fractions. Although many of the fundamental principles underlying DIR are common to both CT- and MR-based ART, the intrinsic properties of MR imaging necessitate additional methodological refinements.

A primary difficulty in CT-to-MR registration arises from the significant contrast differences between the modalities. Unlike CT images, which offer relatively consistent intensity profiles, MR images are subject to a range of artifacts—such as geometric distortions, susceptibility effects, and signal inhomogeneities—that can significantly impact registration accuracy. These MR-specific imaging artifacts often confound conventional similarity metrics and necessitate additional pre-processing steps or specialized loss functions to ensure robust alignment [44,129]. Recent advances in AI have led to the development of deep learning-based registration algorithms that are specifically adapted for the MR images [42]. In these frameworks, network architectures are often augmented with domain adaptation strategies that account for the unique intensity distributions and artifacts encountered in MR imaging. For instance, specialized loss functions that reduce sensitivity to intensity fluctuations and distortions have been integrated into CNN models to more accurately learn complex, nonlinear DVFs. Additionally, multi-modality translation approaches have been proposed whereby GANs or translation models generate sCT images from MR images [130]. Such translation methods serve as an intermediary step that utilize the sCT to achieve the MR-to-CT DIR, thereby facilitating more accurate registration. Moreover, emerging transformer-based architectures have demonstrated an enhanced capacity to capture long-range spatial dependencies via self-attention mechanisms [55,131–133]. These architectures offer a potential advantage over conventional CNNs in modeling the global contextual relationships necessary for compensating MR-induced distortions, thereby yielding more anatomically consistent registrations.

7.3.2.3 Synthetic CT Generation

In current MR-guided radiotherapy workflows, patients undergo both CT and MR simulations prior to treatment planning. This dual-modality approach remains necessary because MR imaging alone cannot directly provide electron density information, which is essential for accurate radiation dose calculation and treatment planning [134]. However, in the context of MRgART—where real-time anatomical changes necessitate rapid plan adaptation—relying on pre-treatment CT scans is impractical. Instead, sCT generation from MRI has emerged as a fundamental component of the MRgART workflow, enabling accurate dose calculation and adaptive planning. Current approaches to sCT generation are broadly categorized into three methodologies: segmentation-based, atlas-based, and learning-based techniques [135–139]. Segmentation-based methods, which assign uniform bulk electron densities to anatomically segmented regions on MR images, are widely adopted in clinical practice due to their simplicity. However, their accuracy is inherently limited by the precision of manual or automated organ segmentation and their inability to account for intra-structural density variations.

Over the past several years, learning-based methods have attracted considerable attention, particularly those leveraging deep learning [140]. These techniques exploit large databases of paired MR and CT images to learn the complex, nonlinear mapping between the two modalities. In deep learning frameworks, CNNs are trained to convert MR images into sCT images without the need for manually extracted features. For example, a U-Net-based architecture was successfully used by Han et al. [141] to generate two-dimensional sCT images from T1-weighted MR images of the brain. Building on this concept, Nie et al. [142] developed a three-dimensional fully convolutional network that utilizes volumetric information to better capture the translation between MR and CT domains. Despite the improvements offered by CNN-based methods, challenges such as sensitivity to voxel-wise registration errors and the potential for image blurriness remain [143]. To overcome these issues, GAN approaches have been introduced [144]. In a GAN framework, a generator network produces sCT images while a discriminator network evaluates their realism, with an adversarial loss function jointly optimizing both networks to enhance image quality.

Conditional GANs further refine this process by constraining the output based on the input MR image [145]. A significant challenge for GAN-based methods is the requirement for perfectly co-registered MR and CT image pairs. To address this, CycleGAN [74] models have been developed; these models use cycle-consistency loss to enable training on unpaired image datasets, and studies have indicated that CycleGAN approaches can even outperform traditional GANs regarding sCT image quality. Recent investigations by multiple research groups have demonstrated that deep learning-based techniques for sCT generation can achieve high dosimetric accuracy for both low- and high-field MR-Linac systems across various anatomical sites [139,140,146,147]. Moreover, advancements in GPU technology have enabled the generation of sCT images in mere seconds per patient, underscoring the efficiency and potential for clinical integration. Indeed, the commercial introduction of an AI-based sCT solution by Siemens marks a significant milestone in this evolving technology.

This synthesis of advanced sCT generation methods illustrates a crucial step in improving the accuracy and efficiency of MRgART. By enabling precise electron density estimation directly from MRI data, sCT generation enhances dose calculation accuracy, ensuring more reliable treatment adaptation.

7.3.2.4 Real-Time MRI and Motion Management

Real-time imaging and dynamic motion management are central to the success of MRgART. These technologies enable continuous visualization of tumor and organ motion during treatment, thereby allowing for on-the-fly adaptations to account for physiological motion and minimize dose to healthy tissues [148]. Recent clinical adoption of MRI-Linac systems makes it possible to perform real-time MRI during treatment delivery [120,149]. Traditional MRI acquisition times are often prohibitive for real-time applications, with single-slice scans lasting up to 2 minutes and whole-volume acquisitions taking significantly longer [150]. To overcome this limitation, cine MRI has been adopted, reducing acquisition times to approximately 15 seconds or less per slice by employing techniques such as undersampling, increased slice thickness, and radial k-space sampling to mitigate motion artifacts. AI has played a promising role in advancing real-time MRI by both accelerating image reconstruction and enhancing the accuracy of motion prediction. Deep learning models—often based on U-Net or its variants—have been effectively deployed to reconstruct high-quality cine MRI images from highly undersampled k-space data [151,152]. These approaches not only shorten the reconstruction time but also improve spatial and temporal resolution, which is critical for precise target localization.

Physiologically induced motion—such as respiratory and cardiac cycles—introduces geometrical uncertainties that can compromise dose delivery, especially in the thorax and upper abdomen. Active motion management strategies, including gating and tracking, utilize real-time imaging data to continuously update the target position during treatment. In contrast to passive approaches or reliance on external surrogate markers, in-room imaging (e.g., cine MRI) allows for direct and accurate target localization. AI methods have been developed to support active motion management [122]. Deep learning models have demonstrated proficiency in automatically segmenting tumors on cine MRI, rapidly delineating targets with high precision [153,154]. In addition, models have been developed to predict organ motion [155,156]. Methods employing autoregressive models and LSTM networks have been used to forecast the movement of key anatomical landmarks [157], such as the diaphragm, thereby facilitating the generation of matching 4D MRI volumes in real time [158,159]. Other studies have focused on direct estimation of DVFs using CNNs or residual network structures, which capture dynamic organ deformations during treatment [120]. In some cases, transformer-based architectures have been integrated to predict subsequent image slices, further enhancing temporal prediction accuracy. Collectively, these AI-driven approaches enable more robust tracking of tumor and organ motion, ultimately contributing to improved treatment precision.

7.4 CONCLUSION

In conclusion, this chapter has demonstrated that the integration of AI into ART is a major advancement to redefine personalized cancer treatment. The evidence presented underscores the potential of AI to enhance treatment precision, streamline clinical workflows, and ultimately improve patient outcomes by enabling real-time adaptation to dynamic anatomical changes. Moving forward, several key strategic imperatives emerge: First, future investigations must prioritize the development of robust, transparent, and adaptable AI algorithms. Second, emphasis should be placed on improving real-time image reconstruction and motion management techniques, and on rigorously validating these models across diverse patient populations. Last, collaborative efforts to establish large, representative datasets and to standardize imaging protocols and data formats are essential for reducing bias and uncertainty in AI performance.

The successful integration of AI into ART relies on close collaboration among radiation oncologists, medical physicists, data scientists, and engineers. Such interdisciplinary partnerships will facilitate the seamless incorporation of AI into routine clinical workflows—from automated segmentation and treatment planning to adaptive dose recalculation and quality assurance—thereby promoting highly personalized and efficient care. Establishing targeted training programs and certification pathways will be critical in equipping healthcare professionals with the necessary expertise to safely and effectively utilize these advanced technologies. Continuous innovation, promoting interdisciplinary collaboration, and rigorously upholding ethical standards will be critical to achieve the full potential of AI. This integrated approach will drive the next generation of personalized cancer care, ensuring that the benefits of AI in ART are realized in ways that enhance both clinical outcomes and the overall quality of patient care.

REFERENCES

1. Schwartz, D.L.; Garden, A.S.; Shah, S.J.; Chronowski, G.; Sejpal, S.; Rosenthal, D.I.; Chen, Y.; Zhang, Y.; Zhang, L.; Wong, P.-F. Adaptive Radiotherapy for Head and Neck Cancer—Dosimetric Results from a Prospective Clinical Trial. *Radiotherapy and Oncology* **2013**, *106*, 80–84.
2. Schwartz, D.L.; Garden, A.S.; Thomas, J.; Chen, Y.; Zhang, Y.; Lewin, J.; Chambers, M.S.; Dong, L. Adaptive Radiotherapy for Head-and-Neck Cancer: Initial Clinical Outcomes from a Prospective Trial. *International Journal of Radiation Oncology, Biology, Physics* **2012**, *83*, 986–993.
3. Castelli, J.; Simon, A.; Louvel, G.; Henry, O.; Chajon, E.; Nassef, M.; Haigron, P.; Cazoulat, G.; Ospina, J.D.; Jegoux, F. Impact of Head and Neck Cancer Adaptive Radiotherapy to Spare the Parotid Glands and Decrease the Risk of Xerostomia. *Radiation Oncology* **2015**, *10*, 1–10.
4. Shen-qu, L. New Advance of Precise Radiotherapy: Image-Guided Adaptive Radiation Therapy. *Chinese Journal of Medical Physics* **2012**, 29(4), 5.
5. Jones, S.; Thompson, K.; Porter, B.; Shepherd, M.; Sapkaroski, D.; Grimshaw, A.; Hargrave, C. Automation and Artificial Intelligence in Radiation Therapy Treatment Planning. *Journal of Medical Radiation Sciences* **2023**, *71*, 290–298, doi:10.1002/jmrs.729.
6. Jeong, C.; Goh, Y.; Kwak, J. Challenges and Opportunities to Integrate Artificial Intelligence in Radiation Oncology: A Narrative Review. *The Ewha Medical Journal* **2024**, doi:10.12771/emj.2024.e49.
7. Kawamura, M.; Kamomae, T.; Yanagawa, M.; Kamagata, K.; Fujita, S.; Ueda, D.; Matsui, Y.; Fushimi, Y.; Fujioka, T.; Nozaki, T.; et al. Revolutionizing Radiation Therapy: The Role of AI in Clinical Practice. *Journal of Radiation Research* **2023**, *65*, 1–9, doi:10.1093/jrr/rrad090.
8. Piperdi, H.; Portal, D.; Neibart, S.; Yue, N.; Jabbour, S.; Reyhan, M. Adaptive Radiation Therapy in the Treatment of Lung Cancer: An Overview of the Current State of the Field. *Frontiers in Oncology* **2021**, *11*, doi:10.3389/fonc.2021.770382.
9. Kashani, R. MO-E-BRC-01: Online Adaptive MR-Guided RT: Workflow and Clinical Implementation. *Medical Physics* **2016**, *436*, doi:10.1118/1.4957269.
10. McDonald, B.A.; Vedam, S.; Yang, J.; Wang, J.; Castillo, P.; Lee, B.; Sobremonte, A.; Ahmed, S.; Ding, Y.; Mohamed, A.S.R.; et al. Initial Feasibility and Clinical Implementation of Daily MR-Guided Adaptive Head and Neck Cancer Radiation Therapy on a 1.5T MR-Linac System: Prospective R-IDEAL 2a/2b Systematic Clinical Evaluation of Technical Innovation. *International Journal of Radiation Oncology*Biology*Physics* **2021**, *109*, 1606–1618, doi:10.1016/j.ijrobp.2020.12.015.

11. Prunaretty, J.; Mekki, F.; Laurent, P.-I.; Morel, A.; Hinault, P.; Bourgier, C.; Azria, D.; Fenoglietto, P. Clinical Feasibility of Ethos Auto-Segmentation for Adaptive Whole-Breast Cancer Treatment. *Frontiers in Oncology* **2024**, *14*, 1507806, doi:10.3389/fonc.2024.1507806.
12. Byrne, M.; Archibald-Heeren, B.; Hu, Y.; Teh, A.; Beserminji, R.; Cai, E.; Liu, G.; Yates, A.; Rijken, J.; Collett, N.; et al. Varian Ethos Online Adaptive Radiotherapy for Prostate Cancer: Early Results of Contouring Accuracy, Treatment Plan Quality, and Treatment Time. *Journal of Applied Clinical Medical Physics* **2021**, *23*, e13479, doi:10.1002/acm2.13479.
13. Guckenberger, M.; Andratschke, N.; Chung, C.; Fuller, D.; Tanadini-Lang, S.; Jaffray, D.A. The Future of MR-Guided Radiation Therapy. *Seminars in Radiation Oncology* **2024** Jan; *34*(1):135–144. doi: 10.1016/j.semradonc.2023.10.015. PMID: 38105088.
14. Cusumano, D.; Boldrini, L.; Dhont, J.; Fiorino, C.; Green, O.; Güngör, G.; Jornet, N.; Klüter, S.; Landry, G.; Mattiucci, G.C. Artificial Intelligence in Magnetic Resonance Guided Radiotherapy: Medical and Physical Considerations on State of Art and Future Perspectives. *Physica Medica* **2021**, *85*, 175–191.
15. Glide-Hurst, C.K.; Lee, P.; Yock, A.D.; Olsen, J.R.; Cao, M.; Siddiqui, F.; Parker, W.; Doemer, A.; Rong, Y.; Kishan, A.U.; et al. Adaptive Radiation Therapy (ART) Strategies and Technical Considerations: A State of the ART Review from NRG Oncology. *International Journal of Radiation Oncology, Biology, Physics* **2021**, *109*, 1054–1075, doi:10.1016/j.ijrobp.2020.10.021.
16. Winkel, D.; Bol, G.H.; Kroon, P.S.; van Asselen, B.; Hackett, S.S.; Werensteijn-Honingh, A.M.; Intven, M.P.W.; Eppinga, W.S.C.; Tijssen, R.H.N.; Kerkmeijer, L.G.W.; et al. Adaptive Radiotherapy: The Elekta Unity MR-Linac Concept. *Clinical and Translational Radiation Oncology* **2019**, *18*, 54–59, doi:10.1016/j.ctro.2019.04.001.
17. Okamoto, H.; Sakasai, T.; Nishioka, S.; Miura, Y.; Aikawa, A.; Kuwahara, J.; Iijima, K.; Abe, Y.; Igaki, H.; Itami, J. [On-Line Adaptive Radiotherapy Using MRI-Guided Technique]. *Igaku butsuri : Nihon Igaku Butsuri Gakkai kikanshi = Japanese Journal of Medical Physics : An Official Journal of Japan Society of Medical Physics* **2019**, *38 4*, 159–165, doi:10.11323/jjmp.38.4_159.
18. Takahashi, N.; Tanaka, S.; Umezawa, R.; Yamamoto, T.; Suzuki, Y.; Kishida, K.; Omata, S.; Arai, K.; Katsuta, Y.; Kadoya, N.; et al. Beginning of Clinical Treatment Using the 1.5 Tesla MR-Linac System in Japan: A Narrative Review. *Translational Cancer Research* **2024**, *13*, 1131–1138, doi:10.21037/tcr-23–1649.
19. Bosse, C.; Narayanasamy, G.; Saenz, D.; Myers, P.; Kirby, N.; Rasmussen, K.; Mavroidis, P.; Papanikolaou, N.; Stathakis, S. Dose Calculation Comparisons between Three Modern Treatment Planning Systems. *Journal of Medical Physics* **2020**, *45*, 143–147, doi:10.4103/jmp.JMP_111_19.
20. Sibolt, P.; Andersson, L.; Calmels, L.; Sjöström, D.; Bjelkengren, U.; Geertsen, P.; Behrens, C. Clinical Implementation of Artificial Intelligence-Driven Cone-Beam Computed Tomography-Guided Online Adaptive Radiotherapy in the Pelvic Region. *Physics and Imaging in Radiation Oncology* **2020**, *17*, 1–7, doi:10.1016/j.phro.2020.12.004.
21. Zhu, L.; Han, Y.; Xi, X.; Fu, H.; Tan, S.; Liu, M.; Yang, S.; Liu, C.; Li, L.; Yan, B. STEDNet: Swin Transformer-Based Encoder-Decoder Network for Noise Reduction in Low-Dose CT. *Medical Physics* **2023**, doi:10.1002/mp.16249.
22. Wortel, G.; Eekhout, D.; Lamers, E.; van der Bel, R.; Kiers, K.; Wiersma, T.; Janssen, T.; Damen, E. Characterization of Automatic Treatment Planning Approaches in Radiotherapy. *Physics and Imaging in Radiation Oncology* **2021**, *19*, 60–65, doi:10.1016/j.phro.2021.07.003.
23. Chung, C.V.; Khan, M.S.; Olanrewaju, A.; Pham, M.; Nguyen, Q.T.; Patel, T.; Das, P.; O'Reilly, M.S.; Reed, V.K.; Jhingran, A.; et al. Knowledge-Based Planning for Fully Automated Radiation Therapy Treatment Planning of 10 Different Cancer Sites. *Radiotherapy and Oncology* **2025**, *202*, 110609, doi:10.1016/j.radonc.2024.110609.
24. Sheng, Y.; Zhang, J.; Ge, Y.; Li, X.; Wang, W.; Stephens, H.; Yin, F.; Wu, Q.; Wu, Q.J. Artificial Intelligence Applications in Intensity Modulated Radiation Treatment Planning: An Overview. *Quantitative Imaging in Medicine and Surgery* **2021**, *11 12*, 4859–4880, doi:10.21037/qims-21–208.
25. Bayat, F.; Ruan, D.; Miften, M.; Altunbas, C. 2D Antiscatter Grid and Scatter Sampling Based CBCT Pipeline for Image Guided Radiation Therapy. *ArXiv* **2023**. https://arxiv.org/pdf/2308.09095
26. Bissonnette, J.-P.; Balter, P.A.; Dong, L.; Langen, K.M.; Lovelock, D.M.; Miften, M.; Moseley, D.J.; Pouliot, J.; Sonke, J.-J.; Yoo, S. Quality Assurance for Image-guided Radiation Therapy Utilizing CT-based Technologies: A Report of the AAPM TG-179. *Medical Physics* **2012**, *39*, 1946–1963.
27. Klein, E.E.; Hanley, J.; Bayouth, J.; Yin, F.-F.; Simon, W.; Dresser, S.; Serago, C.; Aguirre, F.; Ma, L.; Arjomandy, B. Task Group 142 Report: Quality Assurance of Medical Accelerators a. *Medical Physics* **2009**, *36*, 4197–4212.

28. Fung, N.T.C.; Hung, W.M.; Sze, C.K.; Lee, M.C.H.; Ng, W.T. Automatic Segmentation for Adaptive Planning in Nasopharyngeal Carcinoma IMRT: Time, Geometrical, and Dosimetric Analysis. *Medical Dosimetry* **2020**, *45*, 60–65, doi:10.1016/j.meddos.2019.06.002.
29. Ronneberger, O.; Fischer, P.; Brox, T. U-Net: Convolutional Networks for Biomedical Image Segmentation. In Navab, N., Hornegger, J., Wells, W., Frangi, A. (eds) *Medical Image Computing and Computer-Assisted Intervention – MICCAI 2015*. MICCAI 2015. Lecture Notes in Computer Science, Springer, Cham, 2015; Vol. 9351. https://doi.org/10.1007/978-3-319-24574-4_28.
30. He, K.; Zhang, X.; Ren, S.; Sun, J. Deep Residual Learning for Image Recognition. In *2016 IEEE Conference on Computer Vision and Pattern Recognition (CVPR)*, Las Vegas, NV, USA, 2016, pp. 770–778.
31. Isensee, F.; Jaeger, P.F.; Kohl, S.A.A.; Petersen, J.; Maier-Hein, K.H. nnU-Net: A Self-Configuring Method for Deep Learning-Based Biomedical Image Segmentation. *Nature Methods* **2021**, *18*, 203–211, doi:10.1038/s41592-020-01008-z.
32. Sherer, M.V.; Lin, D.; Elguindi, S.; Duke, S.; Tan, L.-T.; Cacicedo, J.; Dahele, M.; Gillespie, E.F. Metrics to Evaluate the Performance of Auto-Segmentation for Radiation Treatment Planning: A Critical Review. *Radiotherapy and Oncology* **2021**, *160*, 185–191, doi:10.1016/j.radonc.2021.05.003.
33. Yashayaeva, A.; MacDonald, R.L.; Cherpak, A. Body Contour Adaptation for Weight-loss and Bolus for Head and Neck Radiotherapy on Ethos Version 2.0 and HyperSight: Synthetic CT versus Direct Calculation. *The Journal of Applied Clinical Medical Physics* **2024**, e14587, doi:10.1002/acm2.14587.
34. Radici, L.; Piva, C.; Casanova Borca, V.; Cante, D.; Ferrario, S.; Paolini, M.; Cabras, L.; Petrucci, E.; Franco, P.; La Porta, M.R.; et al. Clinical Evaluation of a Deep Learning CBCT Auto-Segmentation Software for Prostate Adaptive Radiation Therapy. *Clinical and Translational Radiation Oncology* **2024**, *47*, 100796, doi:10.1016/j.ctro.2024.100796.
35. Sluijter, J.H.; Van De Schoot, A.J.A.J.; Yaakoubi, A.E.; De Jong, M.; Van Der Knaap - Van Dongen, M.S.; Kunnen, B.; Sijtsema, N.D.; Penninkhof, J.J.; De Vries, K.C.; Petit, S.F.; et al. Evaluation of Artificial Intelligence-Based Autosegmentation for a High-Performance Cone-Beam Computed Tomography Imaging System in the Pelvic Region. *Physics and Imaging in Radiation Oncology* **2025**, *33*, 100687, doi:10.1016/j.phro.2024.100687.
36. Chapman, J.W.; Lam, D.; Cai, B.; Hugo, G.D. Robustness and Reproducibility of an Artificial Intelligence-assisted Online Segmentation and Adaptive Planning Process for Online Adaptive Radiation Therapy. *Journal of Applied Clinical Medical Physics* **2022**, *23*, e13702, doi:10.1002/acm2.13702.
37. Ma, C.; Zhou, J.; Xu, X.; Qin, S.; Han, M.; Cao, X.; Gao, Y.; Xu, L.; Zhou, J.; Zhang, W.; et al. Clinical Evaluation of Deep Learning–Based Clinical Target Volume Three-Channel Auto-Segmentation Algorithm for Adaptive Radiotherapy in Cervical Cancer. *BMC Medical Imaging* **2022**, *22*, 123, doi:10.1186/s12880-022-00851-0.
38. Rigaud, B.; Anderson, B.M.; Yu, Z.H.; Gobeli, M.; Cazoulat, G.; Söderberg, J.; Samuelsson, E.; Lidberg, D.; Ward, C.; Taku, N.; et al. Automatic Segmentation Using Deep Learning to Enable Online Dose Optimization During Adaptive Radiation Therapy of Cervical Cancer. *International Journal of Radiation Oncology*Biology*Physics* **2021**, *109*, 1096–1110, doi:10.1016/j.ijrobp.2020.10.038.
39. Moazzezi, M.; Rose, B.; Kisling, K.; Moore, K.L.; Ray, X. Prospects for Daily Online Adaptive Radiotherapy via Ethos for Prostate Cancer Patients without Nodal Involvement Using Unedited CBCT Auto-Segmentation. *Journal Applied Clin Med Phys* **2021**, *22*, 82–93, doi:10.1002/acm2.13399.
40. Mao, W.; Riess, J.; Kim, J.; Vance, S.; Chetty, I.J.; Movsas, B.; Kretzler, A. Evaluation of Auto-Contouring and Dose Distributions for Online Adaptive Radiation Therapy of Patients With Locally Advanced Lung Cancers. *Practical Radiation Oncology* **2022**, *12*, e329–e338, doi:10.1016/j.prro.2021.12.017.
41. Chen, Y.; Gensheimer, M.F.; Bagshaw, H.P.; Butler, S.; Yu, L.; Zhou, Y.; Shen, L.; Kovalchuk, N.; Surucu, M.; Chang, D.T.; et al. Patient-Specific Auto-Segmentation on Daily kVCT Images for Adaptive Radiation Therapy. *International Journal of Radiation Oncology*Biology*Physics* **2023**, *117*, 505–514, doi:10.1016/j.ijrobp.2023.04.026.
42. Fu, Y.; Lei, Y.; Wang, T.; Curran, W.J.; Liu, T.; Yang, X. Deep Learning in Medical Image Registration: A Review. *Physics in Medicine and Biology* **2020**, *65*, 20TR01, doi:10.1088/1361–6560/ab843e.
43. Boveiri, H.R.; Khayami, R.; Javidan, R.; Mehdizadeh, A. Medical Image Registration Using Deep Neural Networks: A Comprehensive Review. *Computers & Electrical Engineering* **2020**, *87*, 106767, doi:10.1016/j.compeleceng.2020.106767.
44. Brock, K.K.; Mutic, S.; McNutt, T.R.; Li, H.; Kessler, M.L. Use of Image Registration and Fusion Algorithms and Techniques in Radiotherapy: Report of the AAPM Radiation Therapy Committee Task Group No. 132. *Medical Physics* **2017**, *44*, e43–e76, doi:10.1002/mp.12256.

45. Lakshmi, K.; Vaithiyanathan, V. Study of Feature Based Image Registration Algorithms for Navigation of Unmanned Aerial Vehicles. *Indian Journal of Science and Technology* **2015**, *8*, 1–7, doi:10.17485/IJST/2015/V8I22/79315.
46. Ito, M.; Ino, F. An Automated Method for Generating Training Sets for Deep Learning Based Image Registration. In *Proceedings of the 11th International Joint Conference on Biomedical Engineering Systems and Technologies – Volume 2: BIOSTEC*, Funchal, Madeira, Portugal, **2018**, pp. 140–147, doi:10.5220/0006634501400147.
47. Kuckertz, S.; Papenberg, N.; Honegger, J.; Morgas, T.; Haas, B.; Heldmann, S. Abstract: Deep Learning Based CT-CBCT Image Registration for Adaptive Radio Therapy. *Proc. SPIE 11313, Medical Imaging 2020: Image Processing*, 113130Q, 2020, Houston, Texas, United States.
48. Balakrishnan, G.; Zhao, A.; Sabuncu, M.R.; Guttag, J.; Dalca, A.V. VoxelMorph: A Learning Framework for Deformable Medical Image Registration. *IEEE Transactions on Medical Imaging* **2019**, *38*, 1788–1800, doi:10.1109/TMI.2019.2897538.
49. Jaderberg, M.; Simonyan, K.; Zisserman, A.; kavukcuoglu, koray Spatial Transformer Networks. In Cortes, C., Lawrence, N.D., Lee, D.D., Sugiyama, M., Garnett, R. (eds.) *Advances in Neural Information Processing Systems 28*; Curran Associates, Inc., 2015; pp. 2017–2025.
50. Xie, H.; Lei, Y.; Wang, T.; Fu, Y.; Tang, X.; Curran, W.; Patel, P.; Liu, T.; Yang, X. Deep Learning-Based Deformable Image Registration of Inter-Fraction CBCT Images for Adaptive Radiation Therapy. **2021**, *11596*, 115962–115962, doi:10.1117/12.2581083.
51. Liang, X.; Bibault, J.-E.; Leroy, T.; Escande, A.; Zhao, W.; Chen, Y.; Buyyounouski, M.K.; Hancock, S.L.; Bagshaw, H.; Xing, L. Automated Contour Propagation of the Prostate from pCT to CBCT Images via Deep Unsupervised Learning. *Medical Physics* **2021**, *48*, 1764–1770, doi:10.1002/mp.14755.
52. Hu, R.; Yan, H.; Nian, F.; Mao, R.; Li, T. Unsupervised Computed Tomography and Cone-Beam Computed Tomography Image Registration Using a Dual Attention Network. *Quantitative Imaging in Medicine and Surgery* **2022**, *12*, 3705–3716, doi:10.21037/qims-21–1194.
53. Cao, Y.; Fu, T.; Duan, L.; Dai, Y.; Gong, L.; Cao, W.; Liu, D.; Yang, X.; Ni, X.; Zheng, J. CDFRegNet: A Cross-Domain Fusion Registration Network for CT-to-CBCT Image Registration. *Computer Methods and Programs in Biomedicine* **2022**, *224*, 107025, doi:10.1016/j.cmpb.2022.107025.
54. Zhu, Y.; Lu, S. Swin-VoxelMorph: A Symmetric Unsupervised Learning Model for Deformable Medical Image Registration Using Swin Transformer. In Wang, L., Dou, Q., Fletcher, P.T., Speidel, S., Li, S. (eds.) *Proceedings of the Medical Image Computing and Computer Assisted Intervention – MICCAI 2022*, Springer Nature: Cham, 2022; pp. 78–87.
55. Chen, J.; Frey, E.C.; He, Y.; Segars, W.P.; Li, Y.; Du, Y. Transmorph: Transformer for Unsupervised Medical Image Registration. *Medical Image Analysis* **2022**, *82*, 102615.
56. Liu, Z.; Lin, Y.; Cao, Y.; Hu, H.; Wei, Y.; Zhang, Z.; Lin, S.; Guo, B. Swin Transformer: Hierarchical Vision Transformer Using Shifted Windows. *2021 IEEE/CVF International Conference on Computer Vision (ICCV)*, Montreal, QC, Canada, **2021**, pp. 9992-10002, doi: 10.1109/ICCV48922.2021.00986.
57. Goodfellow, I.J.; Pouget-Abadie, J.; Mirza, M.; Xu, B.; Warde-Farley, D.; Ozair, S.; Courville, A.; Bengio, Y. Generative Adversarial Networks. *Commun. ACM 63*, 11 (November 2020). **2014**, 139–144. https://doi.org/10.1145/3422622
58. Liang, X.; Morgan, H.; Nguyen, D.; Jiang, S. Deep Learning Based CT-to-CBCT Deformable Image Registration for Autosegmentation in Head and Neck Adaptive Radiation Therapy. *Journal of Artificial Intelligence for Medical Sciences* **2021**, *2*, 62–75.
59. Wang, J.; Li, T.; Xing, L. Iterative Image Reconstruction for CBCT Using Edge-preserving Prior. *Medical Physics* **2009**, *36*, 252–260, doi:10.1118/1.3036112.
60. Zbijewski, W.; Beekman, F.J. Efficient Monte Carlo Based Scatter Artifact Reduction in Cone-Beam Micro-CT. *IEEE Transactions on Medical Imaging* **2006**, *25*, 817–827, doi:10.1109/TMI.2006.872328.
61. Zhang, Y.; Yue, N.; Su, M.; Liu, B.; Ding, Y.; Zhou, Y.; Wang, H.; Kuang, Y.; Nie, K. Improving CBCT Quality to CT Level Using Deep Learning with Generative Adversarial Network. *Medical Physics* **2021**, *48*, 2816–2826, doi:10.1002/mp.14624.
62. Jin, D.S.-C.; Chang, L.-S.; Wang, Y.-H.; Chen, J.-C.; Tseng, S.H.; Liu, T.-Y. Virtual and Real-World Implementation of Deep-Learning-Based Image Denoising Model on Projection Domain in Digital Tomosynthesis and Cone-Beam Computed Tomography Data. *Biomedical Physics & Engineering Express* **2022**, *8*, 065021, doi:10.1088/2057-1976/ac997d.
63. Kurosawa, T.; Nishio, T.; Moriya, S.; Tsuneda, M.; Karasawa, K. Feasibility of Image Quality Improvement for High-Speed CBCT Imaging Using Deep Convolutional Neural Network for Image-Guided Radiotherapy in Prostate Cancer. *Physica Medica* **2020**, *80*, 84–91, doi:10.1016/j.ejmp.2020.10.012.

64. Kofler, A.; Haltmeier, M.; Schaeffter, T.; Kachelrieß, M.; Dewey, M.; Wald, C.; Kolbitsch, C. Neural Networks-Based Regularization for Large-Scale Medical Image Reconstruction. *Physics Medicine and Biology* **2020**, *65*, 135003, doi:10.1088/1361–6560/ab990e.
65. Schnurr, A.-K.; Chung, K.; Russ, T.; Schad, L.R.; Zöllner, F.G. Simulation-Based Deep Artifact Correction with Convolutional Neural Networks for Limited Angle Artifacts. *Zeitschrift für Medizinische Physik* **2019**, *29*, 150–161, doi:10.1016/j.zemedi.2019.01.002.
66. Wang, Y.; Yang, T.; Huang, W. Limited-Angle Computed Tomography Reconstruction Using Combined FDK-Based Neural Network and U-Net. In *Proceedings of the 2020 42nd Annual International Conference of the IEEE Engineering in Medicine & Biology Society (EMBC)*; IEEE: Montreal, QC, Canada, July 2020; pp. 1572–1575.
67. Rossi, M.; Belotti, G.; Paganelli, C.; Pella, A.; Barcellini, A.; Cerveri, P.; Baroni, G. Image-based Shading Correction for narrow-FOV Truncated Pelvic CBCT with Deep Convolutional Neural Networks and Transfer Learning. *Medical Physics* **2021**, *48*, 7112–7126, doi:10.1002/mp.15282.
68. Wang, X.; Jian, W.; Zhang, B.; Zhu, L.; He, Q.; Jin, H.; Yang, G.; Cai, C.; Meng, H.; Tan, X.; et al. Synthetic CT Generation from Cone-Beam CT Using Deep-Learning for Breast Adaptive Radiotherapy. *Journal of Radiation Research and Applied Sciences* **2022**, *15*, 275–282, doi:10.1016/j.jrras.2022.03.009.
69. Cao, Z.; Gao, X.; Chang, Y.; Liu, G.; Pei, Y. A Novel Approach for Eliminating Metal Artifacts Based on MVCBCT and CycleGAN. *Frontiers Oncology* **2022**, *12*, 1024160, doi:10.3389/fonc.2022.1024160.
70. Baroudi, H.; Chen, X.; Cao, W.; El Basha, M.D.; Gay, S.; Gronberg, M.P.; Hernandez, S.; Huang, K.; Kaffey, Z.; Melancon, A.D.; et al. Synthetic Megavoltage Cone Beam Computed Tomography Image Generation for Improved Contouring Accuracy of Cardiac Pacemakers. *Journal of Imaging* **2023**, *9*, 245, doi:10.3390/jimaging9110245.
71. Zhi, S.; Duan, J.; Cai, J.; Mou, X. Artifacts Reduction Method for Phase-Resolved Cone-Beam CT (CBCT) Images via a Prior-Guided CNN. In Bosmans, H., Chen, G.-H., Gilat Schmidt, T. (eds.) *Proceedings of the Medical Imaging 2019: Physics of Medical Imaging*; SPIE: San Diego, USA, March 1 2019; p. 79.
72. Zhang, Z.; Liu, J.; Yang, D.; Kamilov, U.S.; Hugo, G.D. Deep Learning-based Motion Compensation for Four-dimensional Cone-beam Computed Tomography (4D-CBCT) Reconstruction. *Medical Physics* **2023**, *50*, 808–820, doi:10.1002/mp.16103.
73. Thummerer, A.; Seller Oria, C.; Zaffino, P.; Visser, S.; Meijers, A.; Guterres Marmitt, G.; Wijsman, R.; Seco, J.; Langendijk, J.A.; Knopf, A.C.; et al. Deep Learning–Based 4D-synthetic CTs from Sparse-view CBCTs for Dose Calculations in Adaptive Proton Therapy. *Medical Physics* **2022**, *49*, 6824–6839, doi:10.1002/mp.15930.
74. Zhu, J.-Y.; Park, T.; Isola, P.; Efros, A.A. Unpaired Image-to-Image Translation Using Cycle-Consistent Adversarial Networks. *2017 IEEE International Conference on Computer Vision (ICCV)*, Venice, Italy, **2017**, pp. 2242–2251, doi: 10.1109/ICCV.2017.244.
75. Dahiya, N.; Alam, S.R.; Zhang, P.; Zhang, S.; Li, T.; Yezzi, A.; Nadeem, S. Multitask 3D CBCT-to-CT Translation and Organs-at-risk Segmentation Using Physics-based Data Augmentation. *Medical Physics* **2021**, *48*, 5130–5141, doi:10.1002/mp.15083.
76. Kim, J.; Chae, S.-H.; Kim, B.; Baek, J.; Maier, A.; Fahrig, R.; Park, H.-S.; Choi, D.; Choi, J.-H. Multidimensional Noise Reduction in C-Arm Cone-Beam CT via 2D-Based Landweber Iteration and 3D-Based Deep Neural Networks. In Bosmans, H., Chen, G.-H., Gilat Schmidt, T. (eds.) *Proceedings of the Medical Imaging 2019: Physics of Medical Imaging*; SPIE: San Diego, USA, March 1 2019; p. 114.
77. Wei, R.; Liu, B.; Zhou, F.; Bai, X.; Fu, D.; Liang, B.; Wu, Q. A Patient-Independent CT Intensity Matching Method Using Conditional Generative Adversarial Networks (cGAN) for Single X-Ray Projection-Based Tumor Localization. *Physics in Medicine and Biology* **2020**, *65*, 145009, doi:10.1088/1361–6560/ab8bf2.
78. Kida, S.; Kaji, S.; Nawa, K.; Imae, T.; Nakamoto, T.; Ozaki, S.; Ohta, T.; Nozawa, Y.; Nakagawa, K. Visual Enhancement of Cone-beam CT by Use of CycleGAN. *Medical Physics* **2020**, *47*, 998–1010, doi:10.1002/mp.13963.
79. Usui, K.; Ogawa, K.; Goto, M.; Sakano, Y.; Kyougoku, S.; Daida, H. A Cycle Generative Adversarial Network for Improving the Quality of Four-Dimensional Cone-Beam Computed Tomography Images. *Radiation Oncology* **2022**, *17*, 69, doi:10.1186/s13014-022-02042-1.
80. Kurz, C.; Maspero, M.; Savenije, M.H.F.; Landry, G.; Kamp, F.; Pinto, M.; Li, M.; Parodi, K.; Belka, C.; Van Den Berg, C.A.T. CBCT Correction Using a Cycle-Consistent Generative Adversarial Network and Unpaired Training to Enable Photon and Proton Dose Calculation. *Physics in Medicine and Biology* **2019**, *64*, 225004, doi:10.1088/1361–6560/ab4d8c.

81. Stanley, D.N.; Harms, J.; Pogue, J.A.; Belliveau, J.-G.; Marcrom, S.R.; McDonald, A.M.; Dobelbower, M.C.; Boggs, D.H.; Soike, M.H.; Fiveash, J.A. A Roadmap for Implementation of kV-CBCT Online Adaptive Radiation Therapy and Initial First Year Experiences. *Journal of Applied Clinical Medical Physics* **2023**, *24*, e13961.
82. van de Schoot, A.J.; Hoffmans, D.; van Ingen, K.M.; Simons, M.J.; Wiersma, J. Characterization of Ethos Therapy Systems for Adaptive Radiation Therapy: A Multi-machine Comparison. *Journal of Applied Clinical Medical Physics* **2023**, *24*, e13905, doi:10.1002/acm2.13905.
83. Visak, J.; Inam, E.; Meng, B.; Wang, S.; Parsons, D.; Nyugen, D.; Zhang, T.; Moon, D.; Avkshtol, V.; Jiang, S.B.; et al. Evaluating Machine Learning Enhanced Intelligent-optimization-engine (IOE) Performance for Ethos Head-and-Neck (HN) Plan Generation. *Journal of Applied Clinical Medical Physics* **2023**, *24*, doi:10.1002/acm2.13950.
84. Qiu, Z.; Olberg, S.; den Hertog, D.; Ajdari, A.; Bortfeld, T.; Pursley, J. Online Adaptive Planning Methods for Intensity-Modulated Radiotherapy. *Physics in Medicine and Biology* **2023**, *68*, 10TR01, doi:10.1088/1361–6560/accdb2.
85. Lavrova, E.; Garrett, M.D.; Wang, Y.-F.; Chin, C.; Elliston, C.; Savacool, M.; Price, M.; Kachnic, L.A.; Horowitz, D.P. Adaptive Radiation Therapy: A Review of CT-Based Techniques. *Radiology: Imaging Cancer* **2023**, *5*, e230011, doi:10.1148/rycan.230011.
86. Groot Koerkamp, M.L.; Bol, G.H.; Kroon, P.S.; Krikke, L.L.; Harderwijk, T.; Zoetelief, A.J.; Scheeren, A.; van der Vegt, S.; Plat, A.; Hes, J.; et al. Bringing Online Adaptive Radiotherapy to a Standard C-Arm Linac. *Physics and Imaging in Radiation Oncology* **2024**, *31*, 100597, doi:10.1016/j.phro.2024.100597.
87. Li, C.; Guo, Y.; Lin, X.; Feng, X.; Xu, D.; Yang, R. Deep Reinforcement Learning in Radiation Therapy Planning Optimization: A Comprehensive Review. *Physica Medica* **2024**, *125*, 104498, doi:10.1016/j.ejmp.2024.104498.
88. Moreau, G.; François-Lavet, V.; Desbordes, P.; Macq, B. Reinforcement Learning for Radiotherapy Dose Fractioning Automation. *Biomedicines* **2021**, *9*, 214, doi:10.3390/biomedicines9020214.
89. Shen, C.; Nguyen, D.; Chen, L.; Gonzalez, Y.; McBeth, R.; Qin, N.; Jiang, S.B.; Jia, X. Operating a Treatment Planning System Using a Deep-Reinforcement-Learning Based Virtual Treatment Planner for Prostate Cancer Intensity-Modulated Radiation Therapy Treatment Planning. *Medical Physics* **2020**, *47*, 2329–2336, doi:10.1002/mp.14114.
90. Liu, B.; Liu, Y.; Li, Z.; Xiao, J.; Lin, H. Automatic Radiotherapy Treatment Planning with Deep Functional Reinforcement Learning. **2024**, https://doi.org/10.1101/2024.06.23.24309060.
91. Niraula, D.; Cui, S.; Pakela, J.; Wei, L.; Luo, Y.; Ten Haken, R.K.; El Naqa, I. Current Status and Future Developments in Predicting Outcomes in Radiation Oncology. *British Journal of Radiology* **2022**, *95*, 20220239, doi:10.1259/bjr.20220239.
92. Bang, C.; Bernard, G.; Le, W.T.; Lalonde, A.; Kadoury, S.; Bahig, H. Artificial Intelligence to Predict Outcomes of Head and Neck Radiotherapy. *Clinical and Translational Radiation Oncology* **2023**, *39*, 100590, doi:10.1016/j.ctro.2023.100590.
93. Majumder, S.; Katz, S.; Kontos, D.; Roshkovan, L. State of the Art: Radiomics and Radiomics-Related Artificial Intelligence on the Road to Clinical Translation. *BJR Open* **2023**, *6*, tzad004, doi:10.1093/bjro/tzad004.
94. Liang, Z.; Zhou, Q.; Yang, J.; Zhang, L.; Liu, D.; Tu, B.; Zhang, S. Artificial Intelligence-Based Framework in Evaluating Intrafraction Motion for Liver Cancer Robotic Stereotactic Body Radiation Therapy with Fiducial Tracking. *Medical Physics* **2020**, *47*, 5482–5489, doi:10.1002/mp.14501.
95. Lu, K.; Ren, L.; Yin, F.-F. A Geometry-Guided Deep Learning Technique for CBCT Reconstruction. *Physics in Medicine and Biology* **2021**, *66*, doi:10.1088/1361–6560/ac145b.
96. Lei, Y.; Tian, Z.; Wang, T.; Higgins, K.; Bradley, J.D.; Curran, W.J.; Liu, T.; Yang, X. Deep Learning-Based Real-Time Volumetric Imaging for Lung Stereotactic Body Radiation Therapy: A Proof of Concept Study. *Physics in Medicine and Biology* **2020**, *65*, 235003, doi:10.1088/1361–6560/abc303.
97. Salari, E.; Wang, J.; Wynne, J.F.; Chang, C.-W.; Wu, Y.; Yang, X. Artificial Intelligence-Based Motion Tracking in Cancer Radiotherapy: A Review. *Journal of Applied Clinical Medical Physics* **2024**, *25*, e14500, doi:10.1002/acm2.14500.
98. Yoganathan, S.A.; Paloor, S.; Torfeh, T.; Aouadi, S.; Hammoud, R.; Al-Hammadi, N. Predicting Respiratory Motion Using a Novel Patient Specific Dual Deep Recurrent Neural Networks. *Biomedical Physics & Engineering Express* **2022**, *8*, doi:10.1088/2057-1976/ac938f.
99. Yu, S.; Wang, J.; Liu, J.; Sun, R.; Kuang, S.; Sun, L. Rapid Prediction of Respiratory Motion Based on Bidirectional Gated Recurrent Unit Network. *IEEE Access* **2020**, *8*, 49424–49435, doi:10.1109/ACCESS.2020.2980002.

100. Wang, G.; Li, Z.; Li, G.; Dai, G.; Xiao, Q.; Bai, L.; He, Y.; Liu, Y.; Bai, S. Real-Time Liver Tracking Algorithm Based on LSTM and SVR Networks for Use in Surface-Guided Radiation Therapy. *Radiation Oncology* **2021**, *16*, 13, doi:10.1186/s13014-020-01729-7.
101. Edmunds, D.; Sharp, G.; Winey, B. Automatic Diaphragm Segmentation for Real-Time Lung Tumor Tracking on Cone-Beam CT Projections: A Convolutional Neural Network Approach. *Biomedical Physics & Engineering Express* **2019**, *5*, 035005, doi:10.1088/2057-1976/ab0734.
102. Wiersma, R.; Liu, X. A concept study on real-time adaptive radiation therapy optimization through ultra-fast beamlet control. *Biomedical Physics & Engineering Express* **2019,** *5*(5), 055016. doi: 10.1088/2057-1976/ab3ba9. Epub 2019 Aug 30. PMID: 33304619; PMCID: PMC7725270.
103. Xing, Y.; Nguyen, D.; Lu, W.; Yang, M.; Jiang, S.B. A Feasibility Study on Deep Learning-Based Radiotherapy Dose Calculation. *arXiv: Medical Physics* **2019**, doi:10.1002/MP.13953.
104. Kontaxis, C.; Bol, G.; Lagendijk, J.J.W.; Raaymakers, B. DeepDose: Towards a Fast Dose Calculation Engine for Radiation Therapy Using Deep Learning. *Physics in Medicine & Biology* **2020**, *65*, doi:10.1088/1361–6560/ab7630.
105. Wu, C.; Nguyen, D.; Xing, Y.; Montero, A.B.; Schuemann, J.; Shang, H.; Pu, Y.; Jiang, S. Improving Proton Dose Calculation Accuracy by Using Deep Learning. Machine Learn*ing: Science and Technology* **2021**, *2*, 015017, doi:10.1088/2632-2153/abb6d5.
106. Fan, J.; Xing, L.; Dong, P.; Wang, J.; Hu, W.; Yang, Y. Data-Driven Dose Calculation Algorithm Based on Deep U-Net. *Physics in Medicine and Biology* **2020**, *65*, 245035, doi:10.1088/1361–6560/abca05.
107. Liang, B.; Xia, W.; Wei, R.; Xu, Y.; Liu, Z.; Dai, J. A Deep Learning-Based Dose Calculation Method for Volumetric Modulated Arc Therapy. *Radiation Oncology* **2024**, *19*, 141, doi:10.1186/s13014-024-02534-2.
108. Galand, A.; Prunaretty, J.; Mir, N.; Morel, A.; Bourgier, C.; Aillères, N.; Azria, D.; Fenoglietto, P. Feasibility Study of Adaptive Radiotherapy with Ethos for Breast Cancer. *Frontiers Oncology* **2023**, *13*, 1274082, doi:10.3389/fonc.2023.1274082.
109. Kisling, K.; Keiper, T.D.; Branco, D.; Kim, G.G.; Moore, K.L.; Ray, X. Clinical Commissioning of an Adaptive Radiotherapy Platform: Results and Recommendations. *Journal of Applied Clinical Medical Physics* **2022**, *23*, e13801, doi:10.1002/acm2.13801.
110. Kim, J.-Y.; Tawk, B.; Knoll, M.; Hoegen-Saßmannshausen, P.; Liermann, J.; Huber, P.E.; Lifferth, M.; Lang, C.; Häring, P.; Gnirs, R.; et al. Clinical Workflow of Cone Beam Computer Tomography-Based Daily Online Adaptive Radiotherapy with Offline Magnetic Resonance Guidance: The Modular Adaptive Radiotherapy System (MARS). *Cancers* **2024**, *16*, 1210, doi:10.3390/cancers16061210.
111. Lustermans, D.; Fonseca, G.; Taasti, V.; Schoot, A.J. van de; Petit, S.; Elmpt, W. van; Verhaegen, F. Image Quality Evaluation of a New High-Performance Ring-Gantry Cone-Beam Computed Tomography Imager. *Physics in Medicine & Biology* **2024**, *69*, doi:10.1088/1361–6560/ad3cb0.
112. Kim, E.; Park, Y.K.; Zhao, T.; Laugeman, E.; Zhao, X.N.; Hao, Y.; Chung, Y.; Lee, H. Image Quality Characterization of an Ultra-high-speed Kilovoltage Cone-beam Computed Tomography Imaging System on an O-ring Linear Accelerator. *Journal of Applied Clinical Medical Physics* **2024**, *25*, e14337, doi:10.1002/acm2.14337.
113. Gonzalez, Y.; Visak, J.; Overman, L.; Liao, C.-Y.; Yen, A.; Zhuang, T.; Cai, B.; Godley, A.; Zhang, Y.; Timmerman, R.D.; et al. Beyond Conventional Bounds: Surpassing System Limits for Stereotactic Ablative (SAbR) Lung Radiotherapy Using CBCT-based Adaptive Planning System. *Journal of Applied Clinical Medical Physics* **2024**, *25*, doi:10.1002/acm2.14375.
114. Zhao, X.; Stanley, D.N.; Cardenas, C.E.; Harms, J.; Popple, R.A. Do We Need Patient-specific QA for Adaptively Generated Plans? Retrospective Evaluation of Delivered Online Adaptive Treatment Plans on Varian Ethos. *Journal of Applied Clinical Medical Physics* **2022**, *24*, e13876, doi:10.1002/acm2.13876.
115. Nasser, N.; Yang, G.Q.; Koo, J.; Bowers, M.; Greco, K.; Feygelman, V.; Moros, E.G.; Caudell, J.J.; Redler, G. A Head and Neck Treatment Planning Strategy for a CBCT-guided Ring-gantry Online Adaptive Radiotherapy System. *Journal of Applied Clinical Medical Physics* **2023**, *24*, e14134, doi:10.1002/acm2.14134.
116. Raaymakers, B.W.; Lagendijk, J.J.W.; Overweg, J.; Kok, J.G.M.; Raaijmakers, A.J.E.; Kerkhof, E.M.; Van Der Put, R.W.; Meijsing, I.; Crijns, S.P.M.; Benedosso, F. Integrating a 1.5 T MRI Scanner with a 6 MV Accelerator: Proof of Concept. *Physics in Medicine & Biology* **2009**, *54*, N229.
117. Lamb, J.; Cao, M.; Kishan, A.; Agazaryan, N.; Thomas, D.H.; Shaverdian, N.; Yang, Y.; Ray, S.; Low, D.A.; Raldow, A.; et al. Online Adaptive Radiation Therapy: Implementation of a New Process of Care. *Cureus* **2017**, *9*, e1618, doi:10.7759/cureus.1618.

118. Huang, C.-Y.; Yang, B.; Lam, W.W.; Geng, H.; Cheung, K.Y.; Yu, S.K. Magnetic Field Induced Dose Effects in Radiation Therapy Using MR-Linacs. *Medical Physics* **2023**, *50*, 3623–3636, doi:10.1002/mp.16397.
119. Mutic, S.; Dempsey, J.F. The ViewRay System: Magnetic Resonance–Guided and Controlled Radiotherapy. *Seminars in Radiation Oncology* **2014**, *24*, 196–199, doi:10.1016/j.semradonc.2014.02.008.
120. Eidex, Z.; Ding, Y.; Wang, J.; Abouei, E.; Qiu, R.L.; Liu, T.; Wang, T.; Yang, X. Deep Learning in MRI-Guided Radiation Therapy: A Systematic Review. *Journal of Applied Clinical Medical Physics* **2024,** *25*(2), e14155.*arXiv preprint arXiv:2303.11378* **2023**.
121. Liu, Y.; Stojadinovic, S.; Hrycushko, B.; Wardak, Z.; Lau, S.; Lu, W.; Yan, Y.; Jiang, S.B.; Zhen, X.; Timmerman, R.; et al. A Deep Convolutional Neural Network-Based Automatic Delineation Strategy for Multiple Brain Metastases Stereotactic Radiosurgery. *PLoS One* **2017**, *12*, e0185844, doi:10.1371/journal.pone.0185844.
122. Rabe, M.; Kurz, C.; Thummerer, A.; Landry, G. Artificial Intelligence for Treatment Delivery: Image-Guided Radiotherapy. *Strahlentherapie und Onkologie* **2024**, doi:10.1007/s00066-024-02277-9.
123. Ma, Y.; Ma, X.; Li, C.; Jiang, Y.; Zhang, Z.; Xiao, J.; Tian, Y.; Deng, L.; Zhang, T.; Wang, J.; et al. Personalized Auto-Segmentation for Magnetic Resonance Imaging-Guided Adaptive Radiotherapy of Large Brain Metastases. *Radiotherapy and Oncology* **2025**, *205*, 110773, doi:10.1016/j.radonc.2025.110773.
124. Chen, X.; Ma, X.; Yan, X.; Luo, F.; Yang, S.; Wang, Z.; Wu, R.; Wang, J.; Lu, N.; Bi, N.; et al. Personalized Auto-Segmentation for Magnetic Resonance Imaging-Guided Adaptive Radiotherapy of Prostate Cancer. *Medical Physics* **2022**, *49*, 4971–4979, doi:10.1002/mp.15793.
125. Kawula, M.; Hadi, I.; Nierer, L.; Vagni, M.; Cusumano, D.; Boldrini, L.; Placidi, L.; Corradini, S.; Belka, C.; Landry, G.; et al. Patient-Specific Transfer Learning for Auto-Segmentation in Adaptive 0.35 T MRgRT of Prostate Cancer: A Bi-Centric Evaluation. *Medical Physics* **2023**, *50*, 1573–1585, doi:10.1002/mp.16056.
126. Li, Z.; Zhang, W.; Li, B.; Zhu, J.; Peng, Y.; Li, C.; Zhu, J.; Zhou, Q.; Yin, Y. Patient-Specific Daily Updated Deep Learning Auto-Segmentation for MRI-Guided Adaptive Radiotherapy. *Radiotherapy and Oncology* **2022**, *177*, 222–230, doi:10.1016/j.radonc.2022.11.004.
127. Wahid, K.A.; Khriguian, J.; Dede, C.; Khamis, Y.; El-Habashy, D.; Restrepo, N.; Tehami, S.; Sahin, O.; Mohamed, A.S.; Fuller, C.D.; et al. Deep Learning Based Prognostic Prediction in Oropharyngeal Cancer Patients Using Multiparametric MRI Inputs. *International Journal of Radiation Oncology, Biology, Physics* **2023**, *117*, e631, doi:10.1016/j.ijrobp.2023.06.2027.
128. Schmidt, M.A.; Payne, G.S. Radiotherapy Planning Using MRI. *Physics in Medicine and Biology* **2015**, *60*, R323–R361, doi:10.1088/0031–9155/60/22/R323.
129. Heinrich, M.P.; Jenkinson, M.; Bhushan, M.; Matin, T.; Gleeson, F.V.; Brady, S.M.; Schnabel, J.A. MIND: Modality Independent Neighbourhood Descriptor for Multi-Modal Deformable Registration. *Medical Image Analysis* **2012**, *16*, 1423–1435, doi:10.1016/j.media.2012.05.008.
130. McKenzie, E.M.; Santhanam, A.; Ruan, D.; O'Connor, D.; Cao, M.; Sheng, K. Multimodality Image Registration in the Head-and-neck Using a Deep Learning-derived Synthetic CT as a Bridge. *Medical physics* **2020**, *47*, 1094–1104.
131. Zhao, Y.; Chen, X.; McDonald, B.; Yu, C.; Pan, T.; Wang, H.; Wang, X.; Phan, J.; Yang, J. Patch-RegNet: A Hierarchical Deformable Registration Framework for Inter-/Intra-Modality Head-and-Neck Image Registration with ViT-Morph. In *Proceedings of the Medical Imaging 2023: Image Processing*; SPIE, San Diego, California, United States, 2023; Vol. 12464, pp. 9–15.
132. Zhao, Y.; Chen, X.; McDonald, B.; Yu, C.; Mohamed, A.S.; Fuller, C.D.; Court, L.E.; Pan, T.; Wang, H.; Wang, X. A Transformer-Based Hierarchical Registration Framework for Multimodality Deformable Image Registration. *Computerized Medical Imaging and Graphics* **2023**, *108*, 102286.
133. Chen, J.; He, Y.; Frey, E.C.; Li, Y.; Du, Y. ViT-V-Net: Vision Transformer for Unsupervised Volumetric Medical Image Registration. *arXiv:2104.06468 [cs, eess]* **2021**. http://arxiv.org/pdf/2104.06468
134. Edmund, J.M.; Nyholm, T. A Review of Substitute CT Generation for MRI-Only Radiation Therapy. *Radiation Oncology* **2017**, *12*, 28, doi:10.1186/s13014-016-0747-y.
135. Hsu, S.-H.; Cao, Y.; Huang, K.; Feng, M.; Balter, J.M. Investigation of a Method for Generating Synthetic CT Models from MRI Scans of the Head and Neck for Radiation Therapy. *Physics in Medicine and Biology* **2013**, *58*, 8419–8435, doi:10.1088/0031–9155/58/23/8419.
136. Huynh, T.; Gao, Y.; Kang, J.; Wang, L.; Zhang, P.; Lian, J.; Shen, D.; Alzheimer's Disease Neuroimaging Initiative Estimating CT Image From MRI Data Using Structured Random Forest and Auto-Context Model. *IEEE Transactions on Medical Imaging* **2016**, *35*, 174–183, doi:10.1109/TMI.2015.2461533.

137. Andreasen, D.; Van Leemput, K.; Edmund, J.M. A Patch-based pseudo-CT Approach for MRI-only Radiotherapy in the Pelvis. *Medical physics* **2016**, *43*, 4742–4752.
138. Cao, X.; Yang, J.; Gao, Y.; Guo, Y.; Wu, G.; Shen, D. Dual-Core Steered Non-Rigid Registration for Multi-Modal Images via Bi-Directional Image Synthesis. *Medical Image Analysis* **2017**, *41*, 18–31, doi:10.1016/j.media.2017.05.004.
139. Zhao, Y.; Wang, H.; Yu, C.; Court, L.E.; Wang, X.; Wang, Q.; Pan, T.; Ding, Y.; Phan, J.; Yang, J. Compensation Cycle Consistent Generative Adversarial Networks (Comp-GAN) for Synthetic CT Generation from MR Scans with Truncated Anatomy. *Medical Physics* 2023, *50*, 4399–4414.
140. Boulanger, M.; Nunes, J.-C.; Chourak, H.; Largent, A.; Tahri, S.; Acosta, O.; De Crevoisier, R.; Lafond, C.; Barateau, A. Deep Learning Methods to Generate Synthetic CT from MRI in Radiotherapy: A Literature Review. *Physica Medica* **2021**, *89*, 265–281, doi:10.1016/j.ejmp.2021.07.027.
141. Han, X. MR-based Synthetic CT Generation Using a Deep Convolutional Neural Network Method. *Medical Physics* **2017**, *44*, 1408–1419.
142. Nie, D.; Cao, X.; Gao, Y.; Wang, L.; Shen, D. Estimating CT Image from MRI Data Using 3D Fully Convolutional Networks. *Deep Learning and Data Labeling for Medical Applications* **2016**, *2016*, 170–178, doi:10.1007/978-3-319–46976-8_18.
143. Wolterink, J.M.; Dinkla, A.M.; Savenije, M.H.F.; Seevinck, P.R.; van den Berg, C.A.T.; Išgum, I. Deep MR to CT Synthesis Using Unpaired Data. In Tsaftaris, S.A., Gooya, A., Frangi, A.F., Prince, J.L., (eds.) *Proceedings of the Simulation and Synthesis in Medical Imaging*; Springer International Publishing: Cham, 2017; pp. 14–23.
144. Goodfellow, I.; Pouget-Abadie, J.; Mirza, M.; Xu, B.; Warde-Farley, D.; Ozair, S.; Courville, A.; Bengio, Y. Generative Adversarial Nets. In *Proceedings of the Advances in Neural Information Processing Systems*; Curran Associates, Inc., 2014; Vol. 27.
145. Isola, P.; Zhu, J.-Y.; Zhou, T.; Efros, A.A. Image-to-Image Translation with Conditional Adversarial Networks. **2016**, doi:10.48550/arXiv.1611.07004.
146. Chen, X.; Zhao, Y.; Court, L.E.; Wang, H.; Pan, T.; Phan, J.; Wang, X.; Ding, Y.; Yang, J. SC-GAN: Structure-Completion Generative Adversarial Network for Synthetic CT Generation from MR Images with Truncated Anatomy. *Computerized Medical Imaging and Graphics* **2024**, 102353. doi: 10.1016/j.compmedimag.2024.102353. Epub 2024 Feb 10. PMID: 38387114
147. Lei, Y.; Harms, J.; Wang, T.; Liu, Y.; Shu, H.-K.; Jani, A.B.; Curran, W.J.; Mao, H.; Liu, T.; Yang, X. MRI-only Based Synthetic CT Generation Using Dense Cycle Consistent Generative Adversarial Networks. *Medical Physics* **2019**, *46*, 3565–3581.
148. Otazo, R.; Lambin, P.; Pignol, J.-P.; Ladd, M.E.; Schlemmer, H.-P.; Baumann, M.; Hricak, H. MRI-Guided Radiation Therapy: An Emerging Paradigm in Adaptive Radiation Oncology. *Radiology* **2021**, *298*, 248–260, doi:10.1148/radiol.2020202747.
149. Benitez, C.M.; Chuong, M.D.; Künzel, L.A.; Thorwarth, D. MRI-Guided Adaptive Radiation Therapy. *Seminars in Radiation Oncology*, **2024**, *34*, 84–91. doi: 10.1016/j.semradonc.2023.10.013. PMID: 38105097
150. Edelstein, W.A.; Mahesh, M.; Carrino, J.A. MRI: Time Is Dose—and Money and Versatility. *Journal of American College of Radiology* **2010**, *7*, 650–652, doi:10.1016/j.jacr.2010.05.002.
151. Haji-Valizadeh, H.; Guo, R.; Kucukseymen, S.; Tuyen, Y.; Rodriguez, J.; Paskavitz, A.; Pierce, P.; Goddu, B.; Ngo, L.H.; Nezafat, R. Comparison of Complex K-Space Data and Magnitude-Only for Training of Deep Learning–Based Artifact Suppression for Real-Time Cine MRI. *Frontiers in Physics* **2021**, *9*, doi:10.3389/fphy.2021.684184.
152. Li, Z.; Li, S.; Zhang, Z.; Wang, F.; Wu, F.; Gao, S. Radial Undersampled MRI Reconstruction Using Deep Learning With Mutual Constraints Between Real and Imaginary Components of K-Space. *IEEE Journal of Biomedical and Health Informatics* **2024**, *28*, 3583–3596, doi:10.1109/JBHI.2024.3357784.
153. Lin, H.; Xiao, H.; Dong, L.; Teo, K.; Zou, W.; Cai, J.; Li, T. Deep Learning for Automatic Target Volume Segmentation in Radiation Therapy: A Review. *Quantitative Imaging in Medicine and Surgery* **2021**, *11*(12), 4847–4858, doi:10.21037/qims-21–168.
154. Liu, G.; Zhao, Y. A Survey of Deep Learning Methods for MRI Brain Tumor Image Segmentation. In *2022 4th International Conference on Machine Learning, Big Data and Business Intelligence (MLBDBI)*, Shanghai, China, **2022**; pp. 318–323, doi:10.1109/MLBDBI58171.2022.00069.
155. Seregni, M.; Paganelli, C.; Lee, D.; Greer, P.B.; Baroni, G.; Keall, P.J.; Riboldi, M. Motion Prediction in MRI-Guided Radiotherapy Based on Interleaved Orthogonal Cine-MRI. *Physics in Medicine Biology* **2016**, *61*, 872, doi:10.1088/0031–9155/61/2/872.

156. Bourque, A.E.; Carrier, J.-F.; Filion, É.; Bedwani, S. A Particle Filter Motion Prediction Algorithm Based on an Autoregressive Model for Real-Time MRI-Guided Radiotherapy of Lung Cancer. *Biomedical Physics & Engineering Express* **2017**, *3*, 035001, doi:10.1088/2057-1976/aa6b5b.
157. Lombardo, E.; Rabe, M.; Xiong, Y.; Nierer, L.; Cusumano, D.; Placidi, L.; Boldrini, L.; Corradini, S.; Niyazi, M.; Belka, C.; et al. Offline and Online LSTM Networks for Respiratory Motion Prediction in MR-Guided Radiotherapy. *Physics in Medicine & Biology* **2022**, *67*, doi:10.1088/1361–6560/ac60b7.
158. Romaguera, L.V.; Plantefève, R.; Romero, F.P.; Hébert, F.; Carrier, J.-F.; Kadoury, S. Prediction of In-Plane Organ Deformation during Free-Breathing Radiotherapy via Discriminative Spatial Transformer Networks. *Medical Image Analysis* **2020**, *64*, 101754, doi:10.1016/j.media.2020.101754.
159. Terpstra, M.L.; Maspero, M.; Bruijnen, T.; Verhoeff, J.J.C.; Lagendijk, J.J.W.; van den Berg, C.A.T. Real-Time 3D Motion Estimation from Undersampled MRI Using Multi-Resolution Neural Networks. *Medical Physics* **2021**, *48*, 6597–6613, doi:10.1002/mp.15217.

8 Motion Management in Radiation Therapy

Yingzi Liu and Zhen Tian

8.1 INTRODUCTION

During radiation therapy, intra-fractional patient motion—including respiratory, cardiac, and gastrointestinal movement—can lead to tumor localization uncertainty, particularly in the thoracic and abdominal regions.[1–3] To mitigate this, motion management techniques such as respiratory gating, abdominal compression, breath-hold, and surface-guiding are commonly employed to maintain the tumor within a predictable position range. However, studies have shown that even with motion management techniques, the magnitude, frequency, and regularity of motion may deviate from baseline, potentially leading to dosimetric uncertainties.[2,4,5] This tumor localization uncertainty is of particular concern in stereotactic body radiation therapy (SBRT), which has ≤5 fractionation regimen and delivers high doses per fraction with small uncertainty margins, highly conformal dose distributions, steep dose gradients, and often targets tumors in close proximity to organs-at-risk (OARs).[6,7] Real-time tumor or target monitoring is therefore crucial for SBRT treatment sites affected by motion, to ensure accurate dose delivery and minimize exposure to surrounding healthy tissues.

Currently, direct real-time tumor monitoring techniques include two-dimensional (2D) kilovoltage (kV) imaging, radiofrequency/electromagnetic tracking, ultrasound, cine magnetic resonance imaging (MRI), and positron emission tomography (PET)-guided radiotherapy. There are also indirect methods like optical and surface guidance. Those tools make real-time adaptive radiotherapy possible, but effective motion management needs more than just tracking—it also depends on accurate, fast localization, and motion prediction to deal with system delays. Other key factors are spatial resolution and how much of the anatomy can be seen clearly, which is often limited to 2D at high temporal resolution. This chapter will briefly cover the challenges with current major intra-fractional motion management methods. Since these motion management techniques produce large amounts of data and require fast processing, it is no surprise that artificial intelligence (AI) is often suggested as a solution for the future improvement of real-time motion management. Deep learning, a subset of AI, uses neural networks to automatically learn from data. It has gained significant attention and success for its ability to capture complex patterns and fine details through patient-specific training. In this chapter, we will focus on how AI, especially deep learning, can help address key challenges in motion management for radiotherapy.

8.2 AI APPLICATION IN 2D kV-BASED MOTION MANAGEMENT

Triggered or continuous 2D kV (i.e., kV fluoroscopy) imaging enables real-time tumor tracking using implanted markers placed in or near the tumor. But marker implantation is invasive and expensive, and markers can migrate over time. Non-marker tracking avoids these problems but has its own challenges—since the patient's three-dimensional (3D) anatomy is projected onto the 2D image, tumor can be difficult to see, especially in areas like the liver or pancreas,[8] and tumors can be obscured by high-density structures like bone. This highlights the need for real-time 3D imaging during SBRT to improve motion monitoring and support better motion management.

Traditional computed tomography (CT) reconstructs 3D images from multiple 2D projections acquired at different angles, typically using filtered back-projection. These reconstruction methods

 DOI: 10.1201/9781003480365-9

require a sufficient number of 2D angular projections to satisfy the classic Shannon–Nyquist sampling theorem. However, due to collision risks, the rotation speed of the linear accelerator (LINAC) gantry is limited, making real-time volumetric imaging impractical with the traditional methods.[9] The time constraint allows only one or a few X-ray projections to be acquired in real time. Compressed sensing has been used to reduce the number of required projections in iterative image reconstruction.[10–15] It is based on the idea that medical imaging can be represented with relatively a few nonzero coefficients when transformed into a particular domain, meaning that it allows for under-sample and still reconstructs a high-quality image. Accurate generation of volumetric images is possible only if the model is able to learn the semantic representation of the 3D structure from the limited input projections. If not properly implemented or unrealistic, the reconstruction process can introduce artifacts or distortions in the final image, especially when the under-sampling is too aggressive. It has shown that the achievable sparsity in compressed sensing technique still falls short of what is needed for real-time volumetric imaging with uncompromised imaging quality.[9]

Another method estimated 3D tumor location by leveraging machine learning along with patient-specific prior knowledge.[16–19] These approaches typically build a patient-specific motion model from the patient's own four-dimensional CT (4D CT) images using deformable registration and principal component analysis (PCA). The model then estimates the PCA coefficients from a single 2D projection using techniques such as optimization, linear regression, or sparse learning. Real-time deformation vector fields (DVFs) are generated from these PCA coefficients to reconstruct the patient's current 3D anatomy. However, concerns about the robustness of these methods in handling variations and irregularities in patient's positioning, respiratory motion, and anatomical changes limit their routine clinical adoption.[8]

More recently, deep learning has been employed to directly learn the 2D-to-3D transformation in the feature domain, allowing the generation of synthetic 3D CT images from just one or a few 2D kV projections.[9,20,21] Shen et al.[9] and Lei et al.[20] demonstrated the feasibility of reconstructing 3D CT images of the abdomen, lung, and head and neck from a single X-ray projection. But due to limited information available from a single projection, the quality of the reconstructed images can vary depending on the projection angle, which restricts their clinical applicability. To address this, a follow-up study by Lei et al.[22] showed that combining orthogonal kV and megavoltage (MV) projections acquired simultaneously can provide more anatomical information and improve the accuracy for synthetic 3D image reconstruction. For low-contrast tumors like those in the liver, Shao et al.[21] proposed a mesh registration method to enable real-time tumor tracking from a single X-ray projection. Compared to earlier methods, these deep learning techniques have demonstrated improved accuracy and robustness in handling patient positioning, anatomy, and motion. Regardless of the specific model configuration or supplemental training data, the key input remains a 2D kV projection, and the key output is a synthetic 3D image. This section will use Lei et al.'s work[20] as a case study to introduce core deep learning-based 2D-to-3D transformation techniques and explore their potential for clinical integration.

8.2.1 Overview of the Deep Learning-Based 2D-to-3D Transformation Methods

The basic idea of 2D-to-3D transformation networks is to take a single 2D kV projection image from the patient as input and generate synthetic 3D CT image as output. The networks follow a similar structure with two main stages: training and inference. The training data consists of paired 2D projection and 3D CT images, with the 3D CT serving as ground truth. The network is trained under one or more supervision methods by optimizing its parameters. The overall network consists of three modules, including an encoding module, a transformation module, and a decoding module. The encoding module is to learn the feature representation by extracting semantic features from the input 2D projection image. By reshaping the 2D feature map extracted by the encoding module to a 3D feature map, the transformation module bridges the 2D and 3D feature spaces. The decoding module is to learn the transformation from the 3D feature domain to the 3D image domain.

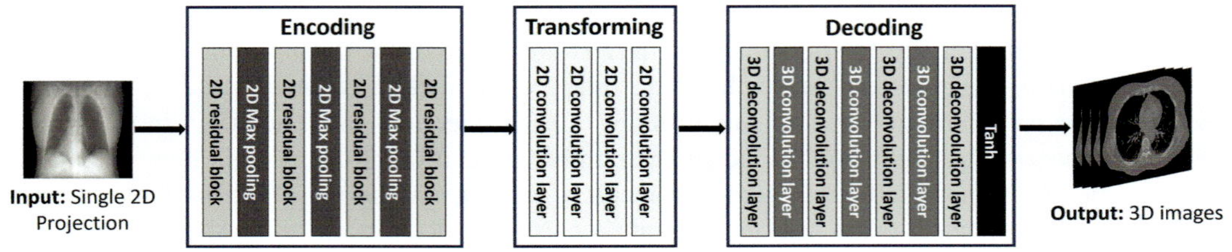

FIGURE 8.1 Schematic of a deep learning-based 2D-to-3D transformation network developed by Lei et al. The network consists of an encoding module, a transforming network, and a decoding network. It takes a single 2D projection as input and outputs 3D synthetic CT images.

During inference, the well-trained network uses the same feed-forward process: it extracts features from a single 2D image and outputs a synthetic 3D CT image quickly enough for real-time application. Figure 8.1 shows the architecture of Lei et al.'s[20] deep learning network, called TransNet.

8.2.2 Data Preparation

Unlike other domains such as computer vision, deep learning in medical imaging faces unique challenges, such as limited annotated data and high inter-patient variability. These factors hinder the generalizability of models across a diverse patient population, particularly due to significant differences in tumor shape, size, location, and motion. However, for an individual patient, anatomical structures tend to remain relatively stable between CT simulation and the subsequent radiation treatments, despite minor variations caused by motion or setup differences. This consistency provides an opportunity to incorporate prior patient-specific information to improve model generalizability issues. Accordingly, Lei et al. trained their deep learning networks in a patient-specific manner, tailoring the learning process to scenarios directly relevant to each individual patient.

Training the network requires a large number of 3D CT images with minimal or no respiratory motion, paired with their corresponding 2D kV X-ray projections acquired by the clinical imaging system on a LINAC. To avoid unnecessary radiation exposure and streamline clinical workflow, these 2D projections were not acquired directly. Instead, synthetic projections were digitally generated from each phase of the patient's own 4D CT, i.e., phase-resolved 3D CT, rather than capturing real 2D projections at multiple angles with the patient holding their breath at various respiratory amplitudes. Ray-tracing algorithms were used to produce these digital 2D projections based on the Cone Beam Computed Tomography (CBCT) imaging geometry.

However, the 4D CT images acquired during CT simulation typically represent only a single treatment scenario. In practice, patient anatomy, treatment setup, and respiratory characteristics such as amplitude, period, and regularity can vary across treatment fractions. To address these variations, a data augmentation strategy was applied to each phase of the 4D CT, introducing translations, rotations, and organ deformations to simulate a broad range of potential clinical variations. This approach not only improved the network's robustness to inter-fraction variability but also mitigated overfitting by effectively expanding the size and diversity of the training dataset.

8.2.3 Supervision and Loss Function

The performance of a deep learning network is highly influenced by the choice of loss function used for supervision during network training. Conventionally, a loss function based on the mean squared error (MSE) between the predicted synthetic 3D image and the corresponding ground truth is employed, emphasizing image-domain voxel-wise intensity differences.[9]

In Lei's work, the loss function extended beyond image-domain supervision by incorporating both perceptual and adversarial components. The total loss was formulated as a weighted sum of four terms:

$$L_{\text{total}}\left(\hat{y}, y\right) = \lambda_{\text{mae}} \cdot L_{\text{mae}}\left(\hat{y}, y\right) + \lambda_{\text{gd}} \cdot L_{\text{gd}}\left(\hat{y}, y\right) + \lambda_p \cdot L_p\left(f_{\hat{y}}, f_y\right) + L_{\text{adv}}\left(\hat{y}\right) \tag{8.1}$$

The first two terms, $L_{\text{mae}}\left(\hat{y}, y\right)$ and $L_{\text{gd}}\left(\hat{y}, y\right)$, are image distance loss between the obtained synthetic $\hat{y}$ and the ground-truth 3D image y. The former computes the mean absolute error (MAE) to capture voxel-wise intensity differences, while the latter calculates the gradient difference to account for structural discrepancies at the gradient level.

The third term, $L_p\left(f_{\hat{y}}, f_y\right)$, is a perceptual loss that measures semantic (content accuracy) and perceptual (imaging quality) differences between the synthetic and ground-truth 3D images. This loss encourages more accurate reconstruction of organ boundaries in synthetic images. To compute this loss, a pre-trained deep neural network named SegNet, which is a conventional end-to-end feature pyramid network (as shown in Figure 8.1), was employed to extract both the low- and high-level feature maps from the synthetic image $\hat{y}$ and the ground-truth 3D image y. Specifically, the combined feature representations are denoted as $f_{\hat{y}} = \bigcup_{i=1}^{N} F_s^i\left(\hat{y}\right)$ and $f_y = \bigcup_{i=1}^{N} F_s^i\left(y\right)$, where N is the number of pyramid levels in SegNet and $F_s^i\left(\cdot\right)$ represents the feature map extracted at the i-th level.

The perceptual loss is then defined as the squared Euclidean distance between the corresponding feature maps:

$$L_p\left(f_{\hat{y}}, f_y\right) = \sum_{i=1}^{N} \frac{\omega_i}{C_i \cdot H_i \cdot W_i \cdot D_i} F_s^i\left(\hat{y}\right) - F_s^i\left(y\right)_2^2 \tag{8.2}$$

where C_i, H_i, W_i, and D_i represent the number of channels, height, width, and depth of the feature map at the i-th pyramid level, respectively. In SegNet, lower-level feature maps capture fine structural details (e.g., edges and textures), while higher-level maps encode more abstract semantic information (e.g., anatomical shapes and organ-level context). Since feature maps at higher levels are spatially coarser, their contribution to the total loss was up-weighted using scale factors ω_i, defined as $\omega_i = 1.2^{i-1}$ in Lei et al.'s implementation.

The fourth term in the total loss function, $L_{\text{adv}}\left(\hat{y}\right)$, is an adversarial loss aimed at improving the realism of the synthetic 3D image so that it closely resembles the ground-truth 3D image. This approach draws on the principles of conditional generative adversarial networks, where a discriminator network is trained to distinguish between synthetic and real images, while a generator (in this case, the 2D-to-3D transformation network) learns to produce output that can fool the discriminator.[23,24] As shown in Figure 8.1, the discriminator was implemented as a conventional fully convolutional network that outputs a binary decision, represented as $F_{\text{dis}}\left(\cdot\right)$. A value of 0 indicates that the input is identified as synthetic, while a value of 1 indicates that it is real. The discriminator loss quantifies the classification error when distinguishing real from synthetic images and is defined as

$$L_{\text{dis}}\left(\hat{y}, y\right) = \text{SCE}\left(F_{\text{dis}}\left(\hat{y}\right), 0\right) + \text{SCE}\left(F_{\text{dis}}\left(y\right), 1\right) \tag{8.3}$$

where the function $\text{SCE}\left(\cdot,\cdot\right)$ denotes the sigmoid cross-entropy (SCE) function between the predicted and target labels. A lower SCE value indicates better alignment between the predicted and target distributions. Conversely, the adversarial loss applied to the generator is defined as

$$L_{\text{adv}}\left(\hat{y}\right) = \text{SCE}\left(F_{\text{dis}}\left(\hat{y}\right), 1\right) \tag{8.4}$$

This loss penalizes the generator when the discriminator successfully identifies the synthetic image as fake. A lower value of $L_{\text{adv}}\left(\hat{y}\right)$ implies a greater ability of the generator to deceive the discriminator, thereby increasing the perceptual realism of the generated image. These two losses form a minimax game: the discriminator aims to minimize L_{dis}, increasing its classification accuracy, while the generator aims to minimize L_{adv}, enhancing the quality and realism of the synthetic image.

Through this adversarial training dynamic, the generator learns to produce synthetic 3D images that are visually and semantically closer to the real images.

A common rule of thumb for determining the weighting factors in a multi-term loss function is to first ensure that the initial numerical values of the individual loss components are within the same order of magnitude. This helps prevent any single term from dominating the optimization process purely due to scale. Subsequently, the weighting factors should be empirically tuned to reflect the relative importance and priority of each loss component in the specific application context. Once the network is sufficiently trained and converged, its performance is typically robust to minor variations in the weighting values.

8.2.4 Evaluation Results

Since real-time volumetric imaging is not currently available in clinical practice, there is no ground truth for a patient's instantaneous 3D anatomy during treatment delivery. Therefore, Lei et al. evaluated their trained networks using digitally reconstructed 2D projections paired with phase-specific 3D CT images from 4D CT datasets that were not included in the training set. This served as proof-of-concept for real-time volumetric imaging. Quantitative evaluation of the generated synthetic 3D images was performed using multiple metrics, including MAE, peak signal-to-noise ratio (PSNR), and structural similarity index (SSIM). Lei et al. demonstrated that incorporating perceptual loss improved the network's ability to accurately recover organ boundaries, while adversarial loss significantly enhanced the realism of the synthetic images. As a result, their method produces 3D images of acceptable image quality (see Figure 8.2), achieving lower MAE (e.g., 90.3 ± 15.8 HU vs. 115.7 ± 23.2 HU using 0° projection, 103.9 ± 12.1 HU vs. 123.5 ± 15.3 HU using 90° projection),

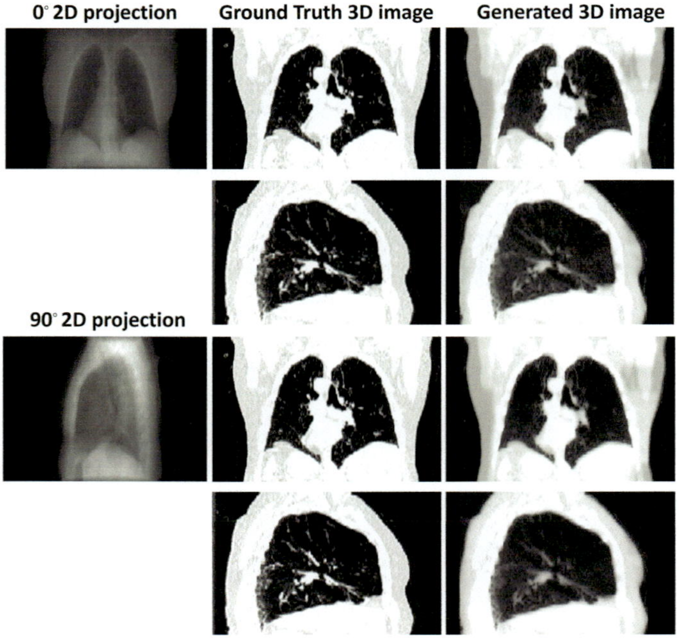

FIGURE 8.2 The 3D synthetic CT images obtained for a patient at inhale (phase 0) using Lei's method,[20] generated from a single 2D kV projection of projection angle 0° and from a single 2D kV projection of projection angle 90°, respectively. The ground-truth 3D CT images are also shown in the figure for comparison.

higher PSNR (e.g., 15.6 ± 2.2 dB vs. 14.5 ± 2.2 dB using 0° projection, 15.2 ± 2.8 dB vs. 14.2 ± 2.8 dB using 90° projection), and higher SSIM (e.g., 0.849 ± 0.081 vs. 0.804 ± 0.100 using 0° projection, 0.832 ± 0.099 vs. 0.780 ± 0.136 using 90° projection) compared to the method developed by Shen et al.[20]

Lei et al. tested the robustness of their 2D-to-3D transformation network to image noise, by adding Gaussian noise with sigma ratio of 0.01, 0.05, and 0.1 to the 2D projection data as testing noisy projection.[20] It is reported that the image qualities of the generated 3D images gradually degrade as the input 2D projection data of 0° projection angle gets more and more noisy (see Figure 8.3). The obtained MAE value of the generated 3D images increases from 90.3 ± 15.8 HU to 110.2 ± 11.9 HU, 115.9 ± 11.4 HU, and 128.2 ± 10.7 HU for these three different noise levels, respectively. PSNR decreases from 15.6 ± 2.2 dB to 15.1 ± 2.1 dB, 14.5 ± 2.1 dB, and 13.5 ± 2.0 dB, and SSIM degrades from 0.849 ± 0.081 to 0.831 ± 0.088, 0.803 ± 0.094, and 0.746 ± 0.105.

Lei et al. also tested the robustness of the 2D-3D generation network to motion and anatomical variations.[20] In this experiment, the original 4D CT images of a patient case were deformed to simulate a challenging scenario with doubled respiratory motion amplitude and 50% tumor shrinkage

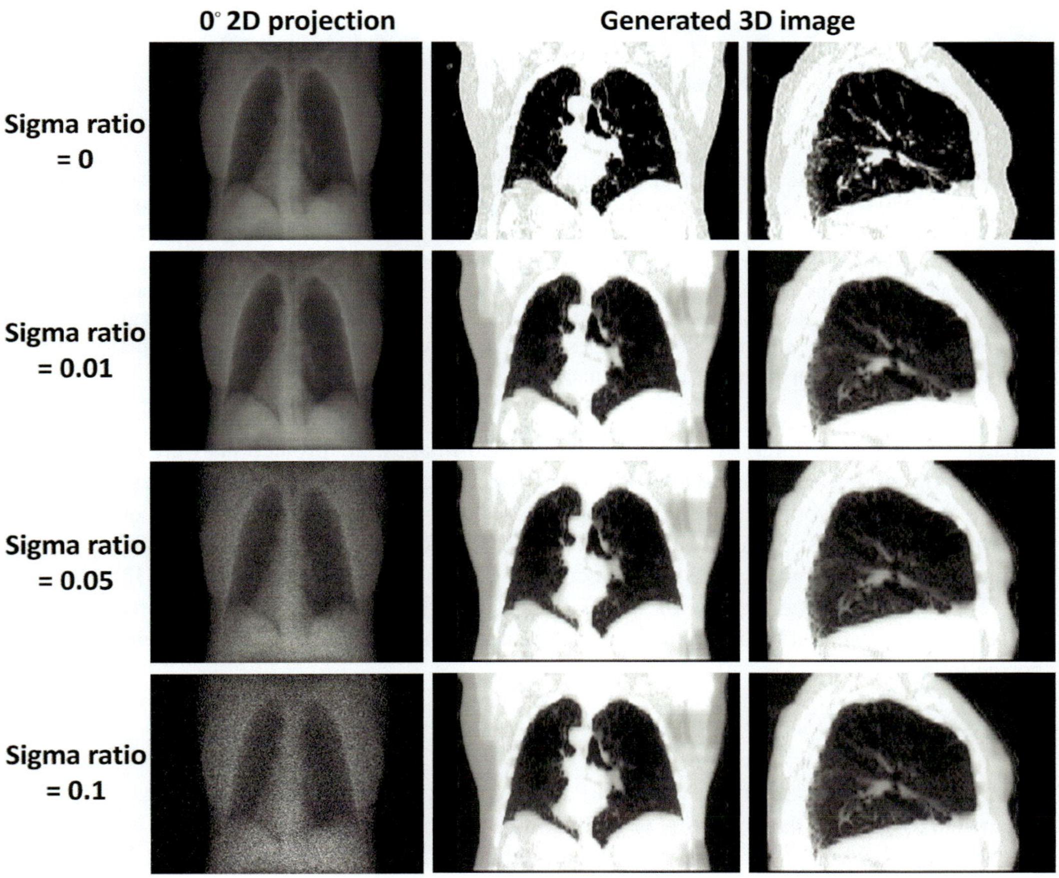

FIGURE 8.3 The 3D synthetic CT images generated from a single 2D kV projection of 0° projection angle with different noise levels. The first column displays the input 2D kV projection. The second and third columns display the generated 3D synthetic CT images in coronal and sagittal views, respectively. The four rows correspond to four different noise levels, that is, sigma ratio equals 0 (no added noise), 0.01, 0.05, and 0.1, respectively.

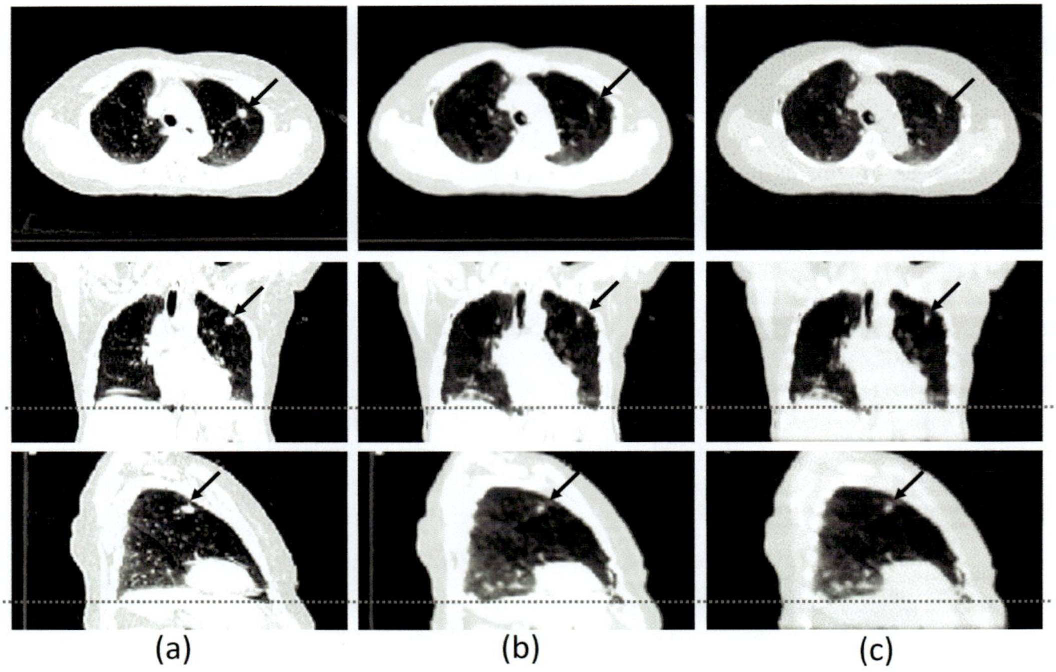

FIGURE 8.4 Visual results from Lei et al.'s simulation of a challenging testing scenario with doubled motion amplitude and approximately 50% tumor shrinkage compared to the original 4D CT. (a) Original CT at inhale (phase 0) in axial, sagittal, and coronal views. (b) Deformed CT images after applying the DVFs to simulate doubled motion amplitude and approximately 50% tumor shrinkage. These deformed CT images were used to generate a testing 2D projection of projection angle 0°. (c) The 3D synthetic CT images generated by Lei's method from this testing 2D projection, with the deformed CT images shown in (b) serving as ground truth. The tumor was pointed by an arrow in the images, and the dashed lines show the relative superior-inferior motion between the original and deformed CT images.

compared to the original 4D CT. From these deformed images, 2D projections were generated at various gantry angles and fed into the trained network to generate synthetic 3D images. As shown in Figure 8.4, the network produced 3D images with acceptable accuracy and image quality even under this challenging scenario. The obtained MAE, PSNR, and SSIM values of the 3D synthetic CT images generated from a single 2D projection of 0° projection angle are 79.0 HU, 15.9 dB, and 0.825. Tumors in the generated synthetic CT images and the corresponding ground-truth images were manually delineated by physicians, and the center of mass distance (COM) between them was reported to be 0.8 mm.

8.2.5 Discussion

2D kV imaging remains the most widely utilized modality for image guidance in radiation therapy, particularly during patient setup. Compared to MV imaging, kV imaging offers significantly better tissue contrast, facilitating more accurate patient alignment. Typically, for a LINAC-based radiation therapy, a pair of orthogonal kV images acquired through 90° gantry rotation is used prior to treatment initiation. However, during treatment delivery, performing 90° gantry rotation for orthogonal kV imaging is impractical. Because kV- and MV-imaging systems are mounted orthogonally on LINACs, both images can be acquired quickly without gantry movement. As a result, intra-fractional position verification is generally limited to a single kV image or a combined kV–MV image pair. Compared to a pair of kV images, a single kV image or a combined kV–MV image pair reduces the amount of anatomical information available, making real-time adaptive motion management during treatment difficult. In many cases, when tumor displacement exceeds predefined tolerance thresholds, radiation therapists often need to manually pause the treatment. Additional imaging is then necessary to quantify the extent and direction of motion, often resulting in workflow delays. For tumors susceptible to motion during treatment or difficult to visualize on kV images, such as those in the lung or abdomen, CBCT is frequently employed to estimate and correct for target movement. CBCT not only provides improved estimation of positional shifts but also offers enhanced visualization and delineation of the tumor relative to surrounding anatomy. In SBRT treatment, where high doses are delivered per fraction, CBCT is often essential for position verification. However, the acquisition and reconstruction of CBCT images substantially extend treatment time. This prolonged duration paradoxically increases the risk of additional patient or tumor motion, potentially undermining the corrective benefits of the imaging. Moreover, compared to 3D CT images, CBCT is more prone to artifacts and generally yields lower image quality. These limitations can obscure the tumor and surrounding tissues, reducing the reliability of tumor localization motion assessment.

Given these challenges, there is a critical need for novel imaging techniques capable of reconstructing 3D CT in real time using minimal input data, such as a single kV image or a kV–MV image pair. Such advancements would enhance the precision of motion tracking and enable more efficient, adaptive radiotherapy without the time penalties currently associated with motion management. In a pioneering study, Shen et al.[9] proposed the use of a deep neural network to learn the mapping from a single 2D kV image to the corresponding 3D CT volume. Building upon this foundational work, Lei et al.[20] introduced a more advanced GAN architecture for the 2D-3D transformation task. Their approach incorporated both perceptual and adversarial loss supervision during training, improving the realism and structural fidelity of the synthetic 3D CT. A subsequent study by Lei et al.[22] demonstrated that combining kV and MV projections added additional tissue information, further enhancing the accuracy of synthetic 3D CT. Their method employed Laplacian loss to suppress noise and capture fine structural details, along with convolution-based reweighting to dynamically adjust feature importance and improve image uniformity throughout the reconstruction process. Accurate real-time tumor tracking still requires additional steps, like image registration or segmentation, to localize the tumor within the synthetic 3D volume. This becomes especially difficult when tumors, such as those in the liver, have low contrast relative to surrounding tissues. To address this issue, Shao et al.[21] proposed a new framework that combines deep learning with biomechanical modeling to track liver tumors in real time from a single kV projection. This method uses a deep neural network to predict liver surface deformation based on features extracted from the kV projection. This predicted deformation serves as a boundary condition for a biomechanical model of the liver to analyze tumor motion through finite element analysis. Compared to earlier methods, these deep learning techniques offer much better accuracy and robustness in handling patient positioning, anatomy, and motion. This demonstrates that deep learning-based 2D-to-3D image transformation has strong potential for clinical use in motion management. However, hardware and technical issues still remain to be solved.

Most deep learning methods are trained on one group of patients and then applied to others, which means the training group must be representative enough. But the 2D-to-3D mapping problem is highly under-sampled and has a heavy dependence on the similarity of the training data and the testing data. Given the large variation between patients, as demonstrated in the works mentioned above, a better approach is to train the patient-specific networks using that patient's own 4D CT images and digitally reconstructed 2D projections. To expand the patient-specific training data, data augmentation techniques like translation, rotation, flipping, and scaling are used. These simulate different scenarios, such as daily setup variations and changes in breathing patterns or anatomy. As long as the patient's anatomy doesn't change significantly between the 4D CT scan and treatment (e.g., major weight loss or lung collapse), the training data should be representative enough for that patient.

However, another challenge arises when patients exhibit abnormal lung function or irregular breathing patterns, which can create unexpected conditions that patient-specific models may not handle well. In liver SBRT, for example, the liver can undergo large motion, which may reduce the robustness of mesh-based deformable registration techniques. Moving forward, it is essential to evaluate the robustness of deep learning methods on a larger cohort of patients, including those with atypical cases.

For clinical implementation, the digitally reconstructed 2D projections from 4D CT used for training must closely match the quality of actual in-treatment kV projections. In practice, kV images acquired by flat-panel detectors are often affected by scatter and noise, in contrast to the ideal, noise-free projections produced by conventional ray-tracing methods. This discrepancy can be mitigated through Monte Carlo simulations, which model individual photon interactions to generate more realistic training data. Another practical challenge is the limited field of view (FOV) of clinical kV panels, which may not fully capture the entire transverse span of the patient's anatomy. This limitation can impact methods that rely on accurate organ boundary deformation during network training.[21] A large FOV kV panel is therefore desirable to enable robust 3D CT reconstruction and ensure sufficient coverage of OARs, particularly for adaptive radiotherapy dose calculations.

Real-time 3D imaging also requires high computational efficiency. The 2D-to-3D transformation must be fast enough for real-time use, which may require high-end Graphics Processing Units (GPUs) or multi-GPU systems. In Lei et al.'s study,[20] generating a synthetic 3D image from a kV/MV pair took 20–30 seconds. With powerful GPUs, this can be reduced to about 1–2 seconds.

For the application online adaptive radiotherapy, follow-up studies on fast and accurate automatic tumor delineation and contour deformation from one phase CT to another need to be carried out and verified. Reliability and safety are critical for clinical adoption, especially if synthetic 3D images will guide motion management during treatment. Quality assurance (QA) should be performed at the start of each treatment fraction, or at regular intervals, or when noticeable anatomical changes occur. For example, before treatment begins, a standard CBCT scan can be taken while the patient holds their breath. A few projections from this scan can be randomly selected to generate synthetic 3D images for QA, using the CBCT image as the ground truth.

8.3 AI APPLICATION IN SURFACE-GUIDED MOTION MANAGEMENT

Optical surface-guiding imaging offers radiation-dose-free, noninvasive, large FOV (up to $110 \times 140 \times 240$ cm^3), high temporal resolution (10–24 Hz), and submillimeter detectability approach for patient setup and continuous intra-treatment monitoring.[25] It has become increasingly adopted in clinical practice for applications such as general patient positioning, breast deep-inspiration breath-hold (DIBH) treatments, and frameless stereotactic radiosurgery (SRS). Recently, surface imaging has also been proposed for real-time adaptive radiotherapy.[26,27] However, for treatment sites affected by tumor motion, several studies have reported that the correlation between surface motion and internal tumor movement is often imperfect.[28–30] More recently, with the advancement of surface-guided Radiation Therapy (RT) (SGRT), deep learning-based studies have emerged to investigate the correlation between surface imaging and the internal target motion, particularly for treatment sites such as lung and liver.[25,31] This section will use Pan et al.'s work[31] as a case study to introduce core deep learning-based surface structure to synthetic 3D CT transformation techniques and explore their potential for clinical integration.

8.3.1 Overview of the Deep Learning-Based Surface Structure to Synthetic 3D CT Transformation Methods

Pan et al.'s study leverages deep learning to investigate the relationship between patients' surface motion and internal tumor motion based on two primary hypotheses. The first hypothesis is that patient-specific deep learning training on volumetric images can provide the essential information

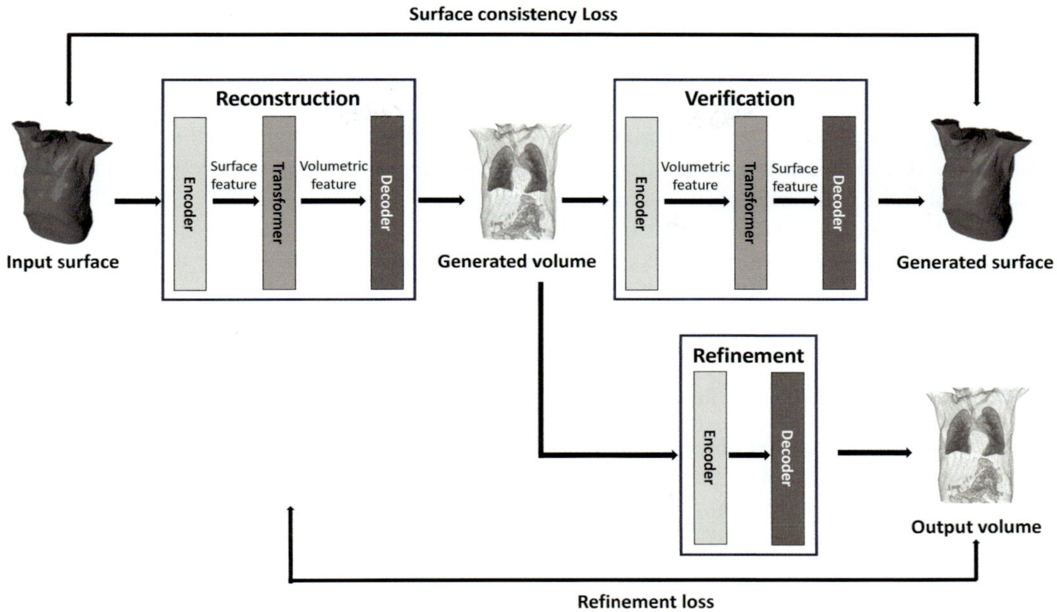

FIGURE 8.5 Illustration of the architecture of the surface-to-volume image synthesis framework. The input is a binary 3D surface volume, and the output is a synthetic 3D CT volume. The model is composed of three modular subnetworks: a reconstruction network, a verification network, and a refinement network.

to bridge the gap between surface imaging and volumetric imaging. The second hypothesis assumes no significant anatomical and breathing pattern changes that occur between the planning CT and treatment delivery, ensuring anatomical consistency. Under these assumptions, the proposed framework aims to generate synthetic CT images that reduce uncertainty in anatomical predictions.

Figure 8.5 illustrates the architecture of the surface-to-volume image synthesis framework. The input is a binary 3D surface volume, and the output is a synthetic 3D CT volume. The model is composed of three modular subnetworks: a reconstruction network, a verification network, and a refinement network (RF). The reconstruction network encodes surface images into feature maps and transforms them into volumetric representations for image reconstruction. During training, this network learns to correlate feature distributions between surface and volumetric data. The verification network maps the reconstructed 3D volume back to a surface representation to ensure consistency with the input surface. The RF network enforces scale invariance in CT values between the predicted and ground-truth CT volumes. It learns high-density tissue representation, noise levels, and contrast by incorporating patient- and machine-specific prior knowledge.

To address the challenge of limited training data, the network is designed to be patient-specific. A separate model is trained for each patient using their own 4DCT data, which is typically acquired during simulation for lung cancer patients to capture respiratory motion. This provides personalized prior knowledge linking external surface motion to internal anatomical structures.

8.3.2 Data Preparation

The model was trained using a large dataset consisting of 500 phase CT images from 50 4DCT scans, each from a different lung cancer patient who underwent radiation therapy at their institution. These 4DCT scans were acquired during treatment simulation and provide rich information on respiratory motion. To improve training efficiency, CT images were cropped to reduce the background air region. In each training experiment, eight respiratory phases were used for training, one randomly selected phase was used for validation, and the remaining phases were reserved for inference. Similar to the 2D-to-3D transformation method described in Section 8.2, patient-specific deep learning models were trained using data augmentation techniques to enhance robustness and performance. This patient-specific training strategy ensures that the model is well adapted to individual anatomy and motion characteristics, enabling accurate generation of volumetric images from surface inputs for use in surface-guided radiation therapy.

Pan et al. assumed that the patient underwent negligible body weight loss/gain, and surface meshes obtained via optical imaging could be accurately translated into surface volumes, specifically binary body masks aligned with the dimensions of ground-truth CT images taken at the simulation.

8.3.3 Supervision and Loss Function

The proposed reconstruction and verification generator networks, G_R and G_V, are trained using the framework of conditional generative adversarial networks (cGANs). In this setup, the generator aims to produce outputs that closely match the ground truth, while a discriminator learns to distinguish between real and synthetic images. The training is guided by a combined loss function:

$$L = L_{\text{vol}} + L_{\text{surf}} = \left[L_{D(S\to V)} + L_{G(S\to V)} + L_{I(V\to V)} + L_{C(V\to S\to V)}\right] + \left[L_{D(V\to S)} + L_{I(S\to S)} + + L_{C(S\to V\to S)}\right] \tag{8.5}$$

Here, V and S denote the volume and surface, respectively.

The term $L_{D(S\to V)} = 100\times \text{MAE}\left(G_R(S{\cdot}N),\ V\right)$ minimizes the HU difference between the synthetic and real 3D volumes. Similarly, $L_{D(V\to S)} = 100\times \text{DICE}\left(G_V(V{\cdot}N),\ S\right)$ measures the overlap between synthetic and ground-truth surface contours.

The generator loss $L_{G(S\to V)} = -\,D_R\left(S{\cdot}G_R(S{\cdot}N)\right)$ enhances visual realism in the reconstructed volume. Identity losses $L_{I(V\to V)} = 5\ \times \text{MAE}\left(G_R(V{\cdot}N),\ V\right)$ and $L_{I(S\to S)} = 5\times \text{DICE}\left(G_V(S{\cdot}N),\ S\right)$ preserve structural details.

Cycle-consistency losses $L_{C(V\to S\to V)}$, $L_{C(S\to V\to S)}$ ensure the reversibility of translation: $L_{C(V\to S\to V)} = 20\times \text{MAE}(G_R\left(G_V(V{\cdot}N){\cdot}N\right),\ V$ and $L_{C(S\to V\to S)} = 20\times \text{DICE}\left(G_V\left(G_R(S{\cdot}N){\cdot}N\right),\ S\right)$, where MAE indicates mean absolute error and DICE indicates dice score.

The discriminator D_R is trained with a gradient penalty term to provide reliable feedback:

$$L_{D_R} = D_R\ \left(S{\cdot}G_R(S{\cdot}N)\right) - \ D_R\ (S{\cdot}V) + 10\times\left(\left\|\nabla\left(D_R\left(S{\cdot}\left[\epsilon\times V + (1-\epsilon)\times G_R(S{\cdot}N)\right]\right)\right)_2^2\right\| - 1\right)^2 \tag{8.6}$$

where ∇ indicates the network gradients to the corresponding inputs and ϵ is a random number sampled from a beta distribution with 2 shape-parameters equal to 0.2. During training, the generator and discriminator networks are updated alternately. Every 10 epochs, performance is evaluated on validation data. After training, only the reconstruction network is used for generating volumes from surface data. Once the reconstruction and verification networks are trained, the down-sampled volumes are up-sampled using trilinear interpolation to obtain intermediate volumes V_I. These are further refined by the refinement network RF, which is trained to minimize the loss:

$$L_{\text{refine}} = \text{MAE}\ \left(\text{RF}(V_I), V_{I,\text{truth}}\right) \tag{8.7}$$

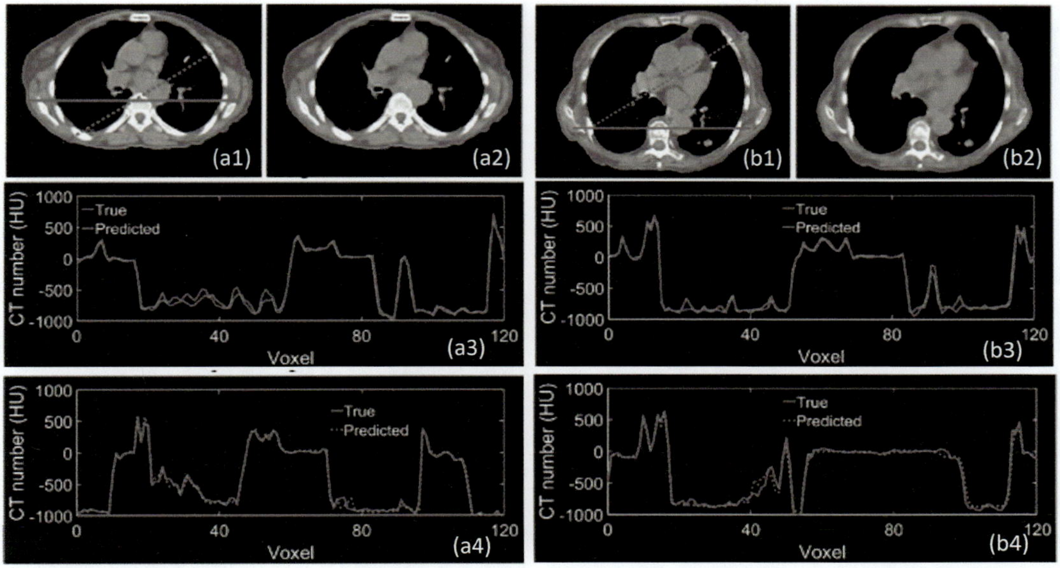

FIGURE 8.6 Comparisons of synthetic and ground-truth CT images for two example cases in transversal view. For Case 1, which achieved the highest SSIM among all the cases, the ground-truth CT images and the synthetic CT images predicted from surface images are shown in (a1) and (a2), respectively. CT number line profiles along the horizontal solid line and oblique dotted line in (a1) are shown in (a3) and (a4). Corresponding results for Case 2, which had the lowest SSIM, are shown in (b1–b4).

8.3.4 Evaluation Results

MAE and PSNR are employed to assess overall image quality in terms of noise, contrast, and CT number accuracy, while SSIM is used to measure structural similarity to ensure anatomical fidelity. To evaluate the predictive performance of the proposed framework, six additional patients who have one initial 4DCT and two follow-up 4DCT scans taken on average 18.0 ± 5.5 and 36.3 ± 9.3 days later were also tested. The model was trained using all phases of the initial 4DCT and tested on the two later scans.

Across the 50 patients who have only one set of 4DCT, the generated CT volumes showed an average MAE of 36.2 ± 7.0 HU, PSNR of 36.4 ± 1.9 dB, and SSIM of 0.94 ± 0.02 within the body contour and an average MAE of 51.8 ± 29.6 HU, PSNR of 35.5 ± 5.0 dB, and SSIM of 0.88 ± 0.09 within gross tumor volume (GTV). Across the six patients who have two resimulated 4DCT sets, the generated CT volumes for resimulated 4DCT set 1 showed an average MAE of 38.8 ± 4.2 HU, PSNR of 35.7 ± 1.4 dB, and SSIM of 0.93 ± 0.01 within the body contour, and an average MAE of 57.0 ± 13.8 HU, PSNR of 34.0 ± 1.5 dB, and SSIM of 0.87 ± 0.05 within GTV; the generated CT volumes for resimulated 4DCT set 2 showed an average MAE of 37.8 ± 4.0 HU, PSNR of 36.3 ± 1.2 dB, and SSIM of 0.94 ± 0.01 within the body contour, and an average MAE of 55.5 ± 13.0 HU, PSNR of 34.5 ± 1.3 dB, and SSIM of 0.89 ± 0.04 within GTV.

Figure 8.6 presents visual comparisons of the synthetic and ground-truth CT images for two example cases in the transverse plane, along with two CT HU line profiles. Figure 8.7 provides the corresponding sagittal view of the synthetic and ground-truth CT images of the two example cases, along with the histogram comparisons of CT numbers.

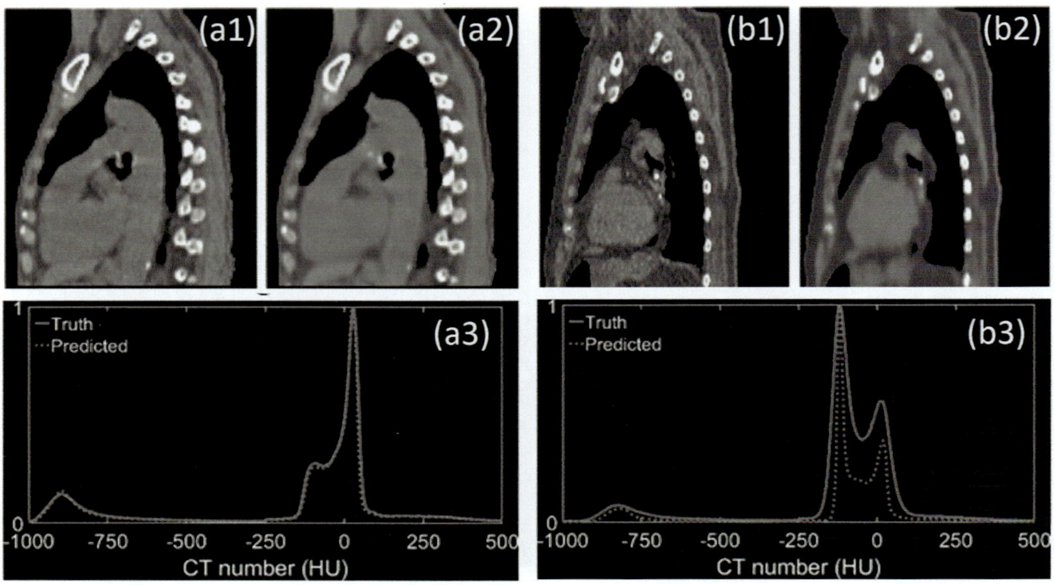

FIGURE 8.7 Comparisons of synthetic and ground-truth CT images for the two example cases in sagittal view. For Case 1, which achieved the highest SSIM among all the cases, the ground-truth CT images and the synthetic CT images predicted from surface images are shown in (a1) and (a2), respectively. The CT number histogram of the two images is shown in (a3). Corresponding results for Case 2, which had the lowest SSIM, are shown in (b1–b3).

8.3.5 Discussion

Surface-guided radiation therapy (SGRT) has seen growing adoption in radiation therapy for monitoring patient motion. However, in treatment sites affected by significant tumor motion, such as the lung, studies have reported that the correlation between external surface motion and internal tumor displacement is often weak or inconsistent.[21–23] In the current clinical practice, radiation delivery is automatically paused when the surface motion exceeds a predefined amplitude threshold. Yet, due to the complex and sometimes obscured relationship between external surface movement and internal tumor motion, being within the surface amplitude tolerance does not necessarily ensure that the tumor remains within its intended position, and vice versa. It is therefore highly desirable to explore the complex relationship between surface imaging and internal tumor motion, under the assumption that some level of correlation exists. Deep learning is well suited for this task due to its ability to learn complex patterns and uncover hidden relationships that traditional methods are often unable to reveal.

In a pioneering study by Pan et al., a cGAN-based deep learning framework was developed to generate synthetic 3D CT images from surface imaging data. Each patient-specific model was individually trained using a patient's own 4D CT phases, allowing training to occur in the background during treatment planning. Once trained, the model enables real-time 3D anatomy prediction with surface imaging devices, supporting patient setup, verification, and continuous monitoring within standard radiation therapy workflows. The synthetic CTs showed strong agreement with ground truth across different regions of interests. The relatively worse results obtained for the resimulated 4DCT set 1 and set 2 of the six patients, compared to the results achieved in the single 4DCT set of the 50 patients, illustrate that variations in patient motion can reduce reconstruction fidelity. This highlights the need for careful motion assessment, especially in patients with significant lung volume changes. Further research is needed to minimize motion-related effects during both image reconstruction and treatment delivery. The results also show uncertainty ranges, suggesting caution when applying the model to new patients. Irregular breathing or poor data quality may widen the error margin, affecting the reliability of synthetic CT predictions.

Although patient-specific training can take several hours, it can be completed during the typical 5- or 10-day planning window before treatment begins, as the 4DCT is acquired beforehand. Once trained, Pan et al.'s model inference time is around 0.4 seconds using a single NVIDIA A100 GPU. A key challenge for clinical adoption is the need for an online training interface. Future work will aim to reduce inference time to under 100 ms and streamline the framework for easier clinical integration.

Pan et al.'s model assumes some correlation between surface imaging and internal tumor motion, though this relationship can be complex. To address residual motion errors, Shao et al.[25] proposed using on-board X-ray imaging to improve accuracy. In their approach, a deep learning model (Surf) first learned the motion correlation between the patient's external surface and liver boundary from respiratory motion and used that to predict boundary motion from on-board surface images. Next, a 2D kV X-ray-based graph neural network (X model) corrected the remaining registration errors from the Surf model. It refined the liver boundary motion using features from a single X-ray projection, assuming that the X-ray and surface images were taken at the same respiratory phase. Finally, a population-based biomechanical model (Bio) used the corrected liver boundary motion as input to estimate the full intra-liver motion. This workflow assumes that the patient's motion during treatment matches the motion seen in 4DCT scans, which still needs further validation—especially for patients with varying inter- or intra-fraction motion. This study has shown accurate liver tumor localization. It is also more robust to scenarios with large motion, as compared to models using the surface imaging or the X-ray projection alone.

A challenge in verifying such models with real patient data is the lack of ground truth for liver tumor motion. Fiducial markers can help track rigid motion but not deformation. Realistic liver phantoms that simulate motion can provide a reference standard for evaluating deformable motion models.

8.4 CHAPTER SUMMARY

In this chapter, we looked at how AI—especially deep learning—is used for motion management in radiation therapy. Since 2D kV imaging and SGRT are the most commonly used techniques in the clinic, we focused on deep learning methods that create synthetic 3D CT images from these inputs. Studies by Lei et al.[20] and Pan et al.[31] show that AI can really help streamline clinical workflows and support adaptive radiotherapy. These methods aren't used in clinics yet, but research is ongoing to improve image accuracy, GPU performance, and hardware integration. Although MRI- and PET-guided radiotherapy are available, they're still used in only a few clinic centers, so we didn't go into detail on those. For more on those, check out review papers.[32–35]

REFERENCES

1. Shirato H, Seppenwoolde Y, Kitamura K, Onimura R, Shimizu S. Intrafractional tumor motion: lung and liver. *Seminars in Radiation Oncology*, 2004; 14(1):10–18. doi: 10.1053/j.semradonc.2003.10.008. PMID: 14752729.
2. Keall PJ, Mageras GS, Balter JM, et al. The management of respiratory motion in radiation oncology report of AAPM Task Group 76 a. *Medical Physics*, 2006;33(10):3874–3900. doi: 10.1118/1.2349696. PMID: 17089851.
3. Mori S, Hara R, Yanagi T, et al. Four-dimensional measurement of intrafractional respiratory motion of pancreatic tumors using a 256 multi-slice CT scanner. 2009;92(2):231–237.

4. Schmidt ML, Hoffmann L, Kandi M, Møller DS, Poulsen PRJAO. Dosimetric impact of respiratory motion, interfraction baseline shifts, and anatomical changes in radiotherapy of non-small cell lung cancer. *Acta Oncologica*, 2013;52(7):1490–1496. doi: 10.3109/0284186X.2013.815798. Epub 2013 Aug 2. PMID: 23905673.
5. Mutaf Y, Scicutella C, Michalski D, et al. A simulation study of irregular respiratory motion and its dosimetric impact on lung tumors. *Physics in Medicine* & Biology, 2011;56(3):845–859. doi: 10.1088/0031-9155/56/3/019. Epub 2011 Jan 17. PMID: 21242627.
6. Liu G, Hu F, Ding X, et al. Simulation of dosimetry impact of 4DCT uncertainty in 4D dose calculation for lung SBRT. *Radiation Oncology*, 2019;14(1):1. doi: 10.1186/s13014-018-1191-y. PMID: 30621744; PMCID: PMC6323842
7. Van den Begin R, Engels B, Gevaert T, et al. Impact of inadequate respiratory motion management in SBRT for oligometastatic colorectal cancer. *Radiation Oncology*, 2014;113(2):235–239. doi: 10.1016/j.radonc.2014.11.005. Epub 2014 Nov 28. PMID: 25441611.
8. Yan H, Tian Z, Shao Y, Jiang SB, Jia X. A new scheme for real-time high-contrast imaging in lung cancer radiotherapy: a proof-of-concept study. *Physics in Medicine & Biology*. 2016;61(6):2372.
9. Shen L, Zhao W, Xing LJNbe. Patient-specific reconstruction of volumetric computed tomography images from a single projection view via deep learning. *Nature Biomedical Engineering*, 2019;3(11):880–888. doi: 10.1038/s41551-019-0466-4
10. Tang J, Nett BE, Chen G-H. Performance comparison between total variation (TV)-based compressed sensing and statistical iterative reconstruction algorithms. *Physics in Medicine & Biology*. 2009;54(19):5781.
11. Jorgensen JS, Sidky EY, Pan X. Quantifying admissible undersampling for sparsity-exploiting iterative image reconstruction in X-ray CT. *IEEE Transactions on Medical Imaging*. 2012;32(2):460–473.
12. Choi K, Wang J, Zhu L, Suh TS, Boyd S, Xing L. Compressed sensing based cone-beam computed tomography reconstruction with a first-order method a. *Medical Physics*. 2010;37(9):5113–5125.
13. Lee H, Xing L, Davidi R, Li R, Qian J, Lee R. Improved compressed sensing-based cone-beam CT reconstruction using adaptive prior image constraints. *Physics in Medicine & Biology*. 2012;57(8):2287.
14. Xu Q, Yu H, Mou X, Zhang L, Hsieh J, Wang G. Low-dose X-ray CT reconstruction via dictionary learning. *IEEE Transactions on Medical Imaging*. 2012;31(9):1682–1697.
15. Tian Z, Jia X, Yuan K, Pan T, Jiang SB. Low-dose CT reconstruction via edge-preserving total variation regularization. *Physics in Medicine & Biology*. 2011;56(18):5949.
16. Li R, Jia X, Lewis JH, et al. Real-time volumetric image reconstruction and 3D tumor localization based on a single x-ray projection image for lung cancer radiotherapy. *Medical Physics*, 2010;37(6Part1):2822–2826. doi: 10.1118/1.3426002. PMID: 20632593.
17. Li R, Lewis JH, Jia X, et al. On a PCA-based lung motion model. *Physics in Medicine & Biology*, 2011;56(18):6009–6030. doi: 10.1088/0031-9155/56/18/015. Epub 2011 Aug 24. PMID: 21865624; PMCID: PMC3915048.
18. Zhao Q, Chou C-R, Mageras G, Pizer S. Local metric learning in 2D/3D deformable registration with application in the abdomen. *IEEE Transactions on Medical Imaging*, 2014;33(8):1592–1600. doi: 10.1109/TMI.2014.2319193. Epub 2014 Apr 22. PMID: 24771575; PMCID: PMC4321725.
19. Xu Y, Yan H, Ouyang L, et al. A method for volumetric imaging in radiotherapy using single x-ray projection. *Medical Physics*. 2015;42(5):2498–2509. doi: 10.1118/1.4918577. PMID: 25979043; PMCID: PMC4409629
20. Lei Y, Tian Z, Wang T, et al. Deep learning-based real-time volumetric imaging for lung stereotactic body radiation therapy: a proof of concept study. Physics in Medicine & Biology. 2020;65(23):235003. doi: 10.1088/1361-6560/abc303. PMID: 33080578; PMCID: PMC11756341.
21. Shao H-C, Wang J, Bai T, et al. Real-time liver tumor localization via a single x-ray projection using deep graph neural network-assisted biomechanical modeling. *Physics in Medicine & Biology*. 2022;67(11):115009.
22. Lei Y, Tian Z, Wang T, et al. Deep learning-based fast volumetric imaging using kV and MV projection images for lung cancer radiotherapy: a feasibility study. *Medical Physics*. 2023;50(9):5518–5527.
23. Nie D, Trullo R, Lian J, et al. Medical image synthesis with deep convolutional adversarial networks. *IEEE Transactions on Biomedical Engineering*. 2018;65(12):2720–2730. doi: 10.1109/TBME.2018.2814538
24. Harms J, Lei Y, Wang T, et al. Paired cycle-GAN-based image correction for quantitative cone-beam computed tomography. *Medical Physics*. 2019;46(9):3998–4009. doi: 10.1002/mp.13656. Epub 2019 Jul 17. PMID: 31206709; PMCID: PMC7771209.
25. Shao H-C, Li Y, Wang J, Jiang S, Zhang Y. Real-time liver tumor localization via combined surface imaging and a single x-ray projection. *Physics in Medicine & Biology*. 2023;68(6):065002.

26. Al-Hallaq HA, Cerviño L, Gutierrez AN, et al. AAPM task group report 302: surface-guided radiotherapy. *Medical Physics.* 2022;49(4):e82–e112.
27. Gierga DP, Turcotte JC, Tong LW, Chen Y-LE, DeLaney TF. Analysis of setup uncertainties for extremity sarcoma patients using surface imaging. *Practical Radiation Oncology.* 2014;4(4):261–266.
28. Stanley DN, McConnell KA, Kirby N, Gutiérrez AN, Papanikolaou N, Rasmussen K. Comparison of initial patient setup accuracy between surface imaging and three point localization: A retrospective analysis. *Journal of Applied Clinical Medical Physics.* 2017;18(6):58–61.
29. Walter F, Freislederer P, Belka C, Heinz C, Söhn M, Roeder F. Evaluation of daily patient positioning for radiotherapy with a commercial 3D surface-imaging system (Catalyst™). *Radiation Oncology.* 2016;11:1–8.
30. Carl G, Reitz D, Schönecker S, et al. Optical surface scanning for patient positioning in radiation therapy: a prospective analysis of 1902 fractions. *Technology in Cancer Research & Treatment.* 2018;17:1533033818806002.
31. Pan S, Chang C-W, Tian Z, et al. Data-driven volumetric computed tomography image generation from surface structures using a patient-specific deep leaning model. *International Journal of Radiation Oncology, Biology, Physics.* 2025;121(5):1349–1360.
32. Zhang X, Yan D, Xiao H, Zhong R. Modeling of artificial intelligence-based respiratory motion prediction in MRI-guided radiotherapy: a review. *Radiation Oncology.* 2024;19(1):140.
33. Zhao W, Shen L, Islam MT, et al. Artificial intelligence in image-guided radiotherapy: a review of treatment target localization. *Quantitative Imaging in Medicine and Surgery.* 2021;11(12):4881.
34. Placidi L, Ruggieri R. Use of artificial intelligence in MR-guided RT. In: Enis Ozyar, Cem Onal, Sara L. Hackett (eds), *Advances in Magnetic Resonance Technology and Applications.* Vol 8. Elsevier; 2023:491–512. ISSN 2666-9099, ISBN 9780323916899, https://doi.org/10.1016/B978-0-323-91689-9.00024-8. (https://www.sciencedirect.com/science/article/pii/B9780323916899000248)
35. Artesani A, Bruno A, Gelardi F, Chiti A. Empowering PET: harnessing deep learning for improved clinical insight. *European Radiology Experimental.* 2024;8(1):17.

9 Proton and FLASH Therapy

Serdar Charyyev, Zi Yang, and Hao Peng

9.1 INTRODUCTION

Artificial intelligence (AI) has emerged as a transformative force across various sectors, with a particularly significant impact in healthcare. This transformation has been enabled by advances in big data, computing power, and machine learning algorithms.[1,2] In radiotherapy specifically, AI has become increasingly relevant as the field progresses toward more precise and personalized cancer treatments, complementing technologies like Intensity-Modulated Radiation Therapy (IMRT), volumetric modulated arc therapy (VMAT), IGRT, SBRT, and proton therapy. The radiotherapy workflow, which encompasses multiple complex stages from imaging to post-treatment follow-up, stands to benefit significantly from AI integration to enhance efficiency.[1–4]

Proton therapy, distinguished from photon therapy by its characteristic Bragg peak, offers superior dose targeting and tissue protection.[5–7] However, this advantage comes with heightened precision requirements, as any delivery errors can result in significant dose deviations. This challenge has spurred AI research in various areas, including image conversion (magnetic resonance imaging (MR) to computed tomography (CT), dual-energy CT (DECT)/cone-beam CT (CBCT) to stopping power ratio (SPR) maps, CBCT to CT), optimization and dose calculation, real-time verification, image guidance, and FLASH therapy. These developments represent promising opportunities for advancing the field of radiation oncology through AI implementation.

9.2 AI FOR TREATMENT PLANNING IN PROTON THERAPY

9.2.1 Stopping Power Ratio and Material Maps

The accurate calculation of SPR is an indispensable component in proton therapy. Dose calculation based on CT images requires the conversion from Hounsfield Units (HU) to SPR. Over the past decade, a widely used approach is a piecewise linear fit based on the HU numbers in a single-energy CT (SECT) measured with tissue surrogates.[8–15] However, using such an empirical fitting for HU–SPR calibration introduces inaccuracies due to three challenges: (1) many-to-one mapping, (2) intrinsic fitting error, and (3) patient-specific tissue heterogeneities. To improve on the abovementioned issues related to SECT, Gao et al.[16] developed a method utilizing deep learning (DL) to enhance SPR estimation from SECT data, aiming to overcome some of the traditional fitting challenges.

Recent advancements have leveraged DECT to enhance SPR estimation and address some of the previously mentioned challenges. Analytical methods using interaction cross-sections (e.g., photoelectric and Compton scattering) derived from DECT images have been integrated into clinical routines for improved accuracy. Some groups adopted AI tools for SPR and material map generation expanding beyond SECT.[17–21] For example, Charyyev et al. proposed generating synthetic DECT (sDECT) from SECT and then deriving SPR from sDECT using a residual attention generative adversarial network (GAN). The SPR maps generated from sDECT were found to be comparable to those from original DECTs (Figure 9.1).[17] Concurrently, Wang et al. integrated a cycle-consistent GAN to predict SPR maps directly from DECTs. Their study, which included 20 head-and-neck cancer patients and employed leave-one-out cross-validation, indicated promising results, though further evaluation with larger patient cohorts and varying DECT acquisition protocols is warranted.[18] Liu et al. proposed using two convolutional neural networks (CNNs), U-Net and ResNet, for deriving elemental concentrations from DECT. While their primary goal was to determine carbon and

DOI: 10.1201/9781003480365-10

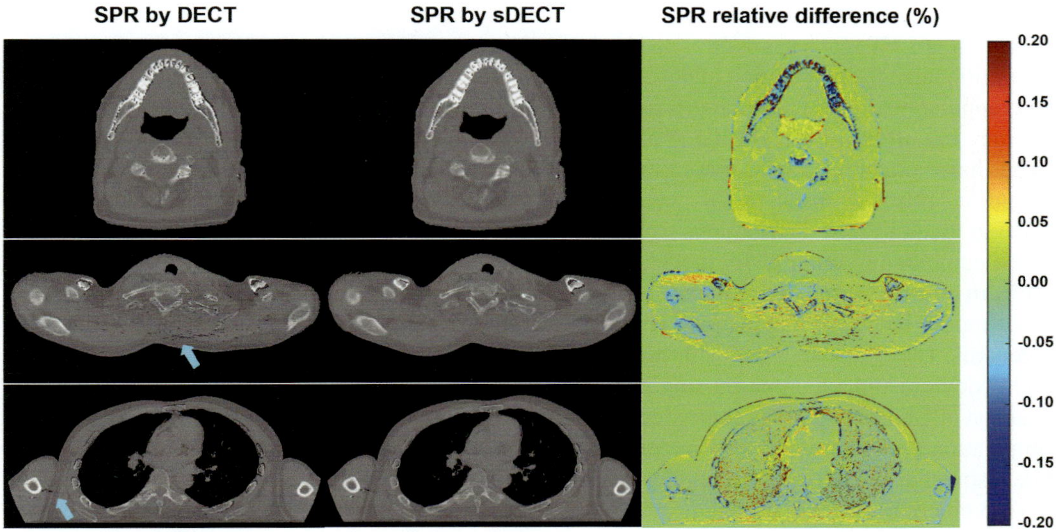

FIGURE 9.1 SPR maps generated from DECT and sDECT, and their relative percent difference maps.

oxygen concentrations, the method is also applicable to hydrogen. They achieved <2% mean absolute errors (MAEs) and <4% root mean-square errors in deriving carbon/oxygen concentrations for brain images when no noise was present.[19] Different accuracy and noise immunity were observed between U-Net and ResNet. Chang et al.[21] further validated a DL-based material estimation model for Monte Carlo (MC) dose calculation in proton therapy, achieving high gamma-passing rates and consistent results with empirical models.

In addition to DECT, recent research highlights the use of other imaging modalities for SPR and material map derivation.[22–24] Harms et al.[22] demonstrated a deep-learning-based approach to generate SPR maps from CBCT images, utilizing a cycle-GAN architecture to predict SPR maps from daily CBCT scans, allowing for online dose calculation and potentially facilitating adaptive radiation therapy. This method, applied to 23 head-and-neck cancer patients, showed high accuracy compared to planning CT, with an MAE of 0.06 and a mean error of −0.01. Scholey et al.[23] utilized DL to map kilovoltage CT (kVCT) HU to megavoltage CT (MVCT) HU, resulting in improved accuracy for relative electron density and SPR. Similarly, Chang et al. introduced a physics-constrained DL-based multimodal imaging framework, integrating magnetic resonance imaging (MRI) and DECT to enhance mass density estimation and reduce proton range uncertainty.[24]

The rationale for these AI-based approaches is elaborated below. Essentially, the role of AI is to map from one domain (CT images) to another (e.g., SPR and elemental concentration). While conventional DECT-based approaches face challenges like ill-posed inverse problems and nonuniqueness, AI models can mitigate these issues. AI models benefit from two key aspects: (1) geometric prior and (2) noise/artifact immunity.[19] Geometric prior refers to the ability of models like U-Net or ResNet to extract both local and global image features, leveraging spatial information to enforce geometrical correlations among voxels. Noise/artifact immunity is also enhanced by AI, as models trained with high-SNR images maintain accuracy when tested with low-SNR images, demonstrating robustness and noise resilience.[19]

9.2.2 Linear Energy Transfer Maps

Linear energy transfer (LET) distributions play a crucial role in enhancing the precision of proton therapy, particularly in understanding the biological effects of proton beams on tissues.[25] The accurate calculation of LET is essential for optimizing treatment plans, as it provides insight into the dose distribution's potential biological impact.[26] This section explores recent advancements in the generation of LET maps using AI.

Traditionally, the calculation of dose-averaged LET (LETd) has relied on MC simulations, which are computationally intensive and time-consuming. These simulations are the gold standard for accuracy but often limit real-time application in clinical settings due to their complexity. Recent studies have sought to address these limitations by leveraging DL techniques to generate LET maps more efficiently. For instance, Gao et al.[27] developed a DL-based framework using a cycle-GAN model to predict LETd distributions from dose maps. Their approach demonstrated superior performance compared to other GAN models, achieving MAE of 0.096 ± 0.019 keV/μm, and promising results in clinical target volumes and surrounding organs.[27] Tang et al.[28] introduced a 3D Cascaded U-Net model for LETd calculation. Their model utilized patient anatomy and dose-to-water data to generate LETd distributions with high accuracy. The model achieved an average MAE of 0.94 ± 0.14 MeV/cm and a gamma-passing rate of 97.4% ± 1.3%, significantly enhancing the speed and precision of LET calculations compared to traditional methods. This DL approach not only reduces computational demands but also integrates seamlessly into proton treatment planning systems.[28] Pirlepesov et al.[29] expanded the application of DL in LET prediction by developing a 3D dose and LETd prediction model using feed-forward neural networks. Their model was trained to accept a prospectively generated beam-path contour and evaluated through dose- and LETd-volume metrics. The accuracy of LETd predictions showed strong agreement with planned distributions, indicating the potential of knowledge-based planning to address biological uncertainties and improve treatment consistency.[29] Starke et al.[30] investigated the use of neural networks as surrogate models for MC simulations to predict LETd based on planned dose distributions and CT images. Their approach, validated through cross-validation on a cohort of brain tumor patients, showed that neural networks could approximate MC-based LETd distributions with reasonable accuracy. This method offers a viable alternative to MC simulations, particularly in resource-constrained settings, and supports the development of more adaptive treatment planning strategies.[30]

In addition to computational methods, experimental validation of LET measurements[31–33] has been explored. Stasica et al.[33] utilized a high-resolution detector, Timepix, to track and identify particles, with the purpose of experimental verification of LET spectra and LETd values for mixed radiation fields produced by the therapeutic proton beam. A CNN was developed for efficient particle track recognition resolving protons from photon and electron events, with recognized protons having high-fidelity LET spectra and LETd values when compared with MC simulations.

9.2.3 MR-Based Planning

Radiation therapy traditionally relies on CT imaging for treatment planning due to its ability to delineate anatomical structures and calculate dosimetric parameters. However, CT images suffer from poor soft tissue contrast, which can complicate the accurate delineation of clinical target volumes (CTVs). MRI, with its superior soft tissue contrast, has been proposed as a complementary modality to address this limitation. To simplify the integration of MRI into treatment planning and reduce the complexities associated with image registration between CT and MRI, MR-only treatment planning has emerged as a promising approach. Central to this process is the generation of synthetic CT (sCT) images from MRI data, so that CT HU numbers from sCT could subsequently be used in treatment planning.

Existing methods for generating sCT images can be broadly categorized into atlas-based, segmentation-based, and AI-based methods. Atlas-based approaches rely on anatomical models to predict CT values but often struggle with irregular anatomical structures and registration errors.[34–40] Segmentation-based methods, which involve manual or semi-automated contouring of anatomical structures, are time-consuming and prone to errors.[41–45]

In recent years, AI-based methods have gained prominence due to their ability to automate and enhance the accuracy of sCT generation. Early AI approaches included dictionary learning[46] and random forests,[47] but DL methods[48–51] have shown significant improvements in feature extraction and image mapping. For instance, Spadea et al. used a U-Net model to predict HU values from MRI data with promising results,[52] and Neppl et al. compared 2-D and 3-D U-Net models for head MRI images.[53] More recently, Florkow et al. demonstrated the feasibility of a U-Net-based method for pediatric abdominal tumors.[54] Their method has shown that the dosimetric differences between standard CT and sCT are minimal, generally within 2%, potentially influenced by interscan differences. Further advancements include the work of Zimmermann et al. who designed MR-only workflow for photon and proton therapy.[55] They proposed an acquisition and stitching protocol for low-field MR scanners to overcome field-of-view limitations, leading to effective sCT generation with high accuracy in delineation and dosimetric comparison. Their approach demonstrated good acceptance and minimal deviations between sCT and conventional CT in treatment plans. Additionally, the same group developed an MRI sequence-independent CNN for generating synthetic head CTs for proton therapy.[56] Their approach utilized a 3D U-Net with ResNet blocks, trained across multiple MRI sequences to enhance sCT generation accuracy. The study achieved excellent structural similarity and minimal differences in dose parameters between original and recalculated treatment plans.

A significant limitation of current sCT generation methods is their reliance on paired MR and CT images, which can introduce errors if the images are misaligned. To address this, GANs have been explored as a solution for synthesizing CT images from unpaired MRI data. Liu et al. employed a 3D dense cycle-GAN for generating abdominal and pelvic sCTs,[57,58] while Kazemifar et al. investigated GANs for brain images.[59] Maspero evaluated conditional GANs for pediatric brain MRI data,[60] and Shafai-Erfani utilized a 3D cycle-GAN for brain MRI images.[61] Chen et al. developed an advanced deep CNN architecture, combining conditional GANs with U-Net models to generate sCTs for intensity-modulated proton therapy (IMPT) in nasopharyngeal carcinoma patients.[62] This study highlighted the effectiveness of GANs in reducing MAEs and improving dosimetric accuracy, with the GAN3D model achieving notable improvements over the GAN2D model. Liu et al.'s[63] proposed a label-GAN model that can generate sDECT images from MRI, effectively simulating both high- and low-energy CT images to estimate SPR. This method achieved MAEs of 79.98 ± 18.11 HU and 80.15 ± 16.27 HU for synthetic low- and high-energy CTs, respectively, and demonstrated a significant improvement over traditional cycle-GANs in generating accurate SPR maps. Li et al. developed an uncertainty-aware framework for MR-based CT synthesis aimed at robust proton therapy planning.[64] Their approach utilized a conditional GAN combined with a Bayesian neural network to predict uncertainties in sCT generation. This framework was tested on 64 brain tumor patients, and the results showed that incorporating uncertainty prediction improved the dosimetric agreement between plans based on sCT and those based on planning CT.

GANs offer the advantage of working with unpaired datasets, reducing the need for perfectly aligned MRI and CT pairs. This capability stems from their bidirectional generator/discriminator workflow and the enforcement of cycle consistency, which helps mitigate voxelwise misalignment issues.[65] Stemming from this flexibility, some groups even trained GANs that derive SPR maps directly from MRI, given that MRI does not inherently provide this information. Gao et al. developed a DL-based framework to estimate both mass density and SPR directly from MRI, bypassing the need for additional imaging modalities like CT.[66] Their models, which utilized T1, T2, and zero echo time MRI sequences, demonstrated high accuracy in predicting mass density and SPR, with mean absolute percentage errors as low as 0.09% for bone tissues. Similarly, Wang et al. focused on synthesizing SPR images from multiple MRI sequences, including T1- and T2-weighted scans, achieving precise SPR estimation with reduced MAEs compared to traditional methods.[67]

MRI-only treatment planning, especially in proton therapy, presents several potential benefits, including the elimination of MR–CT co-registration errors, reduced CT radiation exposure, and a streamlined clinical workflow. Despite these advantages, challenges remain, particularly regarding dataset sizes and the comparison of AI-based methods with conventional approaches. Future research should focus on utilizing larger and more diverse datasets to validate AI methods rigorously and evaluate their performance against traditional techniques in terms of quantitative dosimetric parameters.

9.3 AI FOR DOSE CALCULATION IN PROTON THERAPY

9.3.1 Optimization

AI holds transformative potential throughout the entire spectrum of traditional radiotherapy, from simulation to delivery, including the crucial stage of plan optimization. Recent studies have demonstrated the potential of DL models to enhance optimization aspects of proton therapy planning.[68–70] For example, Kaderka et al. proposed a DL approach for automatic beam angle selection in proton liver treatments, achieving clinically comparable dosimetric outcomes to those manually selected by human planners, with high agreement on beam angles and similar plan quality.[68] Similarly, Cheon et al. developed BAODS-Net, a convolutional neural network-based method for optimizing beam angles in double-scattering proton therapy, which demonstrated high accuracy in beam angle ranking and produced treatment plans with quality comparable to clinical standards.[69] Additionally, Vazquez et al. introduced a DL model to predict percentile dose distributions, enhancing robustness evaluation by providing detailed statistical assessments of dose uncertainty, which outperformed traditional methods.[70]

Building on these innovations, Maes et al. propose a shift away from the traditional iterative planning workflow by utilizing AI for end-to-end optimization. Traditionally, the process involves contouring, beam placement, objective setting, and iterative adjustments to meet clinical goals, which can be time-consuming. In contrast, their approach integrates a 3D U-Net model into the planning system to directly predict dose distributions from regions of interest (ROIs) and beam configurations (Figure 9.2), thereby bypassing iterative adjustments.[71] This method simplifies planning by providing an initial dose distribution estimate, referred to as dose prediction. However, since the 3D U-Net does not incorporate physical constraints, a subsequent Dose Mimicking Optimization step is employed to convert these AI-generated Dose Predictions into clinically deliverable plans. Evaluation of this approach demonstrated that the AI-optimized plans achieved clinical quality comparable to traditional methods while offering enhanced dosimetric coverage.[71]

These advancements collectively highlight the transformative impact of AI on proton therapy planning, specifically on optimization and robustness.

9.3.2 Dose Calculation

Dose calculation is a fundamental aspect of radiotherapy, playing a crucial role in determining the precise delivery of radiation to target tissues while minimizing exposure to surrounding healthy tissues. With rapid advancements in technology, the integration of AI into dose calculation processes

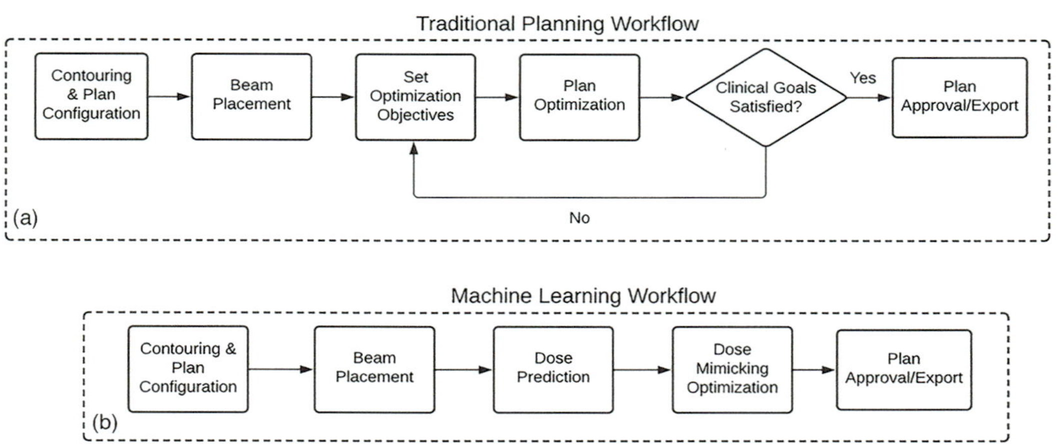

FIGURE 9.2 Workflow for traditional treatment planning (a) and ML-based treatment planning (b).

has reached a point where it is not only feasible but increasingly prevalent in clinical settings. This section explores the various ways in which AI is enhancing proton dose calculation.

In proton therapy, dose calculation is notably more complex than in photon therapy due to the unique physical properties of protons. Two primary approaches have been developed for dose calculation in proton therapy: the Pencil Beam Algorithm (PBA) and Monte Carlo Simulation (MC). The PBA involves tracing individual pencil beams through the patient, which simplifies the process but often falls short in accuracy due to its assumptions of lateral homogeneity and insufficient modeling of tissue heterogeneity and particle interactions.[72–74] Conversely, MC simulations provide a more accurate representation by modeling the detailed interactions of protons with tissues, though they are computationally intensive and time-consuming.[72,75–78] Recent studies have explored the use of graphical processing units (GPUs) to accelerate MC-based calculations, aiming to balance accuracy with computational efficiency.[79–82]

AI has emerged as a transformative tool in dose calculation, particularly through DL models. Early work by the UT Southwestern group demonstrated the potential of densely connected U-Net models for enhancing dose calculation accuracy.[83–85] Their studies utilized DL to bridge the gap between fast but less accurate algorithms like the PBA and the high precision of MC simulations. For instance, one study trained a 3D HD U-Net (a combination of U-Net and DenseNet) model to convert PBA doses into MC doses for a dataset of 290 patients (90 head and neck, 93 liver, 75 prostate, and 32 lung), achieving high gamma (1 mm/1%) passing rates across various tumor sites, 92.8% (head and neck), 92.7% (liver), 89.7% (lung), and 99.6% (prostate), and significantly reducing calculation times to less than 4 seconds.[85] In a similar vein, Javaid et al. explored using DL to "denoise" MC dose distributions. By starting with MC simulations using fewer particles, their approach leveraged U-Net to refine these distributions to match those obtained from simulations with a larger number of particles, thus reducing computation time while maintaining accuracy.[86] Their model demonstrated impressive results, with gamma-index pass rates consistently above 94% and computation times dramatically shorter than traditional MC simulations.[86]

The above examples show how CNNs have been used in the context of proton therapy dose calculation, where less accurate data is boosted to a more accurate level. Rather than inputting less accurate (noisy) data, some researchers have explored using more direct inputs such as CT images and beam masks to improve dose prediction. For example, Zhang et al. adopted a fully connected 3D U-Net model, utilizing a multi-channel 3D matrix as input.[87] This matrix included pre-processed CT matrices, contour bitmask matrices, and beam mask matrices. The model was trained to produce a 3D dose matrix based on ground-truth dose data. To account for the significant impact of beam paths on dose distributions in pencil beam scanning proton therapy (PBSPT), enhancements were made to the beam mask method. This method involved extracting beam-path information from the radiotherapy treatment plan and assigning values to voxels within beam paths, thus improving dose prediction accuracy in target regions and multi-beam overlapped areas. The sliding window technique was also used to focus on local details during model training, further enhancing performance.[87] Similarly, Guerreiro et al. developed a network that predicts 3D dose distributions based on beam segment shapes and patient anatomy.[88] Their approach utilized five different 3D volumes as inputs, including a ray-traced mask of the segment, which encoded field sizes and scattering components. The deep convolutional network was trained with patch-based training and data augmentation, utilizing a root mean squared error (RMSE) loss function and the ADAM optimizer. Chen et al. presented a dose prediction model that utilized CT images and contour data of target volumes and organs at risk. This approach demonstrated the ability to generate detailed and accurate dose predictions by effectively integrating structural and anatomical information.[89]

To add more examples, recent research introduced a DL-based millisecond-speed dose calculation algorithm (DoTA), which utilizes CNNs combined with a transformer self-attention mechanism to accurately predict proton dose distributions from CT and energies as inputs. This method achieved remarkable performance with a gamma pass rate of 99.37% and improved speed and precision compared to traditional methods like analytical pencil beam algorithms and MC simulations.[90] Another notable study employed a 3D CNN for proton dose calculation in head-and-neck cases,

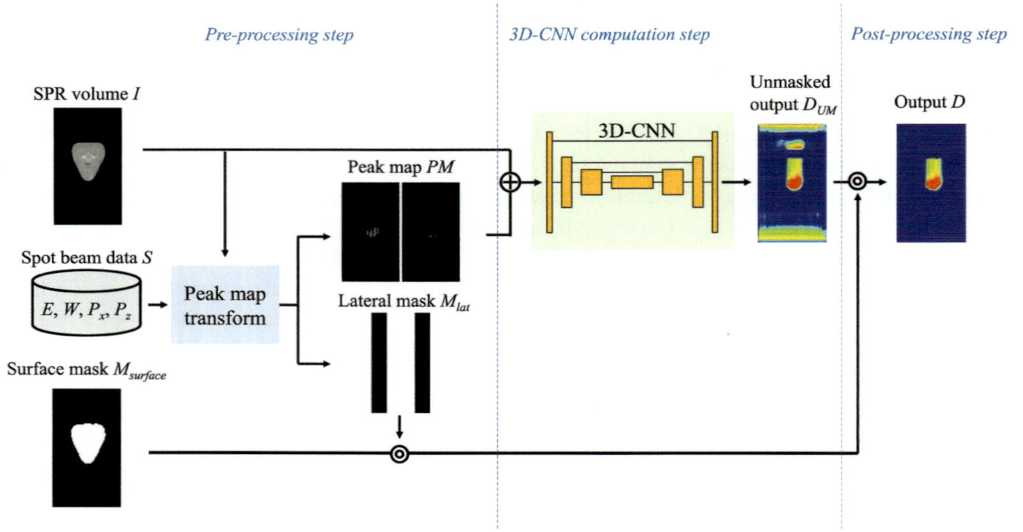

FIGURE 9.3 Diagram of our proton dose calculation method using a 3D CNN, which incorporates beam parameters, such as spot weight, spot position, and beam energies as inputs and MC dose maps as outputs.

incorporating beam parameters, such as spot weight, spot position, and beam energies as inputs and MC dose maps as outputs (Figure 9.3).[91] This study highlighted the potential for improved training efficiency and generalization using transfer learning, although it also noted challenges such as intermediate processing stages and voxel resolution limitations.[91]

Other DL models have been designed to address various challenges in dose prediction for proton therapy. The development of the recurrent U-Net (RU-net) architecture for IMPT exemplifies these advancements. This model, trained using a multi-MU approach, demonstrated superior performance compared to traditional peak-monitor unit models. It achieved an improved gamma-passing rate and reduced MAEs, with predictions made in under half a second.[92] Such models are crucial for real-time dose prediction and plan optimization in clinical settings. Recent advances include the use of Long Short-Term Memory (LSTM) recurrent neural networks (RNNs) by Neishabouri et al., who focused on pencil beams. Their approach showed that LSTM networks could effectively handle the high heterogeneity of lung tissues, providing dose maps with high agreement to MC simulations and significantly faster computation times.[93] Additionally, a hierarchically densely connected U-Net model demonstrated strong performance across various organ sites, showcasing its superiority over the PBA in terms of evaluation metrics such as the gamma-index and dose volume histograms.[94]

GANs have also been explored for dose prediction in proton therapy. For example, recent studies have employed a 3D U-Net trained as a generator within a GAN framework to enhance dose prediction accuracy. This approach has shown promise in predicting dose distributions for proton minibeam therapy, outperforming traditional methods and demonstrating high generalization performance across varying target geometries and proton energies.[95] Furthermore, Zhang et al. introduced a Discovery Cross-Domain Generative Adversarial Network (DiscoGAN) for dose calculation. This innovative approach used GANs to map beam parameters to dose distributions, incorporating auxiliary features like HU values and SP kernels to capture complex relationships in proton therapy. Their model achieved fast computation times and high accuracy, with mean relative errors consistently below 3%.[96] The integration of AI with traditional physics-based models can enhance the interpretability and effectiveness of dose calculations. For example, DiscoGAN models illustrate how AI can refine preliminary dose profiles generated by simpler algorithms like the PBA, incorporating additional physical information to improve accuracy. This synergy between AI and physics highlights the importance of leveraging analytical knowledge to guide AI developments and interpret their results effectively.[96]

9.3.3 Adaptive Proton Therapy

Adaptive proton therapy (APT) represents a significant leap forward in precision radiotherapy, which takes a fair share of benefits from advancements in AI. AI plays a transformative role in APT by addressing two critical tasks: fast dose calculation and fast plan optimization. These tasks are interleaved with various components covered earlier in this chapter, including synthetic CT (sCT) generation, MR-based planning, and optimization. Given the breadth of topics we've discussed, this subsection is shorter and will focus on covering aspects similar to previous ones.

A key advancement in AI for APT is the development of methods for generating synthetic CTs. For instance, Viar-Hernandez et al. demonstrated the efficacy of a 3D vision transformer (ViT3D) for synthesizing head-and-neck CTs from CBCT images,[97] achieving a reduction in the absolute relative error in SPR maps to below 5%. This advancement facilitates more accurate dose calculations essential for adaptive therapy. Building on this, Pang et al. compared various DL models for sCT generation and found that the conditional generative adversarial network (cGAN) provided superior results.[98] The cGAN model not only reduced MAEs but also enhanced dosimetric accuracy, proving its potential for APT in treating nasopharynx cancer. Moreover, Wang et al. applied a self-attention cycle-GAN for generating synthetic CTs in pediatric brain tumor cases. Their approach showed improved dosimetric accuracy, facilitating more precise adaptive planning.[99] This aligns with findings of de Koster et al., who evaluated DL-based sCTs for head-and-neck cancer and found high dosimetric accuracy and minimal differences from planning and repeat CTs.[100]

Thummerer et al. further contributed to this field by employing a DL-based method to correct scatter in CBCT images for lung cancer patients.[101] This method demonstrated high agreement in dose calculations and normal tissue complication probabilities, underscoring its potential clinical utility. In another study[102] by the same group, the focus was on generating 4D-synthetic CTs from sparse-view 4D-CBCTs. Their approach achieved dosimetric accuracy comparable to 4D-CTs, highlighting AI's capability to handle respiratory motion and anatomical variations effectively.

In a novel approach, Kaushik et al. introduced the anatomy-preserving virtual CT (APvCT), which showed high agreement with planning CTs and outperformed corrected CBCT in terms of dose calculation accuracy.[103] This innovation enhances the APT workflow by improving accuracy in the presence of anatomical changes.

In the realm of plan optimization, Zhang et al. introduced SWFT-Net,[104] a neural network capable of fine-tuning spot weights (Figure 9.4).[104] This model can generate adapted plans in

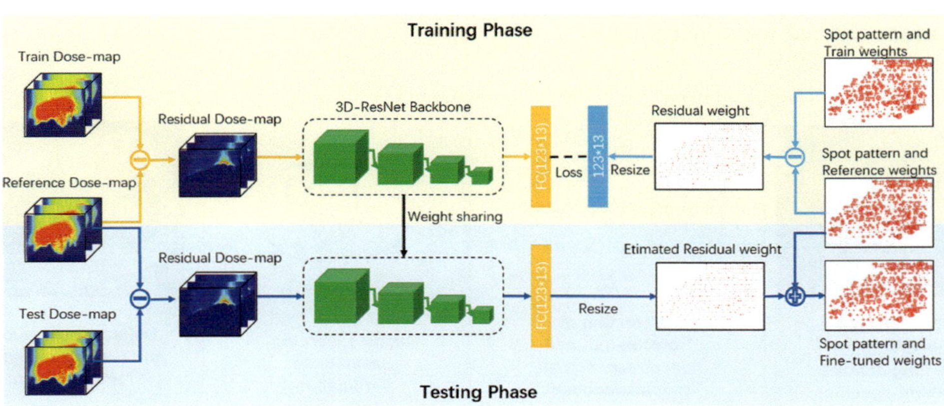

FIGURE 9.4 SFWT-Net, a deep learning framework for spot weight fine-tuning based on residuals of dose maps and spot weights.

under a second, addressing the need for rapid plan optimization in dynamic clinical settings. Similarly, Zhang et al. developed a DL-based MC denoising approach, which drastically cut down the time required for plan verification while maintaining accuracy comparable to traditional methods.[105]

In our perspective, adaptation involves adjustments both prior to and following treatment delivery. If anatomical changes are minimal, the treatment can proceed as originally planned without further modification. However, if there are significant anatomical shifts, recalculating the dose impact and reoptimizing the treatment plan become essential before proceeding with delivery. Post-treatment, verifying the dose is crucial to determine if further adjustments to spot weights are needed between fractions. Section 9.4 will discuss the role of AI in the delivery of proton treatment, where we focus on dose verification using AI tools.

9.4 AI FOR RANGE AND DOSE VERIFICATION IN PROTON THERAPY

Range and dose verification in proton therapy represents a uniquely challenging task (Figure 9.5) that distinguishes itself from other radiotherapy applications in three fundamental ways. First, it involves secondary signals generated by proton beams through distinct physical processes not present in high-energy photon beams. Second, the task is inherently intertwined with instrumentation aspects, including hardware design and signal processing, making it substantially more complex than purely software-oriented tasks. Third, while AI applications in this domain show great promise, the field remains in its early stages with limited published literature available for comprehensive analysis.

A critical challenge in proton therapy centers on the precise monitoring of both the Bragg peak location and actual dose distribution. Multiple factors can introduce uncertainties, including variations in beam profiles, challenges in stopping power conversion from CT images, patient positioning variations, and anatomical modifications over time. The fundamental principle underlying verification methods relies on the correlation between the spatial distribution of secondary signals and the resulting dose distribution. Researchers have explored various secondary signal types, each with distinct advantages and limitations: positron emitter, prompt gamma, secondary electron bremsstrahlung X-ray, acoustic wave, and water luminescence. Among these approaches, Positron Emission Tomography (PET) for detecting positron emitters (such as ^{11}C,^{15}O) has garnered extensive research attention, both with and without AI integration.[106–116] The consensus suggests that PET-based verification shows the most promise for clinical translation. From an AI and machine learning perspective, the underlying principles for implementing AI remain remarkably consistent across different verification approaches. While this chapter emphasizes PET-related studies, readers are encouraged to explore other applications aligned with their interests.

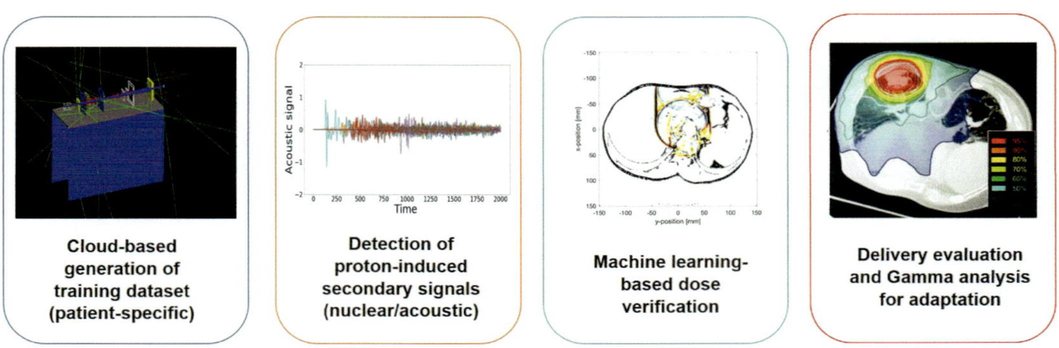

FIGURE 9.5 Clinical workflow of AI-based range and dose verification in proton therapy.

9.4.1 Positron Emitter

In the realm of positron emitter research, Peng and colleagues have made groundbreaking contributions by implementing multiple AI models for range/dose verification in proton therapy.[106–109] Their work demonstrates that AI's effectiveness increases proportionally with the incorporation of physics-related information into the models. The research progression began with Li et al.'s implementation of a simple forward neural network and LSTM RNN for predicting 1D dose distribution in mono-energetic beams.[106] This was followed by Liu et al.'s[107] comprehensive comparison of five RNN models: LSTM, bidirectional LSTM, GRU, bidirectional GRU, and Seq2seq. Their study included the incorporation of anatomical information (HU numbers), revealing that the bidirectional GRU structure achieved superior prediction accuracy and generalization capability, particularly when HU features were included. Building on these foundational studies, the team further enhanced their AI framework across four critical dimensions[108,109]: (1) integrating stopping power alongside HU as prior information to enhance noise immunity and generalization capability, (2) enabling 3D verification capabilities for both center and off-center voxels, (3) expanding analysis to include spread-out Bragg peak (SOBP) cases beyond mono-energetic scenarios, and (4) evaluating performance across two input scenarios—reconstructed PET signals and raw positron emitter signals. However, a notable limitation of these studies was their reliance on a single CT image for model training and testing, highlighting the need for rigorous performance validation across different organ sites, despite the framework's patient-specific verification design.

When conducting AI-related research in proton therapy, or radiotherapy generally, two fundamental questions require attention. First, researchers must clearly articulate the rationale and motivation for introducing AI to a specific task. Second, they must demonstrate tangible benefits compared to non-AI approaches. The significance of addressing these questions often surpasses the actual AI model development. The studies in[106–109] exemplify effective approaches to these considerations. The authors thoroughly explained why mapping from dose profiles to activity profiles (e.g., positron emitter signals) presents significant challenges, noting that while dose profiles depend on stopping power and medium characteristics, proton-induced positron emitter yields additionally depend on nuclear reaction cross-sections. This complexity results in activity-depth profiles showing intricate fluctuation patterns, distinctly different from smooth dose-depth profiles. The selection of RNN-based models was justified by their capability to extract underlying correlations between input sequences (activity profiles) and output sequences (dose profiles) while maintaining parameter efficiency. The authors also provided comprehensive explanations for including HU and/or SP as additional features, noting that without anatomical information, RNN models primarily focus on global features, while the inclusion of HU and SP enables capture of local correlations. They further distinguished between HU and SP contributions, explaining that HU relates to X-ray cross-sections (providing indirect information about tissue carbon and oxygen concentrations) and correlates indirectly with activity profiles, while SP directly influences dose profiles (Figure 9.6).[108]

Regarding comparative advantages over non-AI approaches, the authors presented compelling justifications.[107–109] AI offers ease of use and potential end-to-end solutions, automatically extracting features unlike kernel-based models that rely on preselected functions and fitting routines (such as Gaussian function and power law function convolution).[110–113] The AI approaches demonstrated robust performance, strong generalization capabilities, and enhanced noise immunity. Quantitative comparisons between AI and non-AI methodologies were presented for both dose[114] and range verification.[110,111,114–116] While direct comparisons proved challenging in some cases, even indirect comparisons provided valuable insights for researchers working in this field.

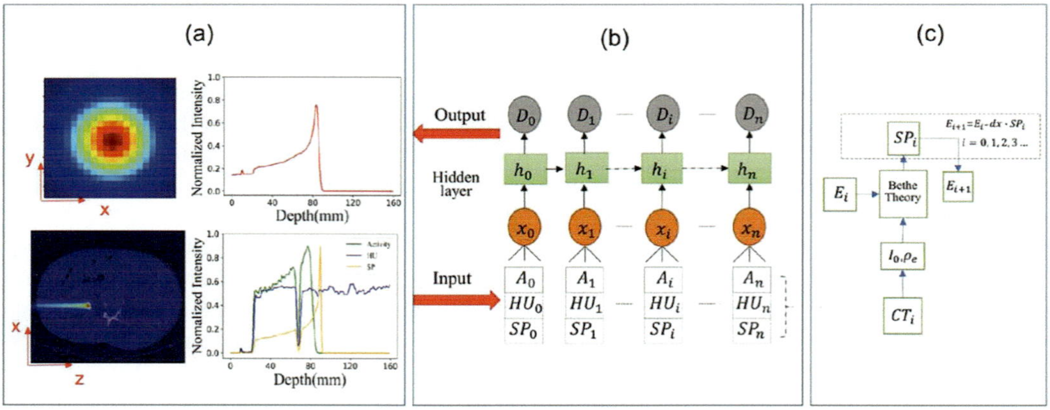

FIGURE 9.6 (a) A CT image based phantom used in simulation and the X/Y/Z coordinate. A dose-depth profile after normalization along the central line (proton energy: 100 MeV), as well as the three other profiles as a function of depth (activity, HU from CT images, and stopping power (SP)). (b) The structure of the RNN model: x is an input vector by concatenating three parts together (Ai, Hui, and SPi), hi represents the hidden unit of the RNN model, and Di is the dose profile at the *i*-th depth (i.e., the predicted dose output). (c) The signal flowchart for analytically modeling the prior of SP at a given depth.

9.4.2 Prompt Gamma

In the domain of prompt gamma (PG) research, scientists have explored the correlation between characteristic photons emitted during charged particle–tissue interactions and dose distribution.[117–120] Gueth et al. developed an approach for detecting discrepancies between planned and delivered doses[118] using a combined classifier that leverages distal falloff and registered correlation features. Liu et al. applied a U-Net model to address similar challenges in brain phantoms,[119] utilizing MC-simulated PG signals as inputs and dose maps as outputs. More recently, Schumann et al. proposed combining a Gaussian-power law convolution filtering procedure with an evolutionary algorithm.[113] However, these studies have yet to fully address various physical factors that can degrade PG signal quality, including counting statistics, limited spatial resolution, and image artifacts.

9.4.3 Secondary Electron Bremsstrahlung X-Rays

Secondary electron bremsstrahlung (SEB) X-rays represent another avenue for range and dose verification,[121–125] with prototype systems already tested in both proton[122] and carbon therapy.[123,124] The primary challenge lies in converting SEB X-ray data to dose images while addressing limited spatial resolution and poor counting statistics. Yamaguchi et al. tackled these challenges by implementing dual U-Net models[125]—one for X-ray to dose conversion and another for resolution enhancement. They innovatively used pre-defined analytical functions with parameters derived from experimental measurements, rather than MC simulations, to streamline data generation. However, significant challenges remain in applying this AI approach to heterogeneous tissues.

9.4.4 Acoustic Signals

The acoustic signal approach has garnered substantial research attention.[126–133] The characteristic pressure wave emission pattern includes signals from both pre-peak and peak dose deposition. Initial research explored the time-of-flight (TOF) method in uniform water media.[126,127] The time-reversal

(TR) reconstruction method was subsequently developed for both 2D and 3D heterogeneous tissues[130,131] to address TOF limitations, including complex arrival time extraction and incomplete dose information. However, the TR method's computational intensity led Yao et al. to develop an AI model (Bi-LSTM RNN) for 2D and 3D scenarios.[132,133] This model effectively correlates acoustic waveforms with dose profiles while incorporating advanced signal processing techniques. The AI approach significantly reduced computational time to mere seconds and required fewer acoustic wave sensors compared to TR methods.

The RNN model's effectiveness in this application stems from its ability to extract sequential correlations while requiring minimal hyper-parameters.[132,133] Each dose profile correlates with a unique 2D map of multi-channel acoustic waveforms, allowing the RNN to analyze time-series signal characteristics effectively. While CNN implementation remains viable, two factors favor RNN: reduced hyperparameter requirements (demanding fewer training samples) and superior temporal correlation identification capabilities. However, data generation for model training remains challenging, particularly since acoustic wave propagation and shapes depend heavily on physical parameters like tissue sound speed. Both AI and non-AI approaches[130–133] rely on simulated datasets for input and output, necessitating careful validation of simulation accuracy against practical signals once prototype systems are developed.

9.4.5 Luminescence

Water luminescence during proton therapy represents another promising research direction.[134–136] This phenomenon, similar to Cerenkov light, can be detected using cooled charge-coupled device (CCD) cameras. Yabe et al. employed a U-Net to predict 2D dose distributions from measured luminescence images in water medium for both proton and carbon beams.[135] However, like SEB X-rays, this approach faces significant challenges when applied to heterogeneous or deep-seated tissues. Importantly, the authors emphasize that the primary challenges in this and related research areas often lie not in AI implementation—as even basic AI models might adequately map detected signals to dose distributions—but rather in instrumentation and signal detection aspects. Consequently, researchers should prioritize justifying AI selection over non-AI approaches and establishing clear performance comparison protocols between these methodologies.

9.5 AI FOR IMAGE GUIDANCE IN PROTON THERAPY

Image guidance plays a crucial role in modern external beam radiotherapy, especially within the context of adaptive radiotherapy. Proton therapy, characterized by its distinct Bragg peak, enables precise tumor targeting with a steep dose falloff. Consequently, accurate patient positioning and continuous monitoring of anatomical changes become even more critical in proton therapy, where variations in tissue composition can lead to beam range uncertainties. As such, image guidance becomes essential in mitigating these uncertainties, making it even more essential in proton therapy than in traditional photon therapy, ultimately ensuring both treatment precision and efficacy.

9.5.1 Image Synthesis

CBCT is extensively used for image guidance in modern radiation therapy systems, including both photon and proton therapy. It plays a critical role in verifying patient positioning and monitoring intrafraction anatomical changes, which allows for timely patient setup adjustments and treatment plan modifications. However, compared to standard CT, the image quality produced by CBCT is compromised due to factors like increased X-ray scatter, limitations in field of view, and variations in patient size, etc. Consequently, one of the primary research areas is focused on leveraging AI for generating synthetic CT (sCT) images from CBCT scans to enhance dose calculation and optimize treatment planning in APT.

GANs are commonly used for generating synthetic CT (sCT) images in proton therapy. Kurz et al.[137] explored the use of cycle-GAN to create sCTs from CBCT scans of prostate cancer patients. They assessed the dosimetric accuracy of sCTs for both VMAT and opposing single-field uniform dose (SFUD) proton plans. Previously, in Section 9.3, we mentioned the use of different networks in the context of APT.[98,101,102] To add few more studies, particularly Hansen et al.[138] developed a 2D U-Net-like architecture called ScatterNet to correct CBCT intensity in the projection space, evaluating its dosimetric accuracy for both IMPT and VMAT plans. While VMAT calculations on corrected CBCTs were highly accurate, results for IMPT were less satisfactory. Similarly, Landry et al.[139] employed a U-Net model to correct CBCT images for prostate cancer treatment, using three different datasets to separate the effects of scatter correction and deformation. Their model, trained on corrected CBCTs generated from deformable image registration (DIR)-based sCTs, showed the best performance among the three datasets for proton pencil beam scanning (PBS) SFUD dose calculations.

The superior soft tissue contrast provided by MRI makes it an ideal modality for image-guided radiation therapy, especially in specific anatomical regions such as the abdomen and brain. However, a significant challenge in implementing MRI-only simulation in proton therapy is the need for electron density and stopping power maps for accurate dose calculations. As a result, a key area of research in image synthesis for proton therapy is the generation of synthetic CTs (sCTs) from MRI scans, opening the door to the possibility of MRI-only proton therapy treatment workflows. We will refer readers to Section 9.2 for more details.[54–57,59,60,99,140]

9.5.2 Image Quality Enhancement

AI has also demonstrated a significant impact on improving and enhancing image quality for image-guided proton radiotherapy, particularly in positioning verification. One major area of research is improving the quality of CBCT images. Uh et al.[141] proposed a DL model for APT CBCT correction, using a combined dataset of adjacent anatomical sites (abdominal and pelvic) and age-dependent body sizes (children and young adults). The results outperformed models trained on site- or age-specific data when comparing dosimetric accuracy for proton dose estimation. Chang et al.[142] proposed an unsupervised learning approach for patient-specific CT metal artifact reduction to assist proton therapy procedures. Their framework employed a DL model for metal artifact reduction combined with a k-means clustering algorithm to correct regions near implants, enhancing overall image quality.

Scatter correction is another crucial task in enhancing CBCT for proton therapy. Compared to conventional methods, AI-based approaches offer promising performance while reducing computational costs, thereby improving efficiency. Lalonde et al.[143] applied a U-Net model for scatter correction on 48 head-and-neck CBCT images and compared the results with Monte Carlo-simulated scatter-free images. Their model demonstrated high accuracy, with minimal mean HU differences from scatter-free images, and the entire CBCT volume could be corrected in less than 5 seconds. Additionally, the proton range calculations were in good agreement with the reference CT data. Similarly, Nomura et al.[144] developed a U-Net-based model for CBCT correction in head-and-neck and lung cases, comparing its performance to conventional kernel superposition methods. The AI-corrected results not only outperformed conventional methods in terms of image quality metrics such as MAE and peak signal-to-noise ratio (PSNR) but also significantly reduced computational costs.

Beyond CBCT/CT quality enhancement, AI has been leveraged to improve other imaging modalities for proton therapy.[145–147] Charyyev et al.[145] employed a residual GAN model to improve the image quality of proton portal imaging (PPI) acquired using a double-scattered proton beam. The model was trained to learn the nonlinear mapping between PPIs and kV digitally reconstructed radiographs (DRR) from CT scans, thereby improving PPI quality for on-board positioning verification in the beam's-eye-view. Compton camera is emerging as a promising technology for real-time imaging for proton therapy, which captures PG rays emitted by proton beams as they travel through a patient's body.[148] However, the nonzero-time resolution of the Compton camera, during which all interactions are recorded simultaneously, produces images that are too noisy for delivery verification. To address this, York et al.[147] proposed a DL approach for Compton camera image correction in proton therapy. Their method featured a compact network design with hyperparameter grid search configuration, reducing computational costs and improving image quality.

9.6 AI FOR FLASH THERAPY

FLASH radiotherapy (FLASH-RT) is an innovative technique that delivers radiation at ultra-high dose rates (typically greater than 40 Gy/s) within a very short time frame (usually under a second). It has been shown to maintain effective tumor control while reducing toxicity to surrounding healthy tissues, a phenomenon known as the "FLASH effect."[149] The underlying reason for this effect is thought to be due to the different ways cancer and normal cells respond to radiation.[150–152] Although the exact mechanisms of the FLASH effect are not yet fully understood, early preclinical studies have shown encouraging results. For example, one study in mice demonstrated that FLASH radiation therapy caused significantly less damage to healthy tissues and reduced side effects such as skin injury, hair loss, and fatigue compared to conventional radiation therapy.[153]

In radiation therapy, the ability to safely deliver an effective dose is often constrained by the potential impact on nearby organs at risk (OARs). FLASH radiotherapy offers several promising advantages over conventional techniques. First, it has the potential to reduce the risk of side effects by providing better protection to healthy tissues. Additionally, the ultra-fast delivery of radiation could significantly shorten treatment times or enable the delivery of higher doses in a single session, allowing for more aggressive cancer treatment while minimizing the overall duration. Ultimately, these benefits could lead to improved patient outcomes and a better quality of life by reducing side effects and streamlining the treatment process.

Despite these potential benefits, further research is necessary to move FLASH radiotherapy from experimental stages[154,155] to clinical application.[156] Most studies so far have been conducted in animal models or small-scale human trials.[157–159] Larger studies are needed to establish long-term safety and efficacy. There is also a need for a deeper understanding of the biological mechanisms involved. Additionally, several technical and logistical challenges must be addressed, such as developing equipment capable of safely delivering ultra-high dose rates,[160] ensuring precise tumor targeting, and establishing reliable dosimetry[161,162] and quality assurance protocols. AI is a powerful tool that has been proved to greatly enhance the quality and efficiency of radiation therapy. While most research on FLASH therapy has focused on understanding its biological mechanisms and developing appropriate equipment, some groups are beginning to explore the use of AI and DL to assist in these investigations.

Much of the research into the radiobiological effects of FLASH therapy remains in the preclinical stage and has been conducted using animal models. A classic model for studying radiation-induced injury is the intestine, where radiation response is evaluated by counting regenerating crypts in histological images of mouse intestines after abdominal irradiation.[158,159] Manual annotation and analysis of these images can be labor-intensive, leading researchers starting to explore AI-based automation. For example, Bell et al.[163] used an AI model to quantify intestinal crypt regeneration 4 days after irradiation, enabling comparisons of normal tissue responses between FLASH and conventional (CONV) irradiation. However, direct crypt number comparison between FLASH and CONV irradiation is insufficient to establish a correlation or modifying factor between FLASH and CONV dose scales.

One can first establish the relationship between crypt count and dose under CONV irradiation and then use this information to estimate the FLASH iso-effective dose (i.e., the dose of CONV irradiation that produces the same normal tissue radiation response as a given dose of FLASH irradiation). To automate this process, Fu and Yang et al.[164,165] developed a DL-based pipeline.

The group implemented an attention-guided cycle-GAN network for stain normalization in histological images, followed by a U-Net model to detect and count crypts, allowing for faster and more automated evaluation of tissue response after FLASH irradiation. Furthermore, the same group developed a DL approach to estimate the FLASH iso-effective dose directly from intestinal cross-section images, using the same dataset from mouse abdominal irradiation.[166] As shown in Figure 9.7,[166] the authors trained a multi-scale ResNet-based model (Figure 9.7a) with CONV data to learn the correlation between image features and the delivered CONV dose, then further tested with FLASH data to project the FLASH dose into the iso-effective CONV dose based on the high-level features extracted from histological images (Figure 9.7b). The DL model achieved a mean squared error of 0.20 Gy^2 on the CONV test set, compared with the classical crypt-counting method (CC), which had a mean squared error of 0.40 Gy^2. Additionally, the DL model estimated iso-effective doses for FLASH doses of 12, 13, 14, 15, and 16 Gy as 12.19 ± 0.46, 12.54 ± 0.37, 12.69 ± 0.26, 12.84 ± 0.26, and 13.03 ± 0.28 Gy, respectively. These results indicated that, except for the 12 Gy

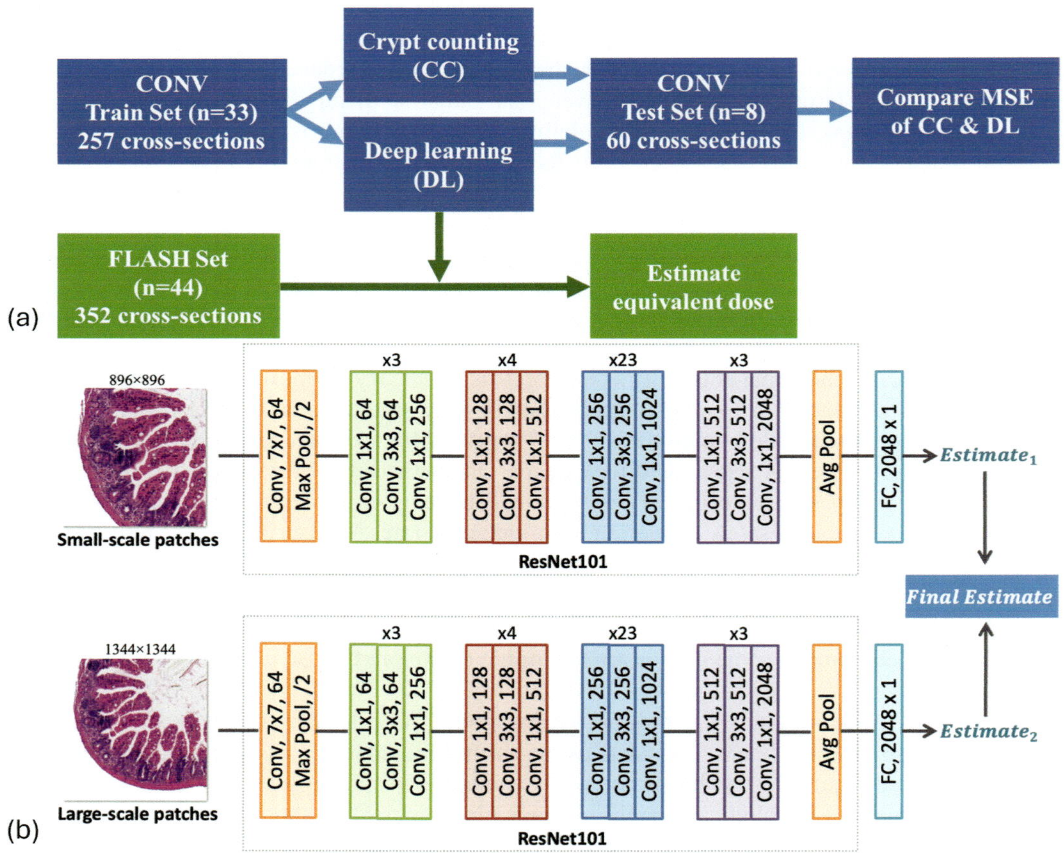

FIGURE 9.7 (a) The overall workflow for deep learning-based FLASH iso-effective dose estimation. The CONV training dataset was used to train the DL model or fit the function from the delivered dose to the crypt number in the CC approach to estimate the delivered dose. The estimation accuracy was assessed using the CONV testing set with mean squared error between estimated and delivered doses. The validated DL model was applied to cross-section images in the entire FLASH dataset to estimate the FLASH iso-effective dose. (b) The architecture and training scheme of the multi-scale ensemble learning for FLASH iso-effective dose estimation. ResNet101-based deep learning models were trained to estimate the delivered dose based on the input patches. Large- and small-scale patches were used to train one large- and one small-scale models, respectively. The multi-scale model is the ensemble of the two models.

dose, FLASH irradiation can reduce intestinal toxicity with iso-effective doses lower than the physical dose ($p < 0.05$). There are, however, several limitations to this work. The FLASH iso-effective dose may vary depending on the tissue type and other factors, such as species and strain, and ideally, it should be determined across a broad range of models. Additionally, this study assumes that tissue responses to CONV and FLASH irradiation are represented similarly in histological analyses, differing only in extent. Nevertheless, this proof-of-concept study demonstrates the potential of applying AI and DL to quantify the iso-effective dose of radiation and assess tissue response following irradiation.

In addition to radiobiology investigations, some groups are beginning to explore the use of AI to facilitate the clinical translation of FLASH therapy. One of the key technical challenges that needs to be addressed is the development of effective image guidance techniques. Due to the ultra-high dose rate of FLASH delivery, fast on-board imaging systems are essential for accurate position verification. However, current systems, particularly CBCT, are not efficient enough for this purpose. Some commercial proton therapy machines are equipped with dual kV sources that enable rapid orthogonal image acquisition, but two projection images are insufficient for providing 3D information on patient positioning and anatomical changes, which is especially critical for FLASH therapy. To address this, Chang et al.[167] developed a DL-based image guidance framework to enable fast volumetric image reconstruction for lung cancer FLASH proton therapy. As illustrated in Figure 9.8,[167] the group created a DL model, InverseNet3D, to reconstruct volumetric images from kV projection pairs. These synthetic images were then compared to reference CT images to assess image quality and evaluate water equivalent thickness (WET) for proton delivery. In their approach, kV projections were simulated from clinical 4D CT data, and the volumetric image generation model was trained using a leave-phase-out, patient-specific training scheme. The reconstructed 3D images demonstrated good performance, with a patient-averaged MAE of 75±22 HU, a PSNR of 19±3.7 dB, and a structural similarity index measure (SSIM) of 0.938±0.044, when compared with clinical reference 4D CT images. Additionally, ray tracing-based WET evaluation yielded a patient-averaged ΔWET of approximately 1 mm, reflecting not only the quality of the reconstructed images but also their potential to monitor anatomical changes along the treatment beam path. This framework demonstrates the potential for fast volumetric image generation, which could play a key role in guiding proton FLASH treatment delivery systems.

Looking ahead, FLASH radiotherapy holds the potential to revolutionize standard radiotherapy practices. However, for this promising modality to become part of routine clinical care, further

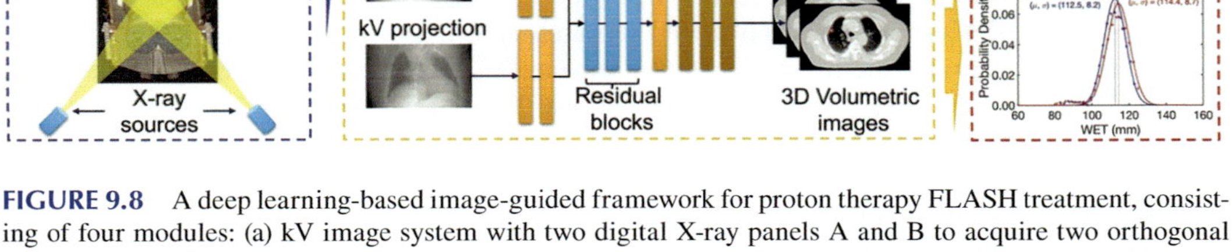

FIGURE 9.8 A deep learning-based image-guided framework for proton therapy FLASH treatment, consisting of four modules: (a) kV image system with two digital X-ray panels A and B to acquire two orthogonal projections simultaneously, (b) deep learning-based volumetric image generation using orthogonal kV projections (InverseNet3D is implemented in this module), (c) image evaluation based on CT numbers to ensure the integrity of generated volumetric images without systematic shift of voxel intensity, and (d) treatment evaluation based on WET to detector potential anatomy changes.

advancements in imaging and treatment technologies are essential. AI, particularly DL, offers great promise in addressing these needs. DL techniques could be leveraged in FLASH-RT for tasks such as rapid volumetric imaging, image synthesis, and in vivo dose verification. That said, the clinical translation of FLASH-RT will also depend on a deeper understanding of its biological mechanisms and effects, as well as the ability to capture these critical biological changes at extremely short timescales. Precise radiobiological quantification is key to fully understanding the FLASH effect, but the scarcity of clinical data makes defining dose constraints a slow and challenging process. One promising approach is to leverage AI and machine learning algorithms to derive FLASH dose-modifying factors from extensive animal studies. These factors could then be applied to existing normal tissue complication probability (NTCP) models and dose constraints from conventional radiotherapy. Additionally, future directions might also include the integration of AI with functional or biologically driven imaging techniques to further study FLASH mechanisms. This integration could help in identifying tissues that are particularly sensitive to FLASH irradiation, enabling better assessments of treatment response and potentially leading to more refined and personalized FLASH-RT protocols.

9.7 PITFALLS AND FUTURE DIRECTIONS

Despite the encouraging advances outlined in this chapter, it's crucial to acknowledge that AI is not a panacea and comes with its own set of challenges. As AI models grow in complexity, understanding the manipulation of inputs and outputs becomes increasingly difficult, as do result interpretation and verification. Riley[168] outlines several common pitfalls to avoid. Drawing from our experience, we identify three prevalent challenges in both proton and photon radiotherapy:

1. The first challenge involves appropriate data generation and splitting. Unlike fields such as computer vision and natural language processing, proton therapy faces significant data scarcity, as evidenced by most examples discussed previously. Limited dataset size can lead to well-documented issues like overfitting. MC simulation-based data augmentation has become a common solution. However, effective dataset generation must be both task-specific and model-specific. Three critical data generation commitments require attention: First, researchers must carefully verify whether MC simulation results accurately reflect practical scenarios (including system setup, beam profile, and image acquisition protocols). Second, patient-specific tasks (such as dose calculation, verification, and Quality Assurance (QA)) require individual data generation for each patient. This raises the challenge of balancing patient specificity with generalization capability, as the latter demands greater sample complexity but offers more efficient data utilization. Transfer learning may offer solutions here. Third, while AI practitioners typically divide data into training, validation, and test sets—whether randomly or systematically—they must always report convergence behaviors and bias/variance tradeoffs. Thorough exploration of different approaches is essential to ensure result consistency.
2. The second challenge concerns feature and hidden variable interpretation. Though often overlooked, this aspect is crucial for AI research and, in our experience, helps prevent overfitting. Consider the infamous "tank problem,"[168,169] where researchers developed a model to identify tanks in military photographs. While the model succeeded with test data, it failed with real-world images because it had learned to recognize incidental features like morning light or clouds rather than tanks themselves. One effective validation approach involves using the same model for different predictions—success in such cases might indicate questionable study design. Additionally, examining hidden variables enables deeper model comparisons, as demonstrated in.[107] Regarding input features and their contributions, multiple rounds of cross-validation are advisable. For instance, in dose verification research utilizing activity profile, CT-derived HU values, and stopping power

as inputs,[108] the researchers systematically altered each input to assess its impact on overall performance—effectively illuminating the black box of their AI model. Similarly, another study randomly permuted acoustic waveform orders to verify whether time differences and sequential information contributed to Bragg peak localization.[131,132] Unfortunately, many proton therapy AI studies omit such crucial validation steps.

3. The third challenge emphasizes starting with the simplest viable model. While researchers often gravitate toward complexity, simpler models—whether non-neural network approaches or shallow neural networks—can sometimes match the performance of deep neural networks. Maintaining focus on the primary objective is crucial to avoid implementing unnecessarily complex solutions or addressing incorrect problems. For instance, basic forward neural networks[106] or regression classifiers[118] suffice for Bragg peak prediction. Advanced models like RNN or GAN[106–109,118] become necessary only for tasks like 3D dose verification. Starting with simple baseline models offers multiple advantages: better dataset understanding, performance baseline establishment, appropriate figure-of-merit selection, and guidance for ablation studies when needed.

Researchers conducting proton therapy AI studies must familiarize themselves with these challenges and pitfalls while maintaining rigorous standards. Thorough soundness checks should be mandatory. The field requires clear standards for performing and reporting research findings, as well as reviewing and publishing AI-related research articles.

9.8 CONCLUSION

The convergence of enhanced computational capabilities, vast datasets, and sophisticated algorithms is revolutionizing the implementation of AI in radiotherapy applications. However, it's crucial to recognize that AI strategies must be specifically tailored to address the fundamental distinctions between photon and particle therapy, particularly regarding their beam interaction physics and delivery mechanisms. The evidence presented throughout this chapter demonstrates that applying AI to proton therapy represents more than merely adapting existing solutions—it offers innovative approaches to address unique challenges in both precision and operational efficiency.

The successful integration of AI in proton therapy hinges on four equally critical pillars: the systematic generation of high-quality data, careful interpretation of outcomes, integration of fundamental physical principles, and thorough validation protocols. These elements carry as much importance as the development of the AI models themselves. Furthermore, there is a pressing need for the scientific community to establish clear, standardized guidelines for conducting and publishing AI research in this field. Looking forward, we can see a well-defined trajectory for advancing AI technologies to enhance the effectiveness of proton therapy treatments.

This expanded narrative does not merely represent an incremental improvement in existing methodologies but rather signals a transformative approach to addressing longstanding challenges in the field. The path forward requires careful attention to both technical development and standardization of practices, ultimately working toward the goal of more effective proton therapy treatments through sophisticated AI implementation.

REFERENCES

1. Thompson RF, Valdes G, Fuller CD, et al. Artificial intelligence in radiation oncology: A specialty-wide disruptive transformation? *Radiother Oncol.* 2018;129(3):421–426. doi:10.1016/j.radonc.2018.05.030
2. Huynh E, Hosny A, Guthier C, et al. Artificial intelligence in radiation oncology. *Nat Rev Clin Oncol.* 2020;17(12):771–781. doi:10.1038/s41571-020-0417–8
3. Meyer P, Noblet V, Mazzara C, Lallement A. Survey on deep learning for radiotherapy. *Comp Biol Med.* 2018;98:126–146. doi:10.1016/j.compbiomed.2018.05.018

4. Kiser KJ, Fuller CD, Reed VK. Artificial intelligence in radiation oncology treatment planning: a brief overview. *J Med Artif Intell*. 2019;2:9. doi:10.21037/jmai.2019.04.02
5. Paganetti H. Range uncertainties in proton therapy and the role of Monte Carlo simulations. *Phys Med Biol*. 2012;57(11):R99–R117. doi:10.1088/0031–9155/57/11/R99
6. Lomax A. Intensity modulation methods for proton radiotherapy. *Phys Med Biol*. 1999;44(1):185–205. doi:10.1088/0031–9155/44/1/014
7. Newhauser WD, Zhang R. The physics of proton therapy. *Phys Med Biol*. 2015;60(8):R155–R209. doi:10.1088/0031–9155/60/8/R155
8. Grant RL, Summers PA, Neihart JL, et al. Relative stopping power measurements to aid in the design of anthropomorphic phantoms for proton radiotherapy. *J Appl Clin Med Phys*. 2014;15(2):4523. doi:10.1120/jacmp.v15i2.4523
9. Taasti VT, Muren LP, Jensen K, et al. Comparison of single and dual energy CT for stopping power determination in proton therapy of head and neck cancer. *Phys Imaging Radiat Oncol*. 2018;6:14–19. doi:10.1016/j.phro.2018.04.002
10. Schneider U, Pedroni E, Lomax A. The calibration of CT Hounsfield units for radiotherapy treatment planning. *Phys Med Biol*. 1996;41(1):111–124. doi:10.1088/0031–9155/41/1/009
11. Hansen DC, Seco J, Sørensen TS, et al. A simulation study on proton computed tomography (CT) stopping power accuracy using dual energy CT scans as benchmark. *Acta Oncol*. 2015;54(9):1638–1642. doi:10.3109/0284186X.2015.1061212
12. Hünemohr N, Krauss B, Tremmel C, Ackermann B, Jäkel O, Greilich S. Experimental verification of ion stopping power prediction from dual energy CT data in tissue surrogates. *Phys Med Biol*. 2014;59(1):83–96. doi:10.1088/0031–9155/59/1/83
13. Yang M, Virshup G, Clayton J, Zhu XR, Mohan R, Dong L. Theoretical variance analysis of single- and dual-energy computed tomography methods for calculating proton stopping power ratios of biological tissues. *Phys Med Biol*. 2010;55(5):1343–1362. doi:10.1088/0031–9155/55/5/006
14. Bourque AE, Carrier JF, Bouchard H. A stoichiometric calibration method for dual energy computed tomography. *Phys Med Biol*. 2014;59(8):2059–2088. doi:10.1088/0031–9155/59/8/2059
15. Zhu J, Penfold SN. Dosimetric comparison of stopping power calibration with dual-energy CT and single-energy CT in proton therapy treatment planning. *Med Phys*. 2016;43(6):2845–2854. doi:10.1118/1.4948683
16. Gao Y, Chang CW, Roper J, et al. Single energy CT-based mass density and relative stopping power estimation for proton therapy using deep learning method. *Front Oncol*. 2023;13:1278180. doi:10.3389/fonc.2023.1278180
17. Charyyev S, Wang T, Lei Y, et al. Learning-based synthetic dual energy CT imaging from single energy CT for stopping power ratio calculation in proton radiation therapy. *Br J Radiol*. 2022;95(1129):20210644. doi:10.1259/bjr.20210644
18. Wang T, Lei Y, Harms J, et al. Learning-based stopping power mapping on dual-energy CT for proton radiation therapy. *Int J Part Ther*. 2021;7(3):46–60. doi:10.14338/IJPT-D-20-00020.1
19. Liu Y, Zhou L, Peng H. Machine learning based oxygen and carbon concentration derivation using dual-energy CT for PET-based dose verification in proton therapy. *Med Phys*. 2022;49(5):3347–3360. doi:10.1002/mp.15581
20. Chang CW, Gao Y, Wang T, et al. Dual-energy CT based mass density and relative stopping power estimation for proton therapy using physics-informed deep learning. *Phys Med Biol*. 2022;67(11). doi:10.1088/1361–6560/ac6ebc
21. Chang CW, Zhou S, Gao Y, et al. Validation of a deep learning-based material estimation model for Monte Carlo dose calculation in proton therapy. *Phys Med Biol*. 2022;67(21). doi:10.1088/1361–6560/ac9663
22. Harms J, Lei Y, Wang T, et al. Cone-beam CT-derived relative stopping power map generation via deep learning for proton radiotherapy. *Med Phys*. 2020;47(9):4416–4427. doi:10.1002/mp.14347
23. Scholey J, Vinas L, Kearney V, et al. Improved accuracy of relative electron density and proton stopping power ratio through CycleGAN machine learning. *Phys Med Biol*. 2022;67(10). doi:10.1088/1361–6560/ac6725
24. Chang CW, Marants R, Gao Y, et al. Multimodal imaging-based material mass density estimation for proton therapy using supervised deep learning. *Br J Radiol*. 2023;96(1152):20220907. doi:10.1259/bjr.20220907
25. Paganetti H. Relative biological effectiveness (RBE) values for proton beam therapy. Variations as a function of biological endpoint, dose, and linear energy transfer. *Phys Med Biol*. 2014;59(22):R419–R472. doi:10.1088/0031–9155/59/22/R419

26. Paganetti H, Blakely E, Carabe-Fernandez A, et al. Report of the AAPM TG-256 on the relative biological effectiveness of proton beams in radiation therapy. *Med Phys*. 2019;46(3):e53–e78. doi:10.1002/mp.13390
27. Gao Y, Chang CW, Pan S, et al. Deep learning-based synthetic dose-weighted LET map generation for intensity modulated proton therapy. *Phys Med Biol*. 2024;69(2):025004. doi:10.1088/1361–6560/ad154b
28. Tang X, Wan Chan Tseung H, Moseley D, et al. Deep learning based linear energy transfer calculation for proton therapy. *Phys Med Biol*. 2024;69(11):115058. doi:10.1088/1361–6560/ad4844
29. Pirlepesov F, Wilson L, Moskvin VP, et al. Three-dimensional dose and LETD prediction in proton therapy using artificial neural networks. *Med Phys*. 2022;49(12):7417–7427. doi:10.1002/mp.16043
30. Starke S, Kieslich A, Palkowitsch M, et al. A deep-learning-based surrogate model for Monte-Carlo simulations of the linear energy transfer in primary brain tumor patients treated with proton-beam radiotherapy. *Phys Med Biol*. 2024;69(16). doi:10.1088/1361–6560/ad64b7
31. Charyyev S, Chang CW, Harms J, et al. A novel proton counting detector and method for the validation of tissue and implant material maps for Monte Carlo dose calculation. *Phys Med Biol*. 2021;66(4):045003. doi:10.1088/1361–6560/abd22e
32. Harrison N, Charyyev S, Oancea C, et al. Characterizing devices for validation of dose, dose rate, and LET in ultra high dose rate proton irradiations. *Medical Physics*. Published online August 17, 2024:mp.17359. doi:10.1002/mp.17359
33. Stasica P, Nguyen H, Granja C, et al. Single proton LET characterization with the Timepix detector and artificial intelligence for advanced proton therapy treatment planning. *Phys Med Biol*. 2023;68(10):104001. doi:10.1088/1361–6560/acc9f8
34. Dowling JA, Sun J, Pichler P, et al. Automatic Substitute Computed Tomography Generation and Contouring for Magnetic Resonance Imaging (MRI)-Alone External Beam Radiation Therapy From Standard MRI Sequences. *Int J Radiat Oncol Biol Phys*. 2015;93(5):1144–1153. doi:10.1016/j.ijrobp.2015.08.045
35. Dowling JA, Lambert J, Parker J, et al. An atlas-based electron density mapping method for magnetic resonance imaging (MRI)-alone treatment planning and adaptive MRI-based prostate radiation therapy. *Int J Radiat Oncol Biol Phys*. 2012;83(1):e5–e11. doi:10.1016/j.ijrobp.2011.11.056
36. Gudur MSR, Hara W, Le QT, Wang L, Xing L, Li R. A unifying probabilistic Bayesian approach to derive electron density from MRI for radiation therapy treatment planning. *Phys Med Biol*. 2014;59(21):6595–6606. doi:10.1088/0031–9155/59/21/6595
37. Uh J, Merchant TE, Li Y, Li X, Hua C. MRI-based treatment planning with pseudo CT generated through atlas registration. *Med Phys*. 2014;41(5):051711. doi:10.1118/1.4873315
38. Sjölund J, Forsberg D, Andersson M, Knutsson H. Generating patient specific pseudo-CT of the head from MR using atlas-based regression. *Phys Med Biol*. 2015;60(2):825–839. doi:10.1088/0031–9155/60/2/825
39. Arabi H, Koutsouvelis N, Rouzaud M, Miralbell R, Zaidi H. Atlas-guided generation of pseudo-CT images for MRI-only and hybrid PET-MRI-guided radiotherapy treatment planning. *Phys Med Biol*. 2016;61(17):6531–6552. doi:10.1088/0031–9155/61/17/6531
40. Burgos N, Guerreiro F, McClelland J, et al. Iterative framework for the joint segmentation and CT synthesis of MR images: application to MRI-only radiotherapy treatment planning. *Phys Med Biol*. 2017;62(11):4237–4253. doi:10.1088/1361–6560/aa66bf
41. Hsu SH, Cao Y, Huang K, Feng M, Balter JM. Investigation of a method for generating synthetic CT models from MRI scans of the head and neck for radiation therapy. *Phys Med Biol*. 2013;58(23):8419–8435. doi:10.1088/0031–9155/58/23/8419
42. Korhonen J, Kapanen M, Keyriläinen J, Seppälä T, Tenhunen M. A dual model HU conversion from MRI intensity values within and outside of bone segment for MRI-based radiotherapy treatment planning of prostate cancer. *Med Phys*. 2014;41(1):011704. doi:10.1118/1.4842575
43. Juttukonda MR, Mersereau BG, Chen Y, et al. MR-based attenuation correction for PET/MRI neurological studies with continuous-valued attenuation coefficients for bone through a conversion from R2* to CT-Hounsfield units. *Neuroimage*. 2015;112:160–168. doi:10.1016/j.neuroimage.2015.03.009
44. Ladefoged CN, Benoit D, Law I, et al. Region specific optimization of continuous linear attenuation coefficients based on UTE (RESOLUTE): application to PET/MR brain imaging. *Phys Med Biol*. 2015;60(20):8047–8065. doi:10.1088/0031–9155/60/20/8047
45. Bredfeldt JS, Liu L, Feng M, Cao Y, Balter JM. Synthetic CT for MRI-based liver stereotactic body radiotherapy treatment planning. *Phys Med Biol*. 2017;62(8):2922–2934. doi:10.1088/1361–6560/aa5059
46. Lei Y, Shu HK, Tian S, et al. Magnetic resonance imaging-based pseudo computed tomography using anatomic signature and joint dictionary learning. *J Med Imaging*. 2018;5(3):034001. doi:10.1117/1.JMI.5.3.034001

47. Huynh T, Gao Y, Kang J, et al. Estimating CT image from MRI Data using structured random forest and auto-context model. *IEEE Trans Med Imaging*. 2016;35(1):174–183. doi:10.1109/TMI.2015.2461533
48. Han X. MR-based synthetic CT generation using a deep convolutional neural network method. *Med Phys*. 2017;44(4):1408–1419. doi:10.1002/mp.12155
49. Nie D, Trullo R, Lian J, et al. Medical image synthesis with context-aware generative adversarial networks. *Med Image Comput Comput Assist Interv*. 2017;10435:417–425. doi:10.1007/978-3-319-66179-7_48
50. Bayisa FL, Liu X, Garpebring A, Yu J. Statistical learning in computed tomography image estimation. *Med Phys*. 2018;45(12):5450–5460. doi:10.1002/mp.13204
51. Xiang L, Wang Q, Nie D, et al. Deep embedding convolutional neural network for synthesizing CT image from T1-weighted MR image. *Med Image Anal*. 2018;47:31–44. doi:10.1016/j.media.2018.03.011
52. Spadea MF, Pileggi G, Zaffino P, et al. Deep convolution neural network (DCNN) multiplane approach to synthetic CT generation from MR images-application in brain proton therapy. *Int J Radiat Oncol Biol Phys*. 2019;105(3):495–503. doi:10.1016/j.ijrobp.2019.06.2535
53. Neppl S, Landry G, Kurz C, et al. Evaluation of proton and photon dose distributions recalculated on 2D and 3D Unet-generated pseudoCTs from T1-weighted MR head scans. *Acta Oncol*. 2019;58(10):1429–1434. doi:10.1080/0284186X.2019.1630754
54. Florkow MC, Guerreiro F, Zijlstra F, et al. Deep learning-enabled MRI-only photon and proton therapy treatment planning for paediatric abdominal tumours. *Radiother Oncol*. 2020;153:220–227. doi:10.1016/j.radonc.2020.09.056
55. Zimmermann L, Buschmann M, Herrmann H, et al. An MR-only acquisition and artificial intelligence based image-processing protocol for photon and proton therapy using a low field MR. *Z Med Phys*. 2021;31(1):78–88. doi:10.1016/j.zemedi.2020.10.004
56. Zimmermann L, Knäusl B, Stock M, Lütgendorf-Caucig C, Georg D, Kuess P. An MRI sequence independent convolutional neural network for synthetic head CT generation in proton therapy. *Z Med Phys*. 2022;32(2):218–227. doi:10.1016/j.zemedi.2021.10.003
57. Liu Y, Lei Y, Wang Y, et al. MRI-based treatment planning for proton radiotherapy: dosimetric validation of a deep learning-based liver synthetic CT generation method. *Phys Med Biol*. 2019;64(14):145015. doi:10.1088/1361–6560/ab25bc
58. Liu Y, Lei Y, Wang Y, et al. Evaluation of a deep learning-based pelvic synthetic CT generation technique for MRI-based prostate proton treatment planning. *Phys Med Biol*. 2019;64(20):205022. doi:10.1088/1361–6560/ab41af
59. Kazemifar S, Barragán Montero AM, Souris K, et al. Dosimetric evaluation of synthetic CT generated with GANs for MRI-only proton therapy treatment planning of brain tumors. *J Appl Clin Med Phys*. 2020;21(5):76–86. doi:10.1002/acm2.12856
60. Maspero M, Bentvelzen LG, Savenije MHF, et al. Deep learning-based synthetic CT generation for paediatric brain MR-only photon and proton radiotherapy. *Radiother Oncol*. 2020;153:197–204. doi:10.1016/j.radonc.2020.09.029
61. Shafai-Erfani G, Lei Y, Liu Y, et al. MRI-based proton treatment planning for base of skull tumors. *Int J Part Ther*. 2019;6(2):12–25. doi:10.14338/IJPT-19–00062.1
62. Chen S, Peng Y, Qin A, et al. MR-based synthetic CT image for intensity-modulated proton treatment planning of nasopharyngeal carcinoma patients. *Acta Oncol*. 2022;61(11):1417–1424. doi:10.1080/0284186X.2022.2140017
63. Liu R, Lei Y, Wang T, et al. Synthetic dual-energy CT for MRI-only based proton therapy treatment planning using label-GAN. *Phys Med Biol*. 2021;66(6):065014. doi:10.1088/1361–6560/abe736
64. Li X, Bellotti R, Meier G, et al. Uncertainty-aware MR-based CT synthesis for robust proton therapy planning of brain tumour. *Radiother Oncol*. 2024;191:110056. doi:10.1016/j.radonc.2023.110056
65. Wolterink JM, Dinkla AM, Savenije MHF, Seevinck PR, Berg CAT van den, Isgum I. Deep MR to CT synthesis using unpaired data. Published online August 3, 2017. Accessed October 23, 2024. https://arxiv.org/abs/1708.01155
66. Gao Y, Chang CW, Mandava S, et al. MRI-only based material mass density and relative stopping power estimation via deep learning for proton therapy: a preliminary study. *Sci Rep*. 2024;14(1):11166. doi:10.1038/s41598-024-61869-8
67. Wang C, Uh J, Patni T, et al. Toward MR-only proton therapy planning for pediatric brain tumors: Synthesis of relative proton stopping power images with multiple sequence MRI and development of an online quality assurance tool. *Med Phys*. 2022;49(3):1559–1570. doi:10.1002/mp.15479
68. Kaderka R, Liu K, Liu L, et al. Toward automatic beam angle selection for pencil-beam scanning proton liver treatments: A deep learning–based approach. *Med Phys*. 2022;49(7):4293–4304. doi:10.1002/mp.15676

69. Cheon W, Ahn SH, Jeong S, et al. Beam angle optimization for double-scattering proton delivery technique using an eclipse application programming interface and convolutional neural network. *Front Oncol.* 2021;11:707464. doi:10.3389/fonc.2021.707464
70. Vazquez I, Gronberg MP, Zhang X, et al. A deep learning-based approach for statistical robustness evaluation in proton therapy treatment planning: a feasibility study. *Phys Med Biol.* 2023;68(9):095014. doi:10.1088/1361–6560/accc08
71. Maes D, Holmstrom M, Helander R, Saini J, Fang C, Bowen SR. Automated treatment planning for proton pencil beam scanning using deep learning dose prediction and dose-mimicking optimization. *J Appl Clin Med Phys.* 2023;24(10):e14065. doi:10.1002/acm2.14065
72. Hong L, Goitein M, Bucciolini M, et al. A pencil beam algorithm for proton dose calculations. *Phys Med Biol.* 1996;41(8):1305–1330. doi:10.1088/0031–9155/41/8/005
73. Newhauser W, Fontenot J, Zheng Y, et al. Monte Carlo simulations for configuring and testing an analytical proton dose-calculation algorithm. *Phys Med Biol.* 2007;52(15):4569–4584. doi:10.1088/0031–9155/52/15/014
74. Paganetti H, Jiang H, Parodi K, Slopsema R, Engelsman M. Clinical implementation of full Monte Carlo dose calculation in proton beam therapy. *Phys Med Biol.* 2008;53(17):4825–4853. doi:10.1088/0031–9155/53/17/023
75. Clasie B, Depauw N, Fransen M, et al. Golden beam data for proton pencil-beam scanning. *Phys Med Biol.* 2012;57(5):1147–1158. doi:10.1088/0031–9155/57/5/1147
76. Grassberger C, Lomax A, Paganetti H. Characterizing a proton beam scanning system for Monte Carlo dose calculation in patients. *Phys Med Biol.* 2015;60(2):633–645. doi:10.1088/0031–9155/60/2/633
77. Schuemann J, Dowdell S, Grassberger C, Min CH, Paganetti H. Site-specific range uncertainties caused by dose calculation algorithms for proton therapy. *Phys Med Biol.* 2014;59(15):4007–4031. doi:10.1088/0031–9155/59/15/4007
78. Ma J, Beltran C, Seum Wan Chan Tseung H, Herman MG. A GPU-accelerated and Monte Carlo-based intensity modulated proton therapy optimization system. *Med Phys.* 2014;41(12):121707. doi:10.1118/1.4901522
79. Gu X, Choi D, Men C, Pan H, Majumdar A, Jiang SB. GPU-based ultra-fast dose calculation using a finite size pencil beam model. *Phys Med Biol.* 2009;54(20):6287–6297. doi:10.1088/0031–9155/54/20/017
80. Fujimoto R, Kurihara T, Nagamine Y. GPU-based fast pencil beam algorithm for proton therapy. *Phys Med Biol.* 2011;56(5):1319–1328. doi:10.1088/0031–9155/56/5/006
81. Jia X, Gu X, Sempau J, Choi D, Majumdar A, Jiang SB. Development of a GPU-based Monte Carlo dose calculation code for coupled electron-photon transport. *Phys Med Biol.* 2010;55(11):3077–3086. doi:10.1088/0031–9155/55/11/006
82. Jia X, Schümann J, Paganetti H, Jiang SB. GPU-based fast Monte Carlo dose calculation for proton therapy. *Phys Med Biol.* 2012;57(23):7783–7797. doi:10.1088/0031–9155/57/23/7783
83. Xing Y, Zhang Y, Nguyen D, Lin MH, Lu W, Jiang S. Boosting radiotherapy dose calculation accuracy with deep learning. *J Appl Clin Med Phys.* 2020;21(8):149–159. doi:10.1002/acm2.12937
84. Xing Y, Nguyen D, Lu W, Yang M, Jiang S. Technical note: A feasibility study on deep learning-based radiotherapy dose calculation. *Med Phys.* 2020;47(2):753–758. doi:10.1002/mp.13953
85. Wu C, Nguyen D, Xing Y, et al. Improving proton dose calculation accuracy by using deep learning. *Mach Learn Sci Technol.* 2021;2(1):015017. doi:10.1088/2632-2153/abb6d5
86. Javaid U, Souris K, Huang S, Lee JA. Denoising proton therapy Monte Carlo dose distributions in multiple tumor sites: A comparative neural networks architecture study. *Phys Med.* 2021;89:93–103. doi:10.1016/j.ejmp.2021.07.022
87. Zhang L, Holmes JM, Liu Z, et al. Beam mask and sliding window-facilitated deep learning-based accurate and efficient dose prediction for pencil beam scanning proton therapy. *Med Phys.* 2024;51(2):1484–1498. doi:10.1002/mp.16758
88. Guerreiro F, Seravalli E, Janssens GO, et al. Deep learning prediction of proton and photon dose distributions for paediatric abdominal tumours. *Radiother Oncol.* 2021;156:36–42. doi:10.1016/j.radonc.2020.11.026
89. Chen M, Pang B, Zeng Y, et al. Evaluation of an automated clinical decision system with deep learning dose prediction and NTCP model for prostate cancer proton therapy. *Phys Med Biol.* 2024;69(11). doi:10.1088/1361–6560/ad48f6
90. Pastor-Serrano O, Perkó Z. Millisecond speed deep learning based proton dose calculation with Monte Carlo accuracy. *Phys Med Biol.* 2022;67(10). doi:10.1088/1361–6560/ac692e

91. Nomura Y, Wang J, Shirato H, Shimizu S, Xing L. Fast spot-scanning proton dose calculation method with uncertainty quantification using a three-dimensional convolutional neural network. *Phys Med Biol.* 2020;65(21):215007. doi:10.1088/1361–6560/aba164
92. Wang W, Chang Y, Liu Y, et al. Feasibility study of fast intensity-modulated proton therapy dose prediction method using deep neural networks for prostate cancer. *Med Phys.* 2022;49(8):5451–5463. doi:10.1002/mp.15702
93. Neishabouri A, Wahl N, Mairani A, Köthe U, Bangert M. Long short-term memory networks for proton dose calculation in highly heterogeneous tissues. *Med Phys.* 2021;48(4):1893–1908. doi:10.1002/mp.14658
94. Nguyen D, Jia X, Sher D, et al. 3D radiotherapy dose prediction on head and neck cancer patients with a hierarchically densely connected U-net deep learning architecture. *Phys Med Biol.* 2019;64(6):065020. doi:10.1088/1361–6560/ab039b
95. Mentzel F, Kröninger K, Lerch M, et al. Small beams, fast predictions: a comparison of machine learning dose prediction models for proton minibeam therapy. *Med Phys.* 2022;49(12):7791–7801. doi:10.1002/mp.16066
96. Zhang X, Hu Z, Zhang G, Zhuang Y, Wang Y, Peng H. Dose calculation in proton therapy using a discovery cross-domain generative adversarial network (DiscoGAN). *Med Phys.* 2021;48(5):2646–2660. doi:10.1002/mp.14781
97. Viar-Hernandez D, Molina-Maza JM, Vera-Sánchez JA, et al. Enhancing adaptive proton therapy through CBCT images: Synthetic head and neck CT generation based on 3D vision transformers. *Med Phys.* 2024;51(7):4922–4935. doi:10.1002/mp.17057
98. Pang B, Si H, Liu M, et al. Comparison and evaluation of different deep learning models of synthetic CT generation from CBCT for nasopharynx cancer adaptive proton therapy. *Med Phys.* 2023;50(11):6920–6930. doi:10.1002/mp.16777
99. Wang C, Uh J, Merchant TE, Hua CH, Acharya S. Facilitating MR-guided adaptive proton therapy in children using deep learning-based synthetic CT. *Int J Part Ther.* 2022;8(3):11–20. doi:10.14338/IJPT-20–00099.1
100. de Koster RJC, Thummerer A, Scandurra D, Langendijk JA, Both S. Technical note: Evaluation of deep learning based synthetic CTs clinical readiness for dose and NTCP driven head and neck adaptive proton therapy. *Med Phys.* 2023;50(12):8023–8033. doi:10.1002/mp.16782
101. Thummerer A, Seller Oria C, Zaffino P, et al. Clinical suitability of deep learning based synthetic CTs for adaptive proton therapy of lung cancer. *Med Phys.* 2021;48(12):7673–7684. doi:10.1002/mp.15333
102. Thummerer A, Seller Oria C, Zaffino P, et al. Deep learning-based 4D-synthetic CTs from sparse-view CBCTs for dose calculations in adaptive proton therapy. *Med Phys.* 2022;49(11):6824–6839. doi:10.1002/mp.15930
103. Kaushik S, Ödén J, Sharma DS, Fredriksson A, Toma-Dasu I. Generation and evaluation of anatomy-preserving virtual CT for online adaptive proton therapy. *Med Phys.* 2024;51(3):1536–1546. doi:10.1002/mp.16941
104. Zhang G, Zhou L, Han Z, Zhao W, Peng H. SWFT-Net: A deep learning framework for efficient fine-tuning spot weights towards adaptive proton therapy. *Phys Med Biol.* 2022;67(24). doi:10.1088/1361–6560/aca517
105. Zhang G, Chen X, Dai J, Men K. A plan verification platform for online adaptive proton therapy using deep learning-based Monte-Carlo denoising. *Phys Med.* 2022;103:18–25. doi:10.1016/j.ejmp.2022.09.018
106. Li Z, Wang Y, Yu Y, Fan K, Xing L, Peng H. Technical note: Machine learning approaches for range and dose verification in proton therapy using proton-induced positron emitters. *Med Phys.* 2019;46(12):5748–5757. doi:10.1002/mp.13827
107. Liu C, Li Z, Hu W, Xing L, Peng H. Range and dose verification in proton therapy using proton-induced positron emitters and recurrent neural networks (RNNs). *Phys Med Biol.* 2019;64(17):175009. doi:10.1088/1361–6560/ab3564
108. Hu Z, Li G, Zhang X, Ye K, Lu J, Peng H. A machine learning framework with anatomical prior for online dose verification using positron emitters and PET in proton therapy. *Phys Med Biol.* 2020;65(18):185003. doi:10.1088/1361–6560/ab9707
109. Ma S, Hu Z, Ye K, Zhang X, Wang Y, Peng H. Feasibility study of patient-specific dose verification in proton therapy utilizing positron emission tomography (PET) and generative adversarial network (GAN). *Med Phys.* 2020;47(10):5194–5208. doi:10.1002/mp.14443
110. Parodi K, Bortfeld T. A filtering approach based on Gaussian–powerlaw convolutions for local PET verification of proton radiotherapy. *Phys Med Biol.* 2006;51(8):1991–2009. doi:10.1088/0031–9155/51/8/003

111. Attanasi F, Knopf A, Parodi K, et al. Extension and validation of an analytical model for *in vivo* PET verification of proton therapy—a phantom and clinical study. *Phys Med Biol.* 2011;56(16):5079–5098. doi:10.1088/0031–9155/56/16/001
112. Remmele S, Hesser J, Paganetti H, Bortfeld T. A deconvolution approach for PET-based dose reconstruction in proton radiotherapy. *Phys Med Biol.* 2011;56(23):7601–7619. doi:10.1088/0031–9155/56/23/017
113. Schumann A, Priegnitz M, Schoene S, Enghardt W, Rohling H, Fiedler F. From prompt gamma distribution to dose: A novel approach combining an evolutionary algorithm and filtering based on Gaussian-powerlaw convolutions. *Phys Med Biol.* 2016;61(19):6919–6934. doi:10.1088/0031–9155/61/19/6919
114. Parodi K, Paganetti H, Shih HA, et al. Patient study of In Vivo verification of beam delivery and range, using positron emission tomography and computed tomography imaging after proton therapy. *International Journal of Radiation Oncology*Biology*Physics.* 2007;68(3):920–934. doi:10.1016/j.ijrobp.2007.01.063
115. Frey K, Bauer J, Unholtz D, et al. TPS $_{PET}$ —A TPS-based approach for *in vivo* dose verification with PET in proton therapy. *Phys Med Biol.* 2014;59(1):1–21. doi:10.1088/0031–9155/59/1/1
116. Hofmann T, Pinto M, Mohammadi A, et al. Dose reconstruction from PET images in carbon ion therapy: a deconvolution approach. *Phys Med Biol.* 2019;64(2):025011. doi:10.1088/1361–6560/aaf676
117. Richter C, Pausch G, Barczyk S, et al. First clinical application of a prompt gamma based in vivo proton range verification system. *Radiotherapy and Oncology.* 2016;118(2):232–237. doi:10.1016/j.radonc.2016.01.004
118. Gueth P, Dauvergne D, Freud N, et al. Machine learning-based patient specific prompt-gamma dose monitoring in proton therapy. *Phys Med Biol.* 2013;58(13):4563–4577. doi:10.1088/0031–9155/58/13/4563
119. Liu CC, Huang HM. A deep learning approach for converting prompt gamma images to proton dose distributions: A Monte Carlo simulation study. *Physica Medica.* 2020;69:110–119. doi:10.1016/j.ejmp.2019.12.006
120. Yamaguchi M, Nagao Y, Ando K, et al. Secondary-electron-bremsstrahlung imaging for proton therapy. *Nucl Instrum Methods Phys Res A.* 2016;833:199–207. doi:10.1016/j.nima.2016.07.034
121. Ando K, Yamaguchi M, Yamamoto S, Toshito T, Kawachi N. Development of a low-energy x-ray camera for the imaging of secondary electron bremsstrahlung x-ray emitted during proton irradiation for range estimation. *Phys Med Biol.* 2017;62(12):5006–5020. doi:10.1088/1361–6560/aa7166
122. Yamaguchi M, Nagao Y, Ando K, et al. Imaging of monochromatic beams by measuring secondary electron bremsstrahlung for carbon-ion therapy using a pinhole x-ray camera. *Phys Med Biol.* 2018;63(4):045016. doi:10.1088/1361–6560/aaa17c
123. Yamamoto S, Yamaguchi M, Akagi T, Sasano M, Kawachi N. Development of a YAP(Ce) camera for the imaging of secondary electron bremsstrahlung x-ray emitted during carbon-ion irradiation toward the use of clinical conditions. *Phys Med Biol.* 2019;64(13):135019. doi:10.1088/1361–6560/ab2072
124. Yamaguchi M, Liu C, Huang H, et al. Dose image prediction for range and width verifications from carbon ion-induced secondary electron bremsstrahlung x-rays using deep learning workflow. *Med Phy.* 2020;47(8):3520–3532. doi:10.1002/mp.14205
125. Jones KC, Nie W, Chu JCH, et al. Acoustic-based proton range verification in heterogeneous tissue: simulation studies. *Phys Med Biol.* 2018;63(2):025018. doi:10.1088/1361–6560/aa9d16
126. Jones KC, Vander Stappen F, Sehgal CM, Avery S. Acoustic time-of-flight for proton range verification in water. *Med Phys.* 2016;43(9):5213–5224. doi:10.1118/1.4961120
127. Hickling S, Xiang L, Jones KC, et al. Ionizing radiation-induced acoustics for radiotherapy and diagnostic radiology applications. *Med Phy.* 2018;45(7). doi:10.1002/mp.12929
128. Nie W, Jones KC, Petro S, Kassaee A, Sehgal CM, Avery S. Proton range verification in homogeneous materials through acoustic measurements. *Phys Med Biol.* 2018;63(2):025036. doi:10.1088/1361–6560/aa9c1f
129. Yu Y, Li Z, Zhang D, Xing L, Peng H. Simulation studies of time reversal-based protoacoustic reconstruction for range and dose verification in proton therapy. *Med Phys.* 2019;46(8):3649–3662. doi:10.1002/mp.13661
130. Yu Y, Qi P, Peng H. Feasibility study of 3D time-reversal reconstruction of proton-induced acoustic signals for dose verification in the head and the liver: A simulation study. *Med Phys.* 2021;48(8):4485–4497. doi:10.1002/mp.15046
131. Yao S, Hu Z, Zhang X, et al. Feasibility study of range verification based on proton-induced acoustic signals and recurrent neural network. *Phys Med Biol.* 2020;65(21):215017. doi:10.1088/1361–6560/abaa5e
132. Yao S, Hu Z, Xie Q, Yang Y, Peng H. Further investigation of 3D dose verification in proton therapy utilizing acoustic signal, wavelet decomposition and machine learning. *Biomed Phys Eng Express.* 2022;8(1):015008. doi:10.1088/2057-1976/ac396d

133. Yamamoto S, Toshito T, Okumura S, Komori M. Luminescence imaging of water during proton-beam irradiation for range estimation. *Med Phy.* 2015;42(11):6498–6506. doi:10.1118/1.4932630
134. Yamamoto S, Komori M, Akagi T, et al. Luminescence imaging of water during carbon-ion irradiation for range estimation: Luminescence imaging of water during carbon-ion irradiation. *Med Phys.* 2016;43(5):2455–2463. doi:10.1118/1.4946821
135. Yabe T, Yamamoto S, Oda M, Mori K, Toshito T, Akagi T. Prediction of dose distribution from luminescence image of water using a deep convolutional neural network for particle therapy. *Med Phys.* 2020;47(9):3882–3891. doi:10.1002/mp.14372
136. Thummerer A, Zaffino P, Meijers A, et al. Comparison of CBCT based synthetic CT methods suitable for proton dose calculations in adaptive proton therapy. *Phys Med Biol.* 2020;65(9):095002. doi:10.1088/1361–6560/ab7d54
137. Kurz C, Maspero M, Savenije MHF, et al. CBCT correction using a cycle-consistent generative adversarial network and unpaired training to enable photon and proton dose calculation. *Phys Med Biol.* 2019;64(22):225004. doi:10.1088/1361–6560/ab4d8c
138. Hansen DC, Landry G, Kamp F, et al. ScatterNet: A convolutional neural network for cone-beam CT intensity correction. *Med Phys.* 2018;45(11):4916–4926. doi:10.1002/mp.13175
139. Landry G, Hansen D, Kamp F, et al. Comparing Unet training with three different datasets to correct CBCT images for prostate radiotherapy dose calculations. *Phys Med Biol.* 2019;64(3):035011. doi:10.1088/1361–6560/aaf496
140. Thummerer A, de Jong BA, Zaffino P, et al. Comparison of the suitability of CBCT- and MR-based synthetic CTs for daily adaptive proton therapy in head and neck patients. *Phys Med Biol.* 2020;65(23):235036. doi:10.1088/1361–6560/abb1d6
141. Uh J, Wang C, Acharya S, Krasin MJ, Hua CH. Training a deep neural network coping with diversities in abdominal and pelvic images of children and young adults for CBCT-based adaptive proton therapy. *Radiother Oncol.* 2021;160:250–258. doi:10.1016/j.radonc.2021.05.006
142. Chang CW, Lei Y, Charyyev S, et al. An unsupervised patient-specific metal artifact reduction framework for proton therapy. In: Linte CA, Siewerdsen JH, eds. *Medical Imaging 2022: Image-Guided Procedures, Robotic Interventions, and Modeling.* SPIE; 2022:31. doi:10.1117/12.2612345
143. Lalonde A, Winey B, Verburg J, Paganetti H, Sharp GC. Evaluation of CBCT scatter correction using deep convolutional neural networks for head and neck adaptive proton therapy. *Phys Med Biol.* 2020;65(24). doi:10.1088/1361–6560/ab9fcb
144. Nomura Y, Xu Q, Shirato H, Shimizu S, Xing L. Projection-domain scatter correction for cone beam computed tomography using a residual convolutional neural network. *Med Phys.* 2019;46(7):3142–3155. doi:10.1002/mp.13583
145. Charyyev S, Lei Y, Harms J, et al. High quality proton portal imaging using deep learning for proton radiation therapy: a phantom study. *Biomed Phys Eng Express.* 2020;6(3):035029. doi:10.1088/2057-1976/ab8a74
146. Krishnamurthy R, Mummudi N, Goda JS, Chopra S, Heijmen B, Swamidas J. Using artificial intelligence for optimization of the processes and resource utilization in radiotherapy. *JCO Global Oncol.* 2022;(8):e2100393. doi:10.1200/GO.21.00393
147. York SA, Ali AM, Lashbrooke DC, et al. Promising hyperparameter configurations for deep fully connected neural networks to improve image reconstruction in proton radiotherapy. In: *2021 IEEE International Conference on Big Data (Big Data).* IEEE, Orlando, FL, USA, 2021:5648–5657. doi:10.1109/BigData52589.2021.9671404
148. Maggi P, Peterson S, Panthi R, et al. Computational model for detector timing effects in Compton-camera based prompt-gamma imaging for proton radiotherapy. *Phys Med Biol.* 2020;65(12):125004. doi:10.1088/1361–6560/ab8bf0
149. Vozenin MC, Hendry JH, Limoli CL. Biological benefits of ultra-high dose rate FLASH Radiotherapy: Sleeping beauty awoken. *Clin Oncol (R Coll Radiol).* 2019;31(7):407–415. doi:10.1016/j.clon.2019.04.001
150. Esplen N, Mendonca MS, Bazalova-Carter M. Physics and biology of ultrahigh dose-rate (FLASH) radiotherapy: A topical review. *Phys Med Biol.* 2020;65(23):23TR03. doi:10.1088/1361–6560/abaa28
151. Gao Y, Liu R, Chang CW, et al. A potential revolution in cancer treatment: A topical review of FLASH radiotherapy. *J Appl Clin Med Phys.* 2022;23(10):e13790. doi:10.1002/acm2.13790
152. Lin B, Gao F, Yang Y, et al. FLASH radiotherapy: History and future. *Front Oncol.* 2021;11:644400. doi:10.3389/fonc.2021.644400

153. Loo BW, Schuler E, Lartey FM, et al. (P003) Delivery of ultra-rapid flash radiation therapy and demonstration of normal tissue sparing after abdominal irradiation of mice. *Int J Radiat Oncol Biol Phys*. 2017;98(2):E16. doi:10.1016/j.ijrobp.2017.02.101
154. Liu R, Charyyev S, Wahl N, et al. An integrated physical optimization framework for proton stereotactic body radiation therapy FLASH treatment planning allows dose, dose rate, and linear energy transfer optimization using patient-specific ridge filters. *Int J Radiat Oncol Biol Phys*. 2023;116(4):949–959. doi:10.1016/j.ijrobp.2023.01.048
155. Harrison N, Kang M, Liu R, et al. A novel inverse algorithm to solve IPO-IMPT of proton FLASH therapy with sparse filters. *Int J Radiat Oncol Biol Phys*. Published online December 2023:S0360301623081877. doi:10.1016/j.ijrobp.2023.11.061
156. Loo BW, Verginadis II, Sørensen BS, et al. Navigating the critical translational questions for implementing FLASH in the clinic. *Semin Radiat Oncol*. 2024;34(3):351–364. doi:10.1016/j.semradonc.2024.04.008
157. Böhlen TT, Germond JF, Bourhis J, et al. Normal tissue sparing by FLASH as a Function of single-fraction dose: A quantitative analysis. *Int J Radiat Oncol Biol Phys*. 2022;114(5):1032–1044. doi:10.1016/j.ijrobp.2022.05.038
158. Marcu LG, Bezak E, Peukert DD, Wilson P. Translational research in FLASH radiotherapy-from radiobiological mechanisms to In Vivo results. *Biomedicines*. 2021;9(2):181. doi:10.3390/biomedicines9020181
159. Ruan JL, Lee C, Wouters S, et al. Irradiation at ultra-high (FLASH) dose rates reduces acute normal tissue toxicity in the mouse gastrointestinal system. *Int J Radiat Oncol Biol Phys*. 2021;111(5):1250–1261. doi:10.1016/j.ijrobp.2021.08.004
160. Charyyev S, Chang CW, Zhu M, Lin L, Langen K, Dhabaan A. Characterization of 250 MeV protons from the varian ProBeam PBS system for FLASH radiation therapy. *Int J Part Ther*. 2023;9(4):279–289. doi:10.14338/IJPT-22–00027.1
161. Charyyev S, Liu R, Yang X, et al. Measurement of the time structure of FLASH beams using prompt gamma rays and secondary neutrons as surrogates. *Phys Med Biol*. 2023;68(14). doi:10.1088/1361–6560/acdc7c
162. Shen J, Ding X, Charyyev S, et al. Time structures of proton pencil beam scanning delivery on a microsecond scale measured with a pixelated semiconductor detector Timepix3. *J Appl Clin Med Phys*. 2024;25(9):e14486. doi:10.1002/acm2.14486
163. Bell BI, Velten C, Pennock M, et al. Whole abdominal pencil beam scanned proton FLASH increases acute lethality. *Int J Radiat Oncol Biol Phys*. Published online September 18, 2024:S0360–3016(24)03327-3. doi:10.1016/j.ijrobp.2024.09.006
164. Yang Z, Melemenidis S, Jiang H, et al. Enhancing histological image analysis and automation through unsupervised attention-guided deep learning for robust stain normalization in H&E-stained images. *Int J Radiat Oncol Biol Phys*. 2024;120(2):e416. doi:10.1016/j.ijrobp.2024.07.927
165. Fu J, Jiang H, Melemenidis S, et al. Deep learning-based pipeline for automatic identification of intestinal regenerating crypts in mouse histological images. *Int J Radiat Oncol Biol Phys*. 2023;117(2):S117–S118. doi:10.1016/j.ijrobp.2023.06.451
166. Fu J, Yang Z, Melemenidis S, et al. Exploring deep learning for estimating the isoeffective dose of FLASH irradiation from mouse intestinal histological images. *Int J Radiat Oncol Biol Phys*. 2024;119(3):1001–1010. doi:10.1016/j.ijrobp.2023.12.032
167. Chang CW, Lei Y, Wang T, et al. Deep learning-based fast volumetric image generation for image-guided proton FLASH radiotherapy. *Res Sq*. Published online July 26, 2023:rs.3.rs-3112632. doi:10.21203/rs.3.rs-3112632/v1
168. Riley P. Three pitfalls to avoid in machine learning. *Nature*. 2019;572(7767):27–29. doi:10.1038/d41586-019-02307-y
169. Kanal LN, Randall NC. Recognition system design by statistical analysis. In: *Proceedings of the 1964 19th ACM National Conference On*. ACM Press, USA; 1964:42.501–42.5020. doi:10.1145/800257.808903

10 Artificial Intelligence in Brachytherapy

Jingchu Chen, Tonghe Wang, and Xiaofeng Yang

10.1 INTRODUCTION

Brachytherapy, a form of internal radiation therapy, delivers high radiation doses directly to the tumor via the placement of radioactive sources within or adjacent to the target tissue. This localized approach, applied through either low-dose rate (LDR) or high-dose rate (HDR) techniques, provides highly conformal dose distributions that minimize exposure to surrounding organs at risk (OARs). Despite its dosimetric advantages and clinical efficacy in treating various malignancies—including gynecologic, prostate, and head and neck cancers—brachytherapy remains a technically demanding and resource-intensive modality [1–5]. Its success depends heavily on expert coordination across a multistep workflow encompassing imaging, applicator placement, segmentation, treatment planning, quality assurance, and delivery.

The complexity and interdependence of these procedural steps, along with significant variability in clinician experience, introduce challenges in standardizing care and ensuring reproducibility. Consequently, there is a growing demand to enhance workflow efficiency, reduce variability, and support clinical decision-making with intelligent automation. Artificial intelligence (AI), encompassing both machine learning (ML) and deep learning (DL) techniques, has emerged as a powerful tool to address these challenges. With its demonstrated capacity to extract meaningful patterns from data, AI is expected to revolutionize how brachytherapy is planned, delivered, and evaluated.

Recent years have witnessed an expanding body of research applying AI to various aspects of brachytherapy [6–8]. These applications range from automatic image registration and segmentation to treatment plan optimization, catheter reconstruction, quality assurance, outcome prediction, and even real-time intraoperative guidance. Using neural network architectures such as convolutional neural networks (CNNs), U-Net variants, and more recently transformer-based models, AI methods are now capable of performing complex clinical tasks with increasing accuracy and speed [9–17]. Figure 10.1 shows the number of AI studies on brachytherapy published from 2015 to August 2024.

This chapter, adapted from "A review of artificial intelligence in brachytherapy" by Chen et al. and used under the CC BY 4.0 license [18], provides a comprehensive overview of AI applications throughout the brachytherapy workflow. Building upon a recent systematic review of over 100 peer-reviewed studies, we summarize the technical innovations, clinical relevance, and practical impact of AI-driven solutions. We also highlight limitations, implementation barriers, and future opportunities, aiming to inform both researchers and clinicians about the evolving role of AI in advancing brachytherapy practice.

10.2 APPLICATIONS OF AI

10.2.1 Imaging Registration

Image registration is critical for aligning multi-modal or multi-temporal images, particularly in workflows involving fractionated treatments or hybrid imaging (e.g., magnetic resonance imaging (MRI) and ultrasound). In gynecologic (GYN) brachytherapy, inter-fractional anatomical changes due to bladder/rectum filling or tumor regression necessitate deformable registration between

 DOI: 10.1201/9781003480365-11

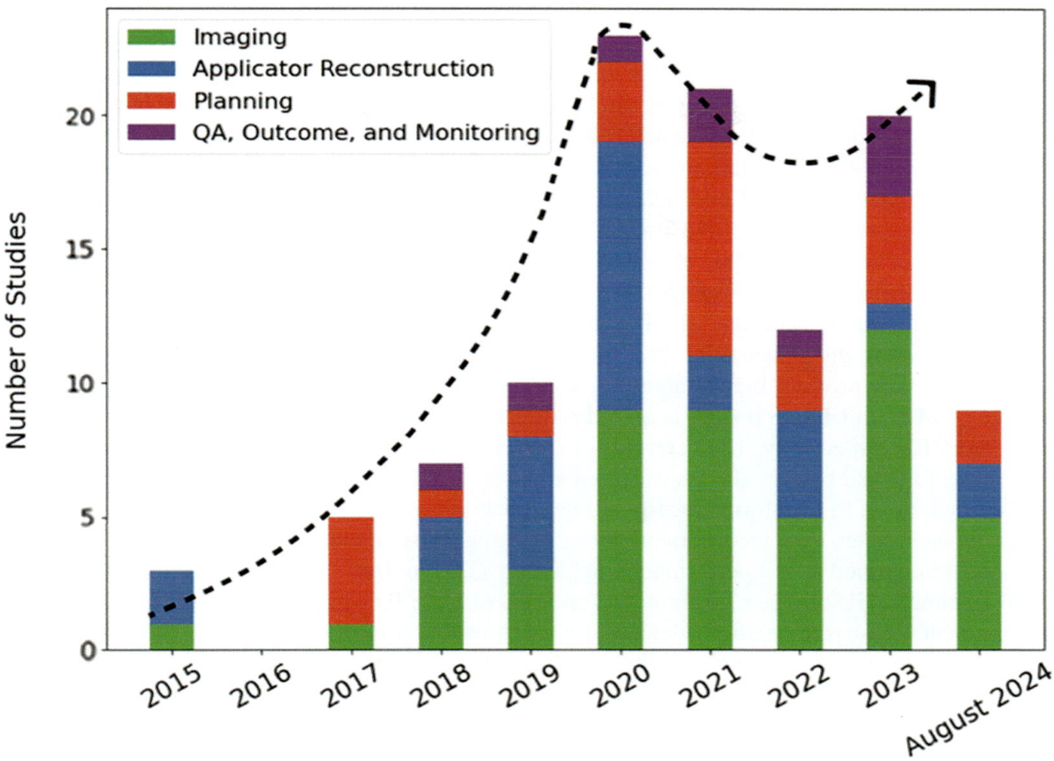

FIGURE 10.1 Overview of the number of studies in applications of AI in brachytherapy from 2015 to August 2024 with an approximate dotted trendline. Reprinted from *JACMP*, A review of artificial intelligence in brachytherapy by Chen et al.

planning and treatment images. Similarly, in prostate brachytherapy, aligning magnetic resonance (MR) images with transrectal ultrasound (TRUS) is essential to fuse high soft-tissue contrast with real-time intraoperative guidance.

To address the inter-fractional anatomical variations commonly observed in GYN brachytherapy, Salehi et al. [19] developed a deep learning-based deformable image registration algorithm known as DIRNet. This non-rigid registration framework was designed to align CT images of the cervix and surrounding OARs, with its performance assessed by comparing the deformed contours to ground-truth annotations. The study demonstrated that DIRNet achieved comparable Dice similarity coefficients (DSC) and significantly outperformed conventional intensity-based methods, such as SimpleElastix, in terms of Jaccard index (JI)—the ratio of intersected to union regions between predicted and reference contours—and mean surface distance (MSD).

In addition to deformable methods, rigid registration techniques can also be applied, particularly when guided by applicator geometry. Ecker et al. [20] proposed a semi-automated approach combining deep learning-based applicator segmentation with conventional rigid registration for MR-guided GYN brachytherapy. A 3D UNETR model was used to segment the applicators, achieving a DSC of 0.70 ± 0.07. The resulting segmentation served as the reference for rigid alignment between fractions. The mean registration error based on predicted segmentation was 2.7 ± 1.4 mm—substantially higher than the 0.7 ± 0.5 mm error observed when using ground-truth contours. This discrepancy was attributed to the limited segmentation accuracy of the applicators. The findings suggest that improving segmentation fidelity could enable accurate and fully automated rigid registration, offering a faster and potentially more reliable alternative to manual methods.

Two distinct deep learning-based methods for MRI-TRUS image registration in prostate brachytherapy were proposed. Zeng et al. [21] introduced a fully automated registration framework using a weakly supervised learning approach, which relies on partially labeled data. The workflow consisted of three stages: initial segmentation of MRI and TRUS images using two fully convolutional networks (FCNs), affine registration via a 2D CNN, and non-rigid registration using a 3D U-Net-based network. The initial segmentation yielded strong agreement with manual contours, with DSC values of 0.88 ± 0.05 for MRI and 0.92 ± 0.03 for TRUS. The model was tested using two input strategies—label-based (SR-L) and image-based (SR-I). The SR-L approach produced the most accurate results, achieving a DSC of 0.91 ± 0.02, a mean target registration error of 2.53 ± 1.39 mm, an MSD of 0.88 mm, and a Hausdorff distance (HD) of 4.41 mm. These findings highlight the efficacy of label-driven registration initialized by DL in achieving high registration accuracy.

Complementing this, Chen et al. [22] proposed a segmentation-based registration method specifically for HDR prostate brachytherapy. Two 3D V-Net models were employed to segment the prostate on MRI and TRUS images acquired post-catheter insertion, achieving DSCs of 0.86 ± 0.05 and 0.90 ± 0.03, respectively. The centroids of the segmented prostate volumes were aligned as an initial step, followed by a spatial transformation network (STN) that applied predicted deformable displacement fields to transform corresponding probability maps. To mitigate overfitting, data augmentation techniques were incorporated during training. Despite the presence of catheter artifacts, the model maintained robust performance, achieving a DSC of 0.87 ± 0.05, a center of mass error of 1.7 ± 0.89 mm, an HD of 7.21 ± 2.07 mm, and an MSD of 1.61 ± 0.64 mm on TRUS images. Although this segmentation-based method yielded slightly lower accuracy compared to the label-based approach, the results remained clinically acceptable. The difference in performance may be attributed to the hierarchical anatomical features emphasized in segmentation-based methods versus intensity-based representations leveraged in label-driven learning.

10.2.2 Image Segmentation

Segmentation of targets and OARs is a prerequisite for treatment planning, dose evaluation, and applicator guidance. Manual contouring remains a major bottleneck, particularly on MRI where visualization is superior but annotation is time-consuming and requires expert knowledge. AI models—particularly CNNs and U-Net variants—have demonstrated high accuracy in segmenting both targets and OARs in GYN and prostate brachytherapy.

Zabihollahy et al. [23] developed a two-stage CNN framework for automatic segmentation of OARs in gynecologic brachytherapy, utilizing a 3D Dense U-Net architecture. The model follows a coarse-to-fine strategy, where an initial 3D U-Net performs coarse segmentation, followed by a refinement stage using a 3D dense block that captures both inter- and intra-slice contextual information. The model was trained and evaluated on two different MRI protocols: MR1 (TR=2,600 ms, TE=95 ms) and MR2 (TR=3,500 ms, TE=97 ms). Improved image contrast in MR2 yielded slightly better performance. Specifically, DSCs for bladder, rectum, and sigmoid were 0.93 ± 0.04, 0.87 ± 0.03, and 0.80 ± 0.10 on MR1 and 0.94 ± 0.05, 0.88 ± 0.04, and 0.80 ± 0.05 on MR2. This hierarchical segmentation approach demonstrated enhanced accuracy across both low- and high-contrast MRI settings, as reflected by improvements in both DSC and Hausdorff distance (HD95), supporting its adaptability across varied imaging conditions.

Several studies have explored the use of neural network-based models to simultaneously segment the high-risk clinical target volume (HR-CTV) and OARs on CT images for gynecologic brachytherapy planning [24–28]. Li et al. [26] and Duprez et al. [27] employed the self-configuring nnU-Net framework to evaluate segmentation performance across various model configurations, including 2D U-Net, 3D U-Net, and 3D Cascade U-Net. Each segmentation task was paired with the architecture that yielded the best results. Both studies consistently found that the 3D Cascade U-Net architecture provided superior performance, achieving higher accuracy in terms of DSC, 95th percentile Hausdorff distance (HD95), and MSD. While Li et al. reported a higher DSC for HR-CTV segmentation (0.836±0.07), Duprez et al. observed a lower HD95 (6.03±2.01 mm), suggesting complementary strengths in segmentation precision. In both studies, the bladder was segmented with the highest accuracy, likely due to its well-defined anatomical boundaries, whereas HR-CTV exhibited the greatest variability, reflecting its less distinct contour definitions. The majority of AI-generated contours were deemed clinically acceptable, with minimal dosimetric deviations from manual contours. These findings reinforce the suitability of 3D Cascade U-Net as a robust and reliable architecture for segmenting critical structures in cervical cancer brachytherapy.

In another CT-based study, Mohammadi et al. [29] introduced a deep convolutional neural network model, ResU-Net, which integrates elements of ResNet and U-Net architectures. Compared to standard U-Net, ResU-Net demonstrated faster processing times and superior segmentation accuracy. The model achieved high performance even for anatomically complex structures such as the sigmoid colon, yielding a median DSC of 0.941, HD95 of 2.82 mm, and MSD of 0.73 mm. Furthermore, the dosimetric differences between ResU-Net-generated contours and manually delineated contours were minimal, typically under 0.5 Gy, supporting its clinical viability for automated planning in brachytherapy.

A dose boost to the dominant intraprostatic lesion (DIL) has been proposed as a strategy to enhance treatment outcomes in prostate HDR brachytherapy [30–32]. Precise segmentation of the DIL is critical to ensure accurate targeting and effective delivery of the boost dose. Positron emission tomography/computed tomography (PET/CT) offers valuable anatomical and functional information for identifying and localizing DILs.

Matkovic et al. [33] developed a Cascaded Regional-Net for automatic segmentation of both the prostate and DIL on PET/CT images. The framework incorporates a Dual Attention Network to extract deep semantic features and isolate the volume-of-interest (VOI) for the prostate, thereby narrowing the search space for DIL localization. Within this VOI, a mask-scoring regional convolutional neural network (MSR-CNN) was used to detect and segment the DIL. The model achieved mean surface distances of 0.666±0.696 and 0.814±1.002 mm and DSCs of 0.932±0.059 and 0.801±0.178 for the prostate and DIL, respectively. While the DIL segmentation yielded a lower DSC due to its small and irregular nature, the results were still considered clinically meaningful.

Wang et al. [34] explored a similar segmentation task using a Cascaded U-Net architecture to segment lesions on both PET-only and PET/CT images. Interestingly, more lesions were detected using PET alone (153 out of 155) compared to PET/CT (144 out of 155), although no statistically significant differences were observed in segmentation accuracy metrics, including DSC (0.68±0.15) and HD95 (4±2 mm). These findings suggest that while CT can enhance anatomical context, it may introduce additional complexity without improving DIL segmentation performance.

Additional efforts have been made to improve lesion segmentation and generalizability. Li et al. [35] validated their DL model on 56 external PET/CT scans and found no significant difference in performance compared to internal datasets, supporting the model's robustness across institutions. Kostyszyn et al. [36] applied a 3D U-Net to PET images acquired with two different PSMA tracers using histological slices as reference standards. Their study aimed to improve both sensitivity and specificity in DIL detection, highlighting the importance of tracer selection and histopathologic validation in advancing AI-based lesion segmentation.

Prostate brachytherapy commonly relies on TRUS imaging to guide needle or catheter placement during implantation. Accurate delineation of the prostate and adjacent OARs is essential for effective treatment planning and dose delivery. A reliable segmentation framework could enable a TRUS-only planning workflow, potentially eliminating the need for supplementary CT or MRI scans and streamlining intraoperative procedures. However, the segmentation task is particularly challenging due to the limited soft-tissue contrast and indistinct boundaries between the prostate and surrounding structures, especially the rectum. As a result, contouring on TRUS is often subjective and highly dependent on the clinician's expertise and experience, leading to variability in target definition.

Several studies have successfully applied DL models to segment the prostate on TRUS images [36–45]. Among these, the most accurate segmentation results were reported by semiautomatic approaches developed by Girum et al. [45] and Peng et al. [36], both achieving DSC exceeding 0.96 on TRUS.

Girum et al. employed a weakly supervised DL framework, consisting of a fully connected CNN integrated with a prior knowledge generator and a segmentation block. This approach, which requires only partial annotations, offers reduced labeling effort and faster training compared to fully supervised methods. The model achieved excellent results on TRUS images (DSC=0.969 ± 0.009; HD=4.25 ± 4.58 mm) and showed promising cross-modality generalization when applied to CT images (DSC=0.954 ± 0.009; HD=5.17 ± 1.41 mm), despite being trained exclusively on ultrasound. This highlights the potential of model adaptation across imaging modalities with limited training data. However, the method requires pseudo-landmarks from users, introducing a dependency on operator input. This can result in inter-observer variability and occasional reductions in segmentation accuracy (e.g., DSC=0.942 in some instances).

Peng et al. proposed A-ProSeg, a semiautomatic model that integrates a closed-principle-curve-based method, a global polygonal contouring strategy, and a memory-based differential evolution algorithm to construct smooth and anatomically accurate prostate boundaries. Trained on a large dataset comprising 226 patients and 945 TRUS slices, the model achieved a DSC of 0.962 ± 0.024 and a reduced HD of 1.9 ± 0.9 mm. Notably, the model demonstrated robustness against imaging noise, maintaining high segmentation accuracy even at low signal-to-noise ratios (SNR=0.8), underscoring its potential for clinical robustness.

While semiautomatic models provide excellent accuracy, they still require some degree of user interaction. In contrast, fully automatic models offer additional workflow efficiency by eliminating the need for manual input. One of the top-performing fully automatic models was introduced by Orlando et al. [46], who developed a 2D modified U-Net to segment radial slices from 3D TRUS volumes and subsequently reconstructed the prostate surface in 3D. This approach yielded a median DSC of 0.94, an HD of 2.89 mm, a volume percent difference (VPD) of 5.78%, and an MSD of 0.89 mm.

In a follow-up study, Orlando et al. [47] systematically investigated the impact of dataset size, image acquisition type (end-fire vs. side-fire), and model architecture (U-Net vs. U-Net++) on segmentation performance. When trained on a large dataset of 7000 2D TRUS slices, the U-Net++ architecture outperformed the original U-Net, achieving improved recall (96.7%) and reduced VPD (4.79%). The study also found that end-fire TRUS images yielded better performance, even with limited training data, whereas side-fire images were more susceptible to degradation in image quality. Interestingly, increasing the dataset size beyond a certain threshold did not significantly improve segmentation accuracy, although it did substantially increase training time.

In prostate brachytherapy, accurate segmentation of OARs—including the rectum, bladder, urethra, and seminal vesicles—is essential to minimize radiation-induced toxicity and ensure optimal dose distribution. Given the anatomical proximity of these structures to the prostate, several research groups have developed deep learning-based models to automate their delineation using TRUS, MRI, and CT imaging modalities.

Sanders et al. [48] conducted an extensive study using T1-, T2-, and combined T1/T2-weighted MRI, training 120 models across combinations of 18 FCNs and multiple convolutional encoders. The most accurate model employed a DenseNet201 encoder, achieving DSCs of 0.90 ± 0.04 (prostate), 0.70 ± 0.15 (external urinary sphincter), 0.80 ± 0.12 (seminal vesicles), 0.91 ± 0.06 (rectum), and 0.96 ± 0.04 (bladder). Despite being trained primarily on T2 and T2/T1-weighted images, the model demonstrated reasonable generalizability to T1-weighted MRI, albeit with slightly reduced accuracy. Notably, segmentation of the external urinary sphincter and seminal vesicles remained suboptimal, reflecting challenges posed by their small size and complex anatomy. In a follow-up study [49], the same group compared contours generated by a commercial DL system (MIM Symphony) to physician-refined contours. They found no statistically significant differences in geometry or dosimetric parameters, further supporting the clinical applicability of deep learning-generated contours.

Duan et al. [50] assessed the performance of commercial deep learning auto-segmentation (DLAS) software on CT images of the male pelvis. The software supports both use of pre-trained models and institutional retraining. Their results showed notable improvements in segmentation accuracy with retraining: DSCs increased from 0.73 to 0.82 for the prostate, from 0.81 to 0.92 for the rectum, and from 0.37 to 0.48 for the seminal vesicles. These findings underscore the importance of site-specific fine-tuning to improve performance in clinical implementation, particularly for anatomically variable or difficult-to-visualize structures.

10.2.3 Other Imaging Applications

Metal artifacts on CT images can significantly hinder the visualization of anatomical structures and brachytherapy applicators. Huang et al. [51] developed a residual learning-based CNNs, termed RL-ARCNN, to reduce metal artifacts on CT images in gynecologic (GYN) cancer brachytherapy. The model was trained on a dataset of 600 simulated artifact-contaminated image slices derived from 20 GYN cancer patients, partitioned into 450 training, 100 validation, and 50 testing slices. By incorporating residual learning, the RL-ARCNN demonstrated superior artifact reduction performance, achieving the highest peak signal-to-noise ratio (PSNR) across various image patch sizes. The optimal result was obtained with a 50×50 patch size, yielding a PSNR of 38.09 dB, indicating effective suppression of metal artifacts and enhanced image quality for treatment planning.

DL techniques have also been employed to enhance image quality by increasing spatial resolution. In clinical practice, 3D TRUS images used in brachytherapy are often acquired with thick slices (2–5 mm) to reduce acquisition time, resulting in lower resolution and limited anatomical detail. To address this limitation, He et al. [52] proposed a generative adversarial network (GAN)-based framework augmented with a deeply supervised attention mechanism to reconstruct high-resolution ultrasound images from low-resolution TRUS data. The model was trained using paired high- and low-resolution datasets from 20 patients, with high-resolution images serving as ground truth. The proposed approach demonstrated strong performance, achieving a mean absolute error (MAE) of 6.5 ± 0.5 and a PSNR of 38.0 ± 2.4 dB, indicating effective resolution enhancement and improved image quality for potential use in treatment planning.

10.2.4 Preplanning

In HDR gynecologic (GYN) brachytherapy, preplanning involves selecting the most appropriate applicator—either intracavitary (IC) or interstitial (IS)—based on the patient's anatomical presentation. With advances in AI, predictive modeling can assist clinicians in this decision-making process.

Stenhouse et al. [11] evaluated 12 ML models to predict the optimal applicator type (IC or IS) for individual patients. To reduce feature dimensionality and avoid overfitting, important anatomical and clinical features—such as needle distribution patterns and contour characteristics—were selected using an F-test. Among the evaluated models, an AdaBoost Classifier, Gradient Boosting Classifier, and Random Forest Classifier demonstrated superior performance and were combined into a weighted voting ensemble. This ensemble model predicted applicator selection with high accuracy ($91.5\pm0.9\%$) and a strong F1 score ($90.6\pm1.1\%$), generating results in under 10 seconds. The model's speed and consistency highlight its potential utility for supporting clinical preplanning workflows.

However, soft-tissue deformation caused by applicator insertion can significantly affect the accuracy of preplanning. Previous studies have shown that applicator insertion can induce an average point-to-point displacement of up to 25 mm in the uterus [53], which can lead to misalignment between preoperative plans and actual anatomy. To address this issue, Ghosh et al. [54] developed a DL model to predict uterine deformation using only pre-insertion MRI. Their framework utilized autoencoders for initial uterus segmentation and a modified U-Net to estimate the deformed uterine position post-applicator insertion. The model achieved a DSC of 0.941±0.033 and a HD of 4.0±3.1 mm for preoperative uterus segmentation. For predicting the deformed anatomy, the model yielded a DSC of 0.881±0.038 and an HD of 5.8±3.6 mm, demonstrating its potential to anticipate anatomical changes and further inform applicator selection.

In LDR prostate brachytherapy, preplanning involves determining both seed placement and the anticipated dose distribution prior to the procedure. Traditionally, this process is manual, time-intensive, and highly dependent on the planner's expertise. Recent advances in DL have enabled rapid, automated planning workflows by learning from prior high-quality plans. Several studies have demonstrated the potential of ML models to streamline and standardize LDR brachytherapy planning.

Nicolae et al. [55,56] developed a machine learning-based prostate implant planning algorithm (PIPA) to automate treatment planning for LDR prostate brachytherapy. In a comparison between PIPA and conventional manual planning, both methods produced plans with similar clinical acceptability—approximately equal proportions required either minor or major modifications. However, PIPA dramatically reduced planning time, generating plans in 2.38±0.96 minutes compared to 43.13±58.70 minutes for manual planning. While these results are promising, the study was conducted on a limited dataset of 41 patients and did not report detailed dose–volume histogram (DVH) comparisons, limiting its generalizability.

In a subsequent and more extensive study, Aleef et al. [57] introduced a two-stage framework combining conditional generative adversarial networks (cGANs) with a simulated annealing optimization algorithm. The model was trained on a large dataset of 961 patients, using cGANs to predict needle distributions and simulated annealing to refine seed locations. Of the automatically generated plans, 90% were deemed clinically acceptable—60% requiring only minor modifications and 30% requiring major adjustments. The planning time was reduced to 3 minutes, compared to 20 minutes for manual plans, while maintaining comparable quality, including a clinical target volume (CTV) V100% of 98.98% versus 99.36% for manual plans.

Building on this work, Aleef et al. [58] later developed the Treatment Planning GAN (TP-GAN), which further accelerated the planning process. This model generated plans with DVH metrics comparable to manual plans while reducing urethral dose. Notably, planning time was reduced to 2.5 minutes per case, or as little as 3 seconds per case without post-processing, demonstrating the potential for real-time, high-quality LDR brachytherapy planning.

10.2.5 Treatment Planning

HDR brachytherapy treatment planning is inherently time-sensitive, often conducted intraoperatively while patients are under anesthesia or immobilized. HDR prostate treatment planning is typically performed in real time using TRUS imaging. One of the key challenges in HDR brachytherapy is that dose distribution is highly dependent on the applicator configuration, which varies from patient to patient, making accurate dose prediction difficult and time-consuming.

AI offers a promising solution by analyzing large datasets to learn complex spatial and dosimetric patterns, thereby enabling rapid prediction of dose–volume histograms (DVHs) for the CTV and OARs. Several studies [52,59–66] have explored the use of DL models to expedite and improve the accuracy of HDR brachytherapy planning.

For instance, Mao et al. [52] developed RapidBrachyDL, a 3D deep convolutional neural network (DCNN) trained to emulate Monte Carlo (MC)-based dose calculations. The model achieved DVH prediction errors of less than 1.5% for both the CTV and OARs, offering accuracy comparable to conventional MC methods. Notably, although the model was trained exclusively on prostate cancer data, it demonstrated promising generalizability when applied to cervical cancer cases, with prediction errors remaining below 3%.

Similarly, Villa et al. [66] trained a DCNN on an MC-generated dose dataset to perform fast inverse planning for LDR brachytherapy. The model achieved low mean percent errors (MPEs) across target and OAR structures, while significantly reducing planning time—delivering dose predictions in just 1.7 seconds.

Li et al. [59] trained a DL model on a cohort of 81 cervical cancer patients, incorporating a range of commonly used applicators, including vaginal cylinders, ovoids, tandem and ovoids (T&O), free needles, and multi-channel applicators. The proposed model, termed the Squeeze-and-Excitation Attention Net (SE_AN), combined a Cascaded U-Net architecture with a Squeeze-and-Excitation module to enhance feature representation and improve dose prediction accuracy. The model's performance was compared with standard U-Net and 3D Cascaded U-Net architectures, with the smallest MAEs of the predicted dose–volume histogram (DVH) metrics. Although SE_AN did not achieve the lowest MAEs for the rectum and HR-CTV compared to the other models, it demonstrated superior clinical relevance by accurately predicting both the number of active sources and the dose gradient for various applicator configurations. Moreover, SE_AN achieved the highest gamma passing rate of 92±10%, indicating strong agreement between predicted and ground-truth dose distributions.

10.2.6 Applicator Reconstruction

Accurate digitization of applicators and catheters is critical in HDR gynecologic (GYN) brachytherapy, as even small localization errors can significantly affect the resulting dose distribution. Several studies have explored deep learning-based approaches to automate the digitization of common applicator types, including T&O, tandem-and-ring (T&R), and Fletcher applicators.

Jung et al. [67] developed a U-Net-based model for automatic segmentation of T&O applicators on CT images, integrating additional spectral clustering and polynomial curve-fitting techniques to refine identification of applicator positions and their central paths. The model achieved high segmentation accuracy, with DSCs of 0.937 for 2D images and 0.931 for 3D volumes. The corresponding HDs were 1.01, 1.21, and 1.18 mm for the tandem, right ovoid, and left ovoid, respectively. Moreover, the tip localization errors were minimal, measured at 0.50, 0.74, and 0.67 mm for the tandem, right ovoid, and left ovoid, respectively. These results highlight the model's potential to provide precise and automated digitization of applicators, reducing manual effort and improving planning efficiency in HDR GYN brachytherapy.

MRI offers superior soft-tissue contrast compared to CT, making it advantageous for visualizing target anatomy in cervical HDR brachytherapy. However, applicator reconstruction on MRI is often challenging due to the inconsistent visibility of contrast-filled fiducial markers within the applicator lumen. An alternative approach involves using manufacturer-provided library models of applicators, which can be rigidly registered to the patient's MRI. This method may offer greater reproducibility and reduce operator dependency compared to manual digitization on CT.

Hrinivich et al. [53] developed an automated reconstruction technique for T&R applicators using T2-weighted MR images. Their method employed a circular Hough transform (CHT) [68] to detect the ring centers, followed by the application of a 3D rotation matrix and 3D translation vector, optimized using a stochastic evolutionary algorithm [69], to align the library model with the imaged applicators. The resulting reconstruction achieved high accuracy, with mean errors of 0.60±0.24 mm for the ring and 0.58±0.24 mm for the tandem. Notably, the variability in reconstruction was lower than typical inter-observer differences, underscoring the method's precision and potential to improve consistency in MRI-based applicator reconstruction.

Plastic catheters pose a significant challenge for MRI-based identification in brachytherapy due to their low hydrogen content, which results in poor signal visibility. To address this, Zaffino et al. [70] developed a 3D U-Net model to automatically segment multiple, closely spaced brachytherapy catheters on MRI. The model demonstrated reasonable performance, achieving an average distance error of 2.0±3.4 mm, a DSC of 0.60±0.17, and a HD of 15.9±20.5 mm. The false positive and false negative catheter rates were 6.7% and 1.5%, respectively.

In prostate brachytherapy, both HDR and LDR offer comparable treatment efficacy, each with distinct advantages [71]. DL has been applied to assist applicator reconstruction in both modalities—HDR (needle and catheter identification) and LDR (needle and seed localization across various imaging modalities). HDR prostate brachytherapy typically uses TRUS, MRI, or CT to guide the insertion of interstitial needles, with TRUS being the most common. Andersén et al. [72] developed a 3D U-Net model trained on 1,102 TRUS-guided HDR procedures (24,422 needles), achieving a root-mean-square distance (RMSD) of 0.55 mm compared to clinical ground truth, outperforming inter-observer variability (0.80 mm). To further enhance needle detection, Zhang et al. explored three DL approaches using 3D TRUS: an ORDL-based method [73], a deeply supervised attention U-Net with total variation (TV) regularization [74], and a large-margin Mask R-CNN with clustering [75]. Among these, the LMMask R-CNN model achieved the best performance, detecting 98% of needles with shaft and tip localization errors of 0.091 ± 0.043 and 0.33 ± 0.363 mm, respectively.

CT images can also be used to reconstruct the needles in HDR prostate brachytherapy. Weishaupt et al. [76] developed a deep learning-based method to automatically digitize HDR prostate needles on CT scans. Using a 2D U-Net architecture, the model first segmented the catheters in 2D slices and then reconstructed their 3D geometries using a density-based linkage clustering algorithm. The model demonstrated high precision, achieving a mean tip distance difference of –0.1 ± 0.6 mm, with a range from –1.8 to 1.4 mm. The mean shaft distance error was 0.13 ± 0.09 mm, with a maximum of 0.96 mm. Notably, the entire reconstruction process was completed in under 1 minute, making it feasible for clinical integration in time-sensitive workflows.

MRI-guided HDR prostate brachytherapy is a more recent approach that offers superior soft-tissue contrast and anatomical visualization compared to TRUS or CT. To facilitate catheter reconstruction in this context, Dai et al. [77] developed a DL model utilizing an attention-gated U-Net combined with TV regularization to suppress excessive image noise. The model achieved a catheter tip localization error of 0.37 ± 1.68 mm, with 87% of catheter tips identified within a localization error of less than ±2.0 mm, and over 71% within an absolute error of ≤1.0 mm. For catheter shaft localization, the error was 0.93 ± 0.50 mm, with 97% of catheters detected within a 2.0 mm error margin, and 63% within 1.0 mm. The shaft localization task yielded precision, recall, and F1 scores of 0.96, 0.86, and 0.91, respectively. These results underscore the potential of AI-assisted catheter digitization to overcome the challenges associated with identifying catheters on MRI, thereby advancing the accuracy and efficiency of MRI-guided HDR prostate brachytherapy.

During LDR prostate brachytherapy procedures, accurate placement of radioactive seeds is guided by TRUS, with adjustments often required based on real-time changes in prostate anatomy. Comparing the implanted seed locations and orientations against the planned positions is essential to ensure optimal dose coverage and make intraoperative plan modifications. To enhance the consistency and efficiency of manual seed segmentation on TRUS images, Golshan et al. [78] developed a CNN model that first employed a coarse sliding window to identify needle tracks and then performed fine segmentation to detect seeds within those tracks. The model achieved a precision of 78% ± 8%, a recall of 64% ± 10%, and an F1 score of 70% ± 8%. The relatively low recall rate suggests that a significant number of seeds were missed, primarily due to the limited quality of ultrasound imaging.

Post-implantation, CT is often used to evaluate seed placement and dosimetry. Nguyen et al. [79] introduced a machine learning-based pipeline to segment individual seeds and clusters of closely spaced ("union") seeds and estimate their orientations. A k-means algorithm was initially used to classify seed groups, followed by modified k-means and Gaussian mixture models with expectation-maximization to resolve clustered seeds. Their dataset included 14 patients with 1,063 implanted seeds and two phantoms containing 1 and 73 seeds, respectively. In phantom studies, the model achieved an angular orientation error of 0.96° ± 0.4° and a distance error of 0.08 ± 0.04 mm. In patient data, the maximum angular orientation error was 3.18° ± 0.9° and the maximum distance error was 0.50 ± 0.16 mm, with a false detection rate ranging from 1.8% to 4.8%.

Although MRI provides superior soft-tissue contrast compared to CT, seed identification remains challenging due to the lack of MR signal from the seeds themselves. The use of an endorectal coil (ERC) can enhance seed visibility but may increase patient discomfort and cost. To automate the identification process, Sanders et al. [80] developed SeedNet, a sliding-window CNN that detects radioactive seeds in prostate MRI. SeedNet demonstrated high accuracy and efficiency, outperforming manual dosimetrist review. When using an ERC, the model achieved recall, precision, and F1 scores of 97.6%, 97.2%, and 97.4%, respectively. Additionally, the model exhibited a low false discovery rate (2.8%), a false negative rate (2.4%), and a root-mean-square error (RMSE) of 0.19 ± 0.04 mm, with an inference time of 56.6 ± 18.2 seconds. These results suggest that SeedNet offers a reliable and efficient solution for seed identification in MRI-based post-implant analysis.

10.2.7 Quality Assurance

Quality assurance (QA) in brachytherapy encompasses multiple components, including safety checks, equipment verification, and treatment plan evaluation. While safety and equipment QA are typically performed manually prior to treatment delivery, plan QA can benefit significantly from AI-driven tools to identify suboptimal plans and enhance overall plan quality. Three studies have explored the use of AI for plan QA. Reijtenbagh et al. [81] developed a random forest (RF) model trained on overlap volume histograms (OVHs) to predict dose–volume histograms (DVHs) for OARs in HDR gynecologic brachytherapy. This model predicted DVHs for the target, bladder, rectum, sigmoid, and small bowel, enabling anatomy-based QA for individual patients. When applied to external datasets from a different institution, the model successfully identified plans that met clinical criteria but were suboptimal, demonstrating its effectiveness in multi-institutional settings. The model's rapid training time—under 1 minute—and prediction time—within seconds—make it highly practical for clinical use. In a subsequent study, Reijtenbagh et al. [89] reported an average dose reduction of 0.62 Gy to all OARs using their AI-based QA model, underscoring its potential to improve treatment safety and plan quality.

In addition, Fan et al. [82] developed a deep neural network model for QA of HDR brachytherapy plans, specifically targeting verification of dwell times and positions. The model was built on the Inception network architecture proposed by Szegedy et al. [83], chosen for its efficient use of parameters, which helps minimize computational load and reduces the risk of overfitting common in traditional CNNs. To address the nonlinear nature of the regression task, the model employed heatmaps to represent the probability distributions of dwell positions, thereby simplifying the prediction process. The model achieved high accuracy, with predicted dwell times deviating less than 2% from the ground truth and dwell positions located within one pixel of the planned values. Although training the model required substantial time, inference was rapid—enabling near real-time QA by providing accurate predictions within seconds.

10.2.8 Outcome Prediction

AI has shown strong potential in predicting clinical outcomes, enabling oncologists and physicists to make more informed decisions regarding patient management. ML models have been applied to three distinct outcome prediction tasks in both prostate and GYN brachytherapy. For locally advanced cervical cancer (LACC), Abdalvand et al. [12] evaluated four ML algorithms—LASSO regression, Ridge regression, support vector machine (SVM), and RF—to predict treatment outcomes. By integrating applicator insertion geometries from 3D MR/CT imaging with physical, dosimetric, radiobiological, and clinical features, and selecting the top ten predictors using LASSO, they found the RF model achieved the best performance (AUC=0.82; accuracy=0.77), though limited by a small dataset ($n = 111$) and the models' ability to handle clinical heterogeneity. In another study, Tian et al. [13] developed a nonlinear kernel-based SVM to predict fistula formation after interstitial brachytherapy. Using sequential feature selection methods, they identified seven key predictors and achieved excellent performance (AUC=0.904, sensitivity=97.1%, specificity=88.5%).

In prostate brachytherapy, ML has also been applied to predict recurrence after treatment. Valdes et al. [84] explored this using MediBoost and CART models on data from 52 patients who underwent salvage HDR brachytherapy. Focusing on key features—such as the percentage of positive biopsy cores and the disease-free interval after initial treatment—the model identified a 5-year recurrence probability of 0.75 when positive cores ^{3}0.35 and disease-free interval <4.12 years. Despite the limited dataset, the findings demonstrated a 70% confidence that the results were not due to random variation, supporting the utility of ML for outcome prediction in prostate cancer.

10.2.9 Discussion

In this chapter, we highlighted the integration of AI across various components of the brachytherapy workflow, emphasizing its ability to match or surpass manual efforts in tasks such as segmentation, classification, and outcome prediction. Across these domains, AI models consistently demonstrated small errors and clinically acceptable performance, offering both efficiency and standardization benefits.

The imaging domain accounts for the majority of AI-related studies, with auto-segmentation emerging as the most impactful application. Manual contouring is labor-intensive and requires extensive expertise, whereas AI-based segmentation can be trained in a matter of hours and perform inference in seconds to minutes—dramatically reducing the time burden compared to the typical 20–40 minutes required by human experts. For instance, King et al. [85] evaluated AI-generated prostate contours on TRUS images using nnU-Net and reported a median DSC of 0.92. The AI contours were preferred by clinical observers in 57.5% of cases, indicating both high geometric accuracy and clinical acceptability. Furthermore, AI models have the potential to reduce inter-observer variability and promote consistency. Andersén et al. [72] demonstrated that their DL model for needle detection produced errors smaller than those observed between clinicians.

Since many AI applications in brachytherapy depend on accurate imaging, improvements in image quality can amplify the overall benefit. Several studies have explored AI-based approaches for enhancing image resolution and reducing artifacts, particularly in TRUS and CT. For example, in prostate brachytherapy, where TRUS is widely used for intraoperative guidance, needle shadows and poor contrast can compromise accuracy. AI models designed for image denoising, super-resolution, and artifact correction help mitigate these limitations, enabling more precise segmentation and applicator reconstruction.

Several studies have shown that high-volume cancer centers tend to produce superior brachytherapy treatment plans, benefiting from more experienced staff and a larger pool of clinical cases. AI models can leverage these high-quality datasets to learn planning strategies more efficiently than human planners, with the potential to generate treatment plans that match or exceed those created manually. While manual planning can achieve excellent results, it is heavily reliant on the planner's expertise and is both time- and resource-intensive. In contrast, AI can generate plans rapidly, consistently, and with reduced dependence on individual experience. Furthermore, AI-based dose prediction models can support real-time QA by identifying suboptimal plans, enabling timely intervention and optimization.

Emerging AI-enabled techniques, such as multi-needle digitization, hold promise for real-time treatment planning and intraoperative dosimetric adjustments. These capabilities can bridge the gap between preplanning and intraoperative execution, minimizing discrepancies that may arise due to anatomical changes or applicator shifts. Despite this promise, key challenges remain—particularly the accuracy of ground-truth contours used during model training and the ability to predict complex needle trajectories in real-time environments. Nevertheless, advancements in these areas could facilitate the adoption of more sophisticated workflows, such as MRI-guided brachytherapy, further enhancing precision and personalization in treatment delivery.

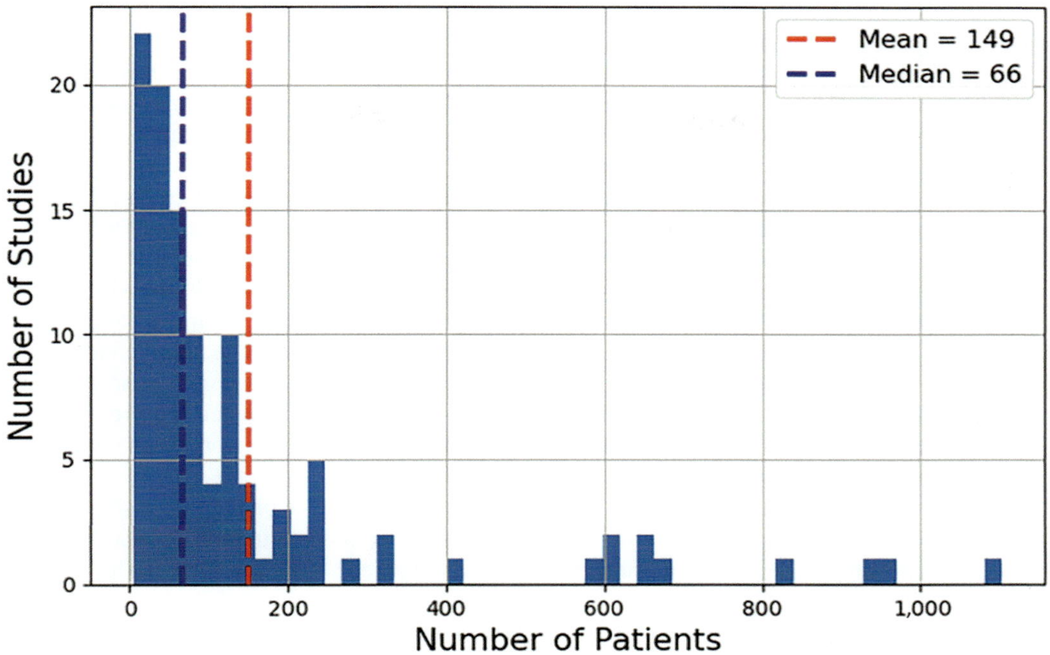

FIGURE 10.2 Distribution of the number of patients in investigated studies. Reprinted from *JACMP*, A review of artificial intelligence in brachytherapy by Chen et al.

Despite encouraging results, the effectiveness and generalizability of current AI models in brachytherapy are constrained by certain limitations. Notably, many studies are based on small, single-institution datasets, raising concerns about model robustness across diverse patient populations and clinical practices. The histogram in Figure 10.2 illustrates the distribution of the number of patients used in the reviewed studies, with most studies having less than 200 patients. An analysis of the reviewed literature reveals that the average and median patient cohort sizes are 153 and 63, respectively. The distribution is skewed by a few outlier studies with exceptionally large datasets, while the majority of studies include fewer than 200 patients. This underscores the need for multi-institutional collaborations and data-sharing initiatives to improve the scalability and clinical applicability of AI models in brachytherapy.

To address the challenge of limited data availability, many studies adopted cross-validation techniques, wherein the dataset is divided into multiple subsets. Each subset is used once for validation while the remaining data are used for training, allowing every data point to contribute to model assessment. This approach maximizes data utility and provides a more robust evaluation of model performance and generalizability. Additionally, data augmentation techniques—such as elastic deformations, rotations, and rescaling—have been widely used, particularly in U-Net-based architectures, to synthetically expand training datasets and enhance model robustness to geometric variations. Transfer learning also presents an effective strategy for small datasets; several studies [23,48,58,63] demonstrated that models pre-trained on large datasets and fine-tuned with limited clinical data can achieve high accuracy, albeit at the cost of increased training time.

A major advancement in the field came with the introduction of the Segment Anything Model (SAM) by Meta AI in April 2023 [86]. SAM is a foundation model trained on over 1 billion segmentation masks from 11 million images, enabling it to perform zero-shot segmentation on unseen objects using prompt-based interaction. Unlike conventional models that require task-specific training, SAM exhibits broad generalization across image types. Building upon this, Ma et al. developed MedSAM [87], a medical imaging counterpart of SAM tailored for universal segmentation across 15 imaging modalities and 30 cancer types. MedSAM is trained on over a million medical image-mask pairs, allowing it to perform cross-modality and cross-organ segmentation without retraining. Its broad adaptability and robust segmentation capability make it a promising candidate for brachytherapy imaging tasks. Integrating MedSAM with domain-specific fine-tuning could further improve segmentation performance in brachytherapy applications where high anatomical precision is required.

Despite the use of techniques such as data augmentation, transfer learning, and cross-validation, the lack of variation in patient anatomy and setup remains a major obstacle for generalizing AI models in brachytherapy. For example, Holupka et al. [88] trained their model using 950 ultrasound images from only ten patients, leading to seed localization errors as high as 2.29 mm when tested on new patient cohorts—highlighting the risk of poor generalizability due to limited anatomical diversity. AI models tend to perform suboptimally on anatomies that deviate significantly from those in the training set, which poses particular risks in HDR brachytherapy where precise planning is critical. Achieving robust and general-purpose brachytherapy dosimetry models requires datasets that are diverse not only in patient anatomy and tumor sites but also in applicator designs, radiation sources, and shielding configurations [52].

Another critical limitation in current AI research is the heavy reliance on data from single institutions. Since brachytherapy workflows are highly sensitive to institutional imaging protocols, models trained on data from one center may not generalize well to others. Although a few studies [35,89] reported no statistically significant drop in performance when tested on external datasets, most lack cross-institutional validation. Even with standardized imaging protocols, the choice of applicator varies significantly between institutions, complicating the transferability of AI models [61,89]. For instance, while most applicator reconstruction studies in cervical cancer brachytherapy focus on T&O applicators, models trained on these may not perform well for T&R or Fletcher applicators. This applicator variability also challenges dose prediction models, as each study often involves only a single applicator type. Moreover, the acceptability of AI-generated treatment plans is influenced by the variability in clinical ground truths, which are dependent on the planning systems and institutional protocols used. Therefore, to achieve broad clinical applicability, future AI models must be developed and validated on large, diverse, and multi-institutional datasets [81].

While AI can significantly enhance the preparation and workflow efficiency of brachytherapy, the quality of treatment ultimately hinges on the technical skill of physicians or surgeons in applicator or needle placement. Brachytherapy presents clear clinical advantages, including a shorter overall treatment duration and outcomes comparable to surgery or external beam radiation therapy (EBRT) [90]. However, its utilization has declined in recent years [91], largely due to procedural complexity and reduced exposure during residency training, which has led to fewer clinicians proficient in performing these treatments [92]. Enhanced training programs can help restore confidence and interest among radiation oncology residents, addressing this gap and revitalizing brachytherapy practice [93]. As the volume of clinical cases increases, AI models will also benefit from more diverse and robust training data, improving their accuracy and generalizability. Ultimately, AI has the potential to simplify workflows, enable real-time planning, and improve treatment precision—contributing to better patient outcomes. Sustained investment in both AI innovation and physician training is therefore critical to ensuring the long-term success and adoption of brachytherapy.

10.3 CONCLUSION

This chapter has summarized the current advancements in AI applied to brachytherapy, with a focus on prostate and gynecologic (GYN) cancer treatments. Compared to EBRT, which benefits from abundant patient data and more streamlined AI integration, brachytherapy presents unique challenges due to its procedural complexity and the need for precise manual interventions. Effective and safe AI integration in brachytherapy will require the inclusion of larger, more diverse patient datasets across multiple institutions, and the adoption of emerging foundation models to improve performance and generalizability.

Despite these challenges, AI holds significant promise in streamlining the brachytherapy workflow—from imaging and segmentation to planning and quality assurance—potentially enhancing treatment precision and operational efficiency. However, a critical gap remains: the lack of clinical trials validating AI applications in brachytherapy. Future research should prioritize rigorous prospective studies to assess the clinical efficacy, safety, and reproducibility of AI-driven approaches.

With continued technological advancement and strategic investment in both AI model development and clinical validation, AI has the potential to substantially improve the quality, consistency, and accessibility of brachytherapy, ultimately leading to better patient outcomes.

REFERENCES

1. Lukens JN, Gamez M, Hu K, Harrison LB, editors. Modern brachytherapy. *Semin Oncol.* 2014; 41(6):831–47. doi: 10.1053/j.seminoncol.2014.09.015. Epub 2014 Oct 31. PMID: 25499641.
2. Chargari C, Deutsch E, Blanchard P, Gouy S, Martelli H, Guérin F, et al. Brachytherapy: An overview for clinicians. *CA Cancer J Clin.* 2019;69(5):386–401.
3. Tanderup K, Ménard C, Polgar C, Lindegaard JC, Kirisits C, Pötter R. Advancements in brachytherapy. *Adv Drug Deliv Rev.* 2017;109:15–25.
4. Demanes DJ, Rege S, Rodriquez RR, Schutz KL, Altieri GA, Wong T. The use and advantages of a multichannel vaginal cylinder in high-dose-rate brachytherapy. *Int J Radiat Oncol Biol Phys.* 1999;44(1):211–9.
5. Skowronek J. Current status of brachytherapy in cancer treatment–short overview. *J Contemp Brachyther.* 2017;9(6):581–9.
6. Fu Y, Zhang H, Morris ED, Glide-Hurst CK, Pai S, Traverso A, et al. Artificial intelligence in radiation therapy. *IEEE Trans Radiat Plasma Med Sci.* 2021;6(2):158–81.
7. Huynh E, Hosny A, Guthier C, Bitterman DS, Petit SF, Haas-Kogan DA, et al. Artificial intelligence in radiation oncology. *Nat Rev Clin Oncol.* 2020;17(12):771–81.
8. Pillai M, Adapa K, Das SK, Mazur L, Dooley J, Marks LB, et al. Using artificial intelligence to improve the quality and safety of radiation therapy. *J Am Coll Radiol.* 2019;16(9):1267–72.
9. El Naqa I, Murphy MJ. *What Is Machine Learning?* Springer; 2015.
10. Wang S, Summers RM. Machine learning and radiology. *Med Image Anal.* 2012;16(5):933–51.
11. Stenhouse K, Roumeliotis M, Ciunkiewicz P, Banerjee R, Yanushkevich S, McGeachy P. Development of a machine learning model for optimal applicator selection in high-dose-rate cervical brachytherapy. *Front Oncol.* 2021;11:611437.
12. Abdalvand N, Sadeghi M, Mahdavi SR, Abdollahi H, Qasempour Y, Mohammadian F, et al. Brachytherapy outcome modeling in cervical cancer patients: A predictive machine learning study on patient-specific clinical, physical and dosimetric parameters. *Brachytherapy.* 2022;21(6):769–82.
13. Tian Z, Yen A, Zhou Z, Shen C, Albuquerque K, Hrycushko B. A machine-learning-based prediction model of fistula formation after interstitial brachytherapy for locally advanced gynecological malignancies. *Brachytherapy.* 2019;18(4):530–8.
14. O'shea K, Nash R. An introduction to convolutional neural networks. arXiv preprint arXiv:151108458. 2015.
15. Goodfellow I, Pouget-Abadie J, Mirza M, Xu B, Warde-Farley D, Ozair S, et al. Generative adversarial networks. *Commun ACM.* 2020;63(11):139–44.
16. Yi X, Walia E, Babyn P. Generative adversarial network in medical imaging: A review. *Med Image Anal.* 2019;58:101552.
17. Hellebust T. Place of modern imaging in brachytherapy planning. *Cancer/Radiothérapie.* 2018;22(4):326–33.
18. Chen J, Qiu RLJ, Wang T, Momin S, Yang X. A review of artificial intelligence in brachytherapy. *J Appl Clin Med Phys.* 2025;26(6):e70034.
19. Salehi M, Vafaei Sadr A, Mahdavi SR, Arabi H, Shiri I, Reiazi R. Deep learning-based non-rigid image registration for high-dose rate brachytherapy in inter-fraction cervical cancer. *J Digit Imaging.* 2023;36(2):574–87.

20. Ecker S, Zimmermann L, Heilemann G, Niatsetski Y, Schmid M, Sturdza AE, et al. Neural network-assisted automated image registration for MRI-guided adaptive brachytherapy in cervical cancer. *Z Med Phys*. 2022;32(4):488–99.
21. Zeng Q, Fu Y, Tian Z, Lei Y, Zhang Y, Wang T, et al. Label-driven magnetic resonance imaging (MRI)-transrectal ultrasound (TRUS) registration using weakly supervised learning for MRI-guided prostate radiotherapy. *Phys Med Biol*. 2020;65(13):135002.
22. Chen Y, Xing L, Yu L, Liu W, Pooya Fahimian B, Niedermayr T, et al. MR to ultrasound image registration with segmentation-based learning for HDR prostate brachytherapy. *Med Phys*. 2021;48(6):3074–83.
23. Zabihollahy F, Viswanathan AN, Schmidt EJ, Morcos M, Lee J. Fully automated multiorgan segmentation of female pelvic magnetic resonance images with coarse-to-fine convolutional neural network. *Med Phys*. 2021;48(11):7028–42.
24. Zhang D, Yang Z, Jiang S, Zhou Z, Meng M, Wang W. Automatic segmentation and applicator reconstruction for CT-based brachytherapy of cervical cancer using 3D convolutional neural networks. *J Appl Clin Med Phys*. 2020;21(10):158–69.
25. Jiang X, Wang F, Chen Y, Yan S. RefineNet-based automatic delineation of the clinical target volume and organs at risk for three-dimensional brachytherapy for cervical cancer. *Ann Transl Med*. 2021;9(23):1721.
26. Li Z, Zhu Q, Zhang L, Yang X, Li Z, Fu J. A deep learning-based self-adapting ensemble method for segmentation in gynecological brachytherapy. *Radiat Oncol*. 2022;17(1):152.
27. Duprez D, Trauernicht C, Simonds H, Williams O. Self-configuring nnU-Net for automatic delineation of the organs at risk and target in high-dose rate cervical brachytherapy, a low/middle-income country's experience. *J Appl Clin Med Phys*. 2023;24(8):e13988.
28. Wang J, Chen Y, Tu Y, Xie H, Chen Y, Luo L, et al. Evaluation of auto-segmentation for brachytherapy of postoperative cervical cancer using deep learning-based workflow. *Phys Med Biol*. 2023;68(5).
29. Mohammadi R, Shokatian I, Salehi M, Arabi H, Shiri I, Zaidi H. Deep learning-based auto-segmentation of organs at risk in high-dose rate brachytherapy of cervical cancer. *Radiother Oncol*. 2021;159:231–40.
30. Vigneault E, Mbodji K, Racine L-G, Chevrette E, Lavallée M-C, Martin A-G, et al. Image-guided high-dose-rate brachytherapy boost to the dominant intraprostatic lesion using multiparametric magnetic resonance imaging including spectroscopy: Results of a prospective study. *Brachytherapy*. 2016;15(6):746–51.
31. Wang T, Press RH, Giles M, Jani AB, Rossi P, Lei Y, et al. Multiparametric MRI-guided dose boost to dominant intraprostatic lesions in CT-based high-dose-rate prostate brachytherapy. *Br J Radiol*. 2019;92(1097):20190089.
32. Goodman CD, Fakir H, Pautler S, Chin J, Bauman GS. Dosimetric evaluation of PSMA PET-delineated dominant intraprostatic lesion simultaneous infield boosts. *Adv Radiat Oncol*. 2020;5(2):212–20.
33. Matkovic LA, Wang T, Lei Y, Akin-Akintayo OO, Abiodun Ojo OA, Akintayo AA, et al. Prostate and dominant intraprostatic lesion segmentation on PET/CT using cascaded regional-net. *Phys Med Biol*. 2021;66(24).
34. Wang T, Lei Y, Schreibmann E, Roper J, Liu T, Schuster DM, et al. Lesion segmentation on (18) F-fluciclovine PET/CT images using deep learning. *Front Oncol*. 2023;13:1274803.
35. Li Y, Imami MR, Zhao L, Amindarolzarbi A, Mena E, Leal J, et al. An automated deep learning-based framework for uptake segmentation and classification on PSMA PET/CT imaging of patients with prostate cancer. *J Imaging Inform Med*. 2024; 37(5):2206–2215. doi: 10.1007/s10278-024-01104-y. Epub 2024 Apr 8. PMID: 38587770; PMCID: PMC11522269.
36. Kostyszyn D, Fechter T, Bartl N, Grosu AL, Gratzke C, Sigle A, Mix M, Ruf J, Fassbender TF, Kiefer S, Bettermann AS, Nicolay NH, Spohn S, Kramer MU, Bronsert P, Guo H, Qiu X, Wang F, Henkenberens C, Werner RA, Baltas D, Meyer PT, Derlin T, Chen M, Zamboglou C. Intraprostatic Tumor Segmentation on PSMA PET Images in Patients with Primary Prostate Cancer with a Convolutional Neural Network. J Nucl Med. 2021 Jun 1;62(6):823-828. doi: 10.2967/jnumed.120.254623. Epub 2020 Oct 30. PMID: 33127624; PMCID: PMC8729869..
37. Girum KB, Lalande A, Hussain R, Crehange G. A deep learning method for real-time intraoperative US image segmentation in prostate brachytherapy. *Int J Comput Assist Radiol Surg*. 2020;15(9):1467–76.
38. Lei Y, Tian S, He X, Wang T, Wang B, Patel P, et al. Ultrasound prostate segmentation based on multidirectional deeply supervised V-Net. *Med Phys*. 2019;46(7):3194–206.
39. Karimi D, Zeng Q, Mathur P, Avinash A, Mahdavi S, Spadinger I, et al. Accurate and robust deep learning-based segmentation of the prostate clinical target volume in ultrasound images. *Med Image Anal*. 2019;57:186–96.

40. Anas EMA, Nouranian S, Mahdavi SS, Spadinger I, Morris WJ, Salcudean SE, et al., editors. *Clinical Target-Volume Delineation in Prostate Brachytherapy Using Residual Neural Networks*, 2017; Cham: Springer International Publishing.
41. Nouranian S, Ramezani M, Spadinger I, Morris WJ, Salcudean SE, Abolmaesumi P. Learning-based multi-label segmentation of transrectal ultrasound images for prostate brachytherapy. *IEEE Trans Med Imaging*. 2016;35(3):921–32.
42. Xu X, Sanford T, Turkbey B, Xu S, Wood BJ, Yan P. Polar transform network for prostate ultrasound segmentation with uncertainty estimation. *Med Image Anal*. 2022;78:102418.
43. Hampole P, Harding T, Gillies D, Orlando N, Edirisinghe C, Mendez LC, et al. Deep learning-based ultrasound auto-segmentation of the prostate with brachytherapy implanted needles. *Med Phys*. 2024;51(4):2665–77.
44. Zeng Q, Samei G, Karimi D, Kesch C, Mahdavi SS, Abolmaesumi P, et al. Prostate segmentation in transrectal ultrasound using magnetic resonance imaging priors. *Int J Comput Assist Radiol Surg*. 2018;13(6):749–57.
45. Girum KB, Créhange G, Hussain R, Lalande A. Fast interactive medical image segmentation with weakly supervised deep learning method. *Int J Comput Assist Radiol Surg*. 2020;15:1437–44.
46. Orlando N, Gillies DJ, Gyacskov I, Romagnoli C, D'Souza D, Fenster A. Automatic prostate segmentation using deep learning on clinically diverse 3D transrectal ultrasound images. *Med Phys*. 2020;47(6):2413–26.
47. Orlando N, Gyacskov I, Gillies DJ, Guo F, Romagnoli C, D'Souza D, et al. Effect of dataset size, image quality, and image type on deep learning-based automatic prostate segmentation in 3D ultrasound. *Phys Med Biol*. 2022;67(7):074002. doi: 10.1088/1361-6560/ac5a93. PMID: 35240585.
48. Sanders JW, Lewis GD, Thames HD, Kudchadker RJ, Venkatesan AM, Bruno TL, et al. Machine segmentation of pelvic anatomy in MRI-assisted radiosurgery (MARS) for prostate cancer brachytherapy. *Int J Radiat Oncol Biol Phys*. 2020;108(5):1292–303.
49. Sanders JW, Kudchadker RJ, Tang C, Mok H, Venkatesan AM, Thames HD, et al. Prospective evaluation of prostate and organs at risk segmentation software for MRI-based prostate radiation therapy. *Radiol Artif Intell*. 2022;4(2):e210151.
50. Duan J, Vargas CE, Yu NY, Laughlin BS, Toesca DS, Keole S, et al. Incremental retraining, clinical implementation, and acceptance rate of deep learning auto-segmentation for male pelvis in a multiuser environment. *Med Phys*. 2023;50(7):4079–91.
51. Huang X, Wang J, Tang F, Zhong T, Zhang Y. Metal artifact reduction on cervical CT images by deep residual learning. *Biomed Eng Online*. 2018;17(1):175.
52. Mao X, Pineau J, Keyes R, Enger SA. RapidBrachyDL: Rapid radiation dose calculations in brachytherapy via deep learning. *Int J Radiat Oncol Biol Phys*. 2020;108(3):802–12.
53. Hrinivich WT, Morcos M, Viswanathan A, Lee J. Automatic tandem and ring reconstruction using MRI for cervical cancer brachytherapy. *Med Phys*. 2019;46(10):4324–32.
54. Ghosh S, Punithakumar K, Huang F, Menon G, Boulanger P. Deep learning using pre-brachytherapy MRI to automatically predict applicator induced complex uterine deformation. *Annu Int Conf IEEE Eng Med Biol Soc*. 2022;2022:3826–9.
55. Nicolae A, Morton G, Chung H, Loblaw A, Jain S, Mitchell D, et al. Evaluation of a machine-learning algorithm for treatment planning in prostate low-dose-rate brachytherapy. *Int J Radiat Oncol Biol Phys*. 2017;97(4):822–9.
56. Nicolae A, Semple M, Lu L, Smith M, Chung H, Loblaw A, et al. Conventional vs machine learning–based treatment planning in prostate brachytherapy: results of a phase I randomized controlled trial. *Brachytherapy*. 2020;19(4):470–6.
57. Aleef TA, Spadinger IT, Peacock MD, Salcudean SE, Mahdavi SS. Centre-specific autonomous treatment plans for prostate brachytherapy using cGANs. *Int J Comput Assist Radiol Surg*. 2021;16(7):1161–70.
58. Aleef TA, Spadinger IT, Peacock MD, Salcudean SE, Mahdavi SS, editors. Rapid treatment planning for low-dose-rate prostate brachytherapy with TP-GAN. *International Conference on Medical Image Computing and Computer-Assisted Intervention*, Strasbourg, France; 2021: Springer.
59. Li Z, Yang Z, Lu J, Zhu Q, Wang Y, Zhao M, et al. Deep learning-based dose map prediction for high-dose-rate brachytherapy. *Phys Med Biol*. 2023;68(17):175015 . doi: 10.1088/1361-6560/acecd2. PMID: 37589292.
60. Akhavanallaf A, Mohammadi R, Shiri I, Salimi Y, Arabi H, Zaidi H. Personalized brachytherapy dose reconstruction using deep learning. *Comput Biol Med*. 2021;136:104755.
61. Cortes KG, Kallis K, Simon A, Mayadev J, Meyers SM, Moore KL. Knowledge-based three-dimensional dose prediction for tandem-and-ovoid brachytherapy. *Brachytherapy*. 2022;21(4):532–42.

62. Zhang HW, Zhong XM, Zhang ZH, Pang HW. Dose prediction of organs at risk in patients with cervical cancer receiving brachytherapy using needle insertion based on a neural network method. *BMC Cancer.* 2023;23(1):385.
63. Zhen X, Chen J, Zhong Z, Hrycushko B, Zhou L, Jiang S, et al. Deep convolutional neural network with transfer learning for rectum toxicity prediction in cervical cancer radiotherapy: a feasibility study. *Phys Med Biol.* 2017;62(21):8246–63.
64. Chen J, Chen H, Zhong Z, Wang Z, Hrycushko B, Zhou L, et al. Investigating rectal toxicity associated dosimetric features with deformable accumulated rectal surface dose maps for cervical cancer radiotherapy. *Radiat Oncol.* 2018;13(1):125.
65. Jaberi R, Siavashpour Z, Aghamiri MR, Kirisits C, Ghaderi R. Artificial neural network based gynaecological image-guided adaptive brachytherapy treatment planning correction of intra-fractional organs at risk dose variation. *J Contemp Brachytherapy.* 2017;9(6):508–18.
66. Villa M, Bert J, Valeri A, Schick U, Visvikis D. Fast Monte Carlo-based inverse planning for prostate brachytherapy by using deep learning. *IEEE Trans Radiat Plasma Med Sci.* 2021;6(2):182–8.
67. Jung H, Gonzalez Y, Shen C, Klages P, Albuquerque K, Jia X. Deep-learning-assisted automatic digitization of applicators in 3D CT image-based high-dose-rate brachytherapy of gynecological cancer. *Brachytherapy.* 2019;18(6):841–51.
68. Duda RO, Hart PE. Use of the Hough transformation to detect lines and curves in pictures. *Commun ACM.* 1972;15(1):11–5.
69. Styner M, Brechbuhler C, Szekely G, Gerig G. Parametric estimate of intensity inhomogeneities applied to MRI. *IEEE Trans Med Imaging.* 2000;19(3):153–65.
70. Zaffino P, Pernelle G, Mastmeyer A, Mehrtash A, Zhang H, Kikinis R, et al. Fully automatic catheter segmentation in MRI with 3D convolutional neural networks: application to MRI-guided gynecologic brachytherapy. *Phys Med Biol.* 2019;64(16):165008.
71. Zaorsky NG, Davis BJ, Nguyen PL, Showalter TN, Hoskin PJ, Yoshioka Y, et al. The evolution of brachytherapy for prostate cancer. *Nat Rev Urol.* 2017;14(7):415–39.
72. Andersen C, Ryden T, Thunberg P, Lagerlof JH. Deep learning-based digitization of prostate brachytherapy needles in ultrasound images. *Med Phys.* 2020;47(12):6414–20.
73. Zhang Y, He X, Tian Z, Jeong JJ, Lei Y, Wang T, et al. Multi-needle detection in 3D ultrasound images using unsupervised order-graph regularized sparse dictionary learning. *IEEE Trans Med Imaging.* 2020;39(7):2302–15.
74. Zhang Y, Lei Y, Qiu RLJ, Wang T, Wang H, Jani AB, et al. Multi-needle localization with attention U-Net in US-guided HDR prostate brachytherapy. *Med Phys.* 2020;47(7):2735–45.
75. Zhang Y, Tian Z, Lei Y, Wang T, Patel P, Jani AB, et al. Automatic multi-needle localization in ultrasound images using large margin mask RCNN for ultrasound-guided prostate brachytherapy. *Phys Med Biol.* 2020;65(20):205003.
76. Weishaupt LL, Sayed HK, Mao X, Choo R, Stish BJ, Enger SA, et al. Approaching automated applicator digitization from a new angle: Using sagittal images to improve deep learning accuracy and robustness in high-dose-rate prostate brachytherapy. *Brachytherapy.* 2022;21(4):520–31.
77. Dai X, Lei Y, Zhang Y, Qiu RLJ, Wang T, Dresser SA, et al. Automatic multi-catheter detection using deeply supervised convolutional neural network in MRI-guided HDR prostate brachytherapy. *Med Phys.* 2020;47(9):4115–24.
78. Golshan M, Karimi D, Mahdavi S, Lobo J, Peacock M, Salcudean SE, et al. Automatic detection of brachytherapy seeds in 3D ultrasound images using a convolutional neural network. *Phys Med Biol.* 2020;65(3):035016.
79. Nguyen HG, Fouard C, Troccaz J. Segmentation, separation and pose estimation of prostate brachytherapy seeds in CT images. *IEEE Trans Biomed Eng.* 2015;62(8):2012–24.
80. Sanders JW, Frank SJ, Kudchadker RJ, Bruno TL, Ma J. Development and clinical implementation of SeedNet: A sliding-window convolutional neural network for radioactive seed identification in MRI-assisted radiosurgery (MARS). *Magn Reson Med.* 2019;81(6):3888–900.
81. Reijtenbagh D, Godart J, de Leeuw A, Seppenwoolde Y, Jürgenliemk-Schulz I, Mens J-W, et al. Multi-center analysis of machine-learning predicted dose parameters in brachytherapy for cervical cancer. *Radiother Oncol.* 2022;170:169–75.
82. Fan J, Xing L, Yang Y. Independent verification of brachytherapy treatment plan by using deep learning inference modeling. *Phys Med Biol.* 2021;66(12):125014.
83. Szegedy C, Liu W, Jia Y, Sermanet P, Reed S, Anguelov D, et al., editors. Going deeper with convolutions. *Proceedings of the IEEE Conference on Computer Vision and Pattern Recognition (CVPR),* Boston, MA, USA, 2015, pp. 1–9.

84. Valdes G, Chang AJ, Interian Y, Owen K, Jensen ST, Ungar LH, et al. Salvage HDR brachytherapy: Multiple hypothesis testing versus machine learning analysis. *Int J Radiat Oncol Biol Phys.* 2018;101(3):694–703.
85. King MT, Kehayias CE, Chaunzwa T, Rosen DB, Mahal AR, Wallburn TD, et al. Observer preference of artificial intelligence-generated versus clinical prostate contours for ultrasound-based high dose rate brachytherapy. *Med Phys.* 2023;50(10):5935–43.
86. Kirillov A, Mintun E, Ravi N, Mao H, Rolland C, Gustafson L, et al., editors. Segment anything. *2023 IEEE/CVF International Conference on Computer Vision (ICCV)*, Paris, France, 2023, pp. 3992–4003.
87. Ma J, He Y, Li F, Han L, You C, Wang B. Segment anything in medical images. *Nat Commun.* 2024;15(1):654.
88. Holupka EJ, Rossman J, Morancy T, Aronovitz J, Kaplan ID. The detection of implanted radioactive seeds on ultrasound images using convolution neural networks. Medical Imaging with Deep Learning 2018, Amsterdam, Netherland, 2022.
89. Reijtenbagh DM, Godart J, de Leeuw AA, Jürgenliemk-Schulz IM, Mens J-WM, Huge M, et al. Multi-center dosimetric predictions to improve plan quality for brachytherapy for cervical cancer treatment. *Radiother Oncol.* 2023;182:109518.
90. Grimm P, Billiet I, Bostwick D, Dicker AP, Frank S, Immerzeel J, et al. Comparative analysis of prostate-specific antigen free survival outcomes for patients with low, intermediate and high risk prostate cancer treatment by radical therapy. Results from the Prostate Cancer Results Study Group. *BJU Int.* 2012;109:22–9.
91. Petereit DG, Frank SJ, Viswanathan AN, Erickson B, Eifel P, Nguyen PL, et al. Brachytherapy: where has it gone? *J Clin Oncol.* 2015;33(9):980.
92. Williams VM, Kahn JM, Thaker NG, Beriwal S, Nguyen PL, Arthur D, et al. The case for brachytherapy: why it deserves a renaissance. *Adv Radiat Oncol.* 2021;6(2):100605.
93. Williams VM, Mansoori B, Young L, Mayr NA, Halasz LM, Dyer BA. Simulation-based learning for enhanced gynecologic brachytherapy training among radiation oncology residents. *Brachytherapy.* 2021;20(1):128–35.

11 Treatment Response Assessment and Prediction

Sunan Cui,[*] Jie Fu,[*] Faisal Yaseen, Clemens Grassberger, and Stephen R. Bowen

11.1 CLINICAL GUIDELINES FOR ASSESSING TUMOR RESPONSE USING IMAGING

Evaluating tumor response using medical imaging is a crucial aspect of oncological practice and clinical trials (Chukwueke and Wen 2019; Sorace et al. 2020). Medical imaging allows for non-invasive monitoring of tumor change in response to therapy, providing valuable information about treatment efficacy. Imaging modalities such as Computed Tomography (CT), Magnetic Resonance Imaging (MRI), and Positron Emission Tomography (PET) offer objective measures of tumor size, morphology, metabolic activity, and other properties of cancer cells and the surrounding tumor microenvironment. These imaging-based evaluations are essential for identifying whether a treatment is causing tumor shrinkage, stabilization, or progression.

Imaging has been used in clinical trials to assess tumor response to treatment, accelerating the discovery of new cancer therapies (Ruchalski et al. 2021; Wen et al. 2017). Overall survival (OS) is considered the gold standard endpoint in clinical trials for demonstrating the benefits of new cancer therapies (Driscoll and Rixe 2009). However, OS can take a long time to observe, particularly in early-stage cancers or when treatments lead to long survival times. Surrogate endpoints for OS, such as progression-free survival, time to progression, and objective response rate, are commonly used to provide earlier prediction of treatment effectiveness (Delgado and Guddati 2021). These surrogate endpoints are determined in part via imaging assessments of tumor response. To ensure consistency across clinical trials, several standardized guidelines have been developed for evaluating imaging-based tumor response.

11.1.1 Response Evaluation Criteria in Solid Tumors

The Response Evaluation Criteria in Solid Tumors (RECIST) guideline has been widely used to evaluate the solid tumor response to treatment in oncology clinical trials (Therasse et al. 2000). This evidence- and consensus-based guideline was introduced in 2000 and revised in 2009 to RECIST version 1.1 (RECIST 1.1) (Eisenhauer et al. 2009). It classifies patients into four response categories (complete response, partial response, progressive disease, and stable disease) based on changes of unidimensional tumor size that can be measured on chest X-ray, CT, or MRI.

Baseline imaging is acquired before treatment initiation. Tumor lesions and pathological lymph nodes can be classified as measurable or non-measurable. Measurable lesions are tumor lesions with the longest diameter of ≥ 10 mm and pathological lymph nodes with the short axis of ≥ 15 mm. A maximum of five measurable lesions (a maximum of two per organ) can be selected as target lesions. The sum of diameters for target lesions can be measured at baseline and tracked on during- or post-treatment images to evaluate tumor response at different time points. Table 11.1 summarizes the definition of each response category.

RECIST 1.1 has several limitations. For example, it does not account for changes in tumor density, which may indicate tumor response to certain targeted therapies, especially for gastrointestinal

[*] The first two authors contributed equally as co-first authors.

DOI: 10.1201/9781003480365-12

TABLE 11.1
Definition of Response Categories Using RECIST 1.1, PERCIST, and EORTC

	RECIST Definitions
Complete response (CR)	Disappearance of all target lesions. Any pathological lymph nodes have the short axis of <10 mm
Partial response (PR)	≥30% decrease in the sum of diameters of the target lesions compared with baseline sum value
Progressive disease (PD)	≥20% and ≥5 mm increase in the sum of diameters of the target lesions compared with the smallest sum value on study, appearance of one or more new lesions, or unequivocal progression of non-target lesions
Stable disease (SD)	Neither CR, PR, or PD
	EORTC Definitions
Complete metabolic response (CMR)	Disappearance of FDG uptake in all target lesions
Partial metabolic response (PMR)	≥25% decrease in SUVmean
Progressive metabolic disease (PMD)	≥25% increase in SUVmean or the appearance of new FDG-avid lesions
Stable disease (SD)	Neither CMR, PMR, or PMD
	PERCIST Definitions
Complete metabolic response (CMR)	Disappearance of FDG uptake in all target lesions
Partial metabolic response (PMR)	≥30% decrease in SUL_{peak}, and an absolute decrease of at least 0.8 SUL units
Progressive metabolic disease (PMD)	≥30% increase in SUL_{peak} and an absolute increase of at least 0.8 SUL units, or the appearance of new lesions
Stable disease (SD)	Neither CMR, PMR, or PMD

stromal tumor (GIST). The Choi response criteria for GIST have been proposed to consider the changes in both tumor size and CT tumor density (Choi et al. 2007). Moreover, RECIST's reliance on size thresholds for progression does not always correlate with actual treatment efficacy. For example, tumors may have a pseudoprogression response pattern, an initial increase in tumor size followed by a delayed response, when treated with immunotherapy (Chiou and Burotto 2015). The modified RECIST 1.1 for immune-based therapeutics (iRECIST) was developed specifically for cancer immunotherapy trials (Seymour et al. 2017). The major change is the introduction of unconfirmed progressive disease response category that requires further confirmation with follow-up images.

11.1.2 Response Assessment in Neuro-Oncology

The Response Assessment in Neuro-Oncology (RANO) Working Group published response criteria for adult patients with high-grade gliomas (RANO-HGG) in 2010 and low-grade gliomas (RANO-LGG) in 2011(Wen et al. 2010; Bent et al. 2011). These criteria have been widely used in glioma clinical trials over the last decade. Challenges posed by pseudoprogression from the advent of immunotherapy or cytostatic chemoradiotherapy have led to the introduction of the modified criteria, including the immunotherapy RANO criteria (iRANO) and the modified RANO criteria (mRANO) (Okada et al. 2015; Ellingson, Wen, and Cloughesy 2017). The existence of different guidelines has resulted in variations of response assessment across clinical trials, making interpretations of studies more difficult. In 2023, RANO 2.0 was introduced to be used for all gliomas regardless of the treatment modalities being evaluated (Wen et al. 2023).

Unlike RECIST 1.1 that is based on unidimensional measurements, RANO 2.0 relied on two-dimensional measurements (the product of the maximal cross-sectional diameters) of tumor on MRI.

As contrast enhancement can be influenced by many factors, such as antiangiogenic agents and radiation effects, changes in contrast-enhancing tumor size may not always reflect tumor response. RANO 2.0 includes criteria for enhancing tumor, nonenhancing tumor, and both components.

RANO has been expanded to include guidelines for other central nervous system (CNS) tumor types, including brain metastases, leptomeningeal metastases, and pediatric brain tumors (Lin et al. 2015; Chamberlain et al. 2017; Bhatia et al. 2023; Wen et al. 2017). These guidelines aim to standardize response assessment in clinical trials and provide more accurate criteria for determining disease progression and treatment efficacy. This expansion also includes efforts like the Neurologic Assessment in Neuro-Oncology (NANO) criteria, which integrates neurologic function into response assessments, addressing other clinical outcomes that are crucial for patients with CNS tumors (Nayak et al. 2017). Despite these advancements, challenges remain, particularly in investigating the values of advanced imaging techniques such as dynamic contrast-enhanced MRI and MR spectroscopy, as well as the ongoing need for validation of the proposed criteria in large clinical trials.

11.1.3 Positron Emission Tomography Response Criteria in Solid Tumors

The European Organisation for Research and Treatment of Cancer (EORTC) criteria (Kim et al. 2017), developed in 1999, was the first to evaluate tumor response using [^{18}F] FDG-PET imaging. Positron Emission Tomography Response Criteria in Solid Tumors (PERCIST) was developed in 2009 to provide a more robust and systematic framework for tumor response assessment (Nayak et al. 2017). A summary of the EORTC and PERCIST criteria is presented in Table 11.1. The following sections will focus specifically on more recent PERCIST.

PERCIST focuses on metabolic changes in tumors, offering an alternative to the anatomy-based RECIST 1.1. For cancer therapies that are more cytostatic than cytotoxic, a good tumor response could be indicated by a reduction in tumor metabolism without a major decrease in tumor size (Tirkes et al. 2013). Changes in tumor metabolism may occur earlier than changes in tumor size.

PERCIST relies on the measurement of the peak standardized uptake value corrected for lean body mass (SUL_{peak}) in the most FDG-avid tumor lesion. A 1 cm^3 spherical volume is typically used to find the highest mean SUL, i.e., $SUL_{peak.}$ Normalizing FDG uptake to lean body mass reduces variability due to patient differences in body composition. Additionally, by focusing on the most FDG-avid lesion at each time point, it minimizes the impact of subjective lesion selection. This offers more consistent and reliable response assessments. PERCIST classifies patients into four response categories (complete metabolic response, partial metabolic response, stable metabolic disease, and progressive metabolic disease) based on the changes in SUL_{peak} between baseline and follow-up PET scans.

The adoption of PERCIST has expanded its clinical utility, especially in cases where metabolic changes may be more predictive of patient outcomes than anatomic changes. A few studies (Riedl et al. 2017; Velez et al. 2020) have shown that PERCIST may be more strongly correlated with patient prognosis compared to RECIST 1.1 in patients with metastatic breast cancer and metastatic castrate-resistant prostate cancer. Nevertheless, more studies are needed to compare the prognostic values of PET-based PERCIST and RECIST 1.1. While PERCIST requires further validation through large trials, its ability to detect early metabolic responses makes it a promising tool for both clinical trials and routine patient care.

Additionally, FDG-PET-based Deauville criteria (Gallamini et al. 2014) have been internationally recommended for clinical reporting and clinical trials in Hodgkin lymphoma and certain types of non-Hodgkin lymphomas. This scale has been shown (Lee et al. 2020) to be associated with OS as well as local recurrence and distant metastasis.

11.1.4 Limitations of Response Criteria Guidelines

These guidelines, despite being widely adopted to assess tumor response, have several notable limitations. First, all three guidelines rely on manual measurements, which lead to intra- and inter-observer variability (Yoon et al. 2016; Provenzale, Ison, and DeLong 2009; Provenzale and Mancini 2012; Turgeon et al. 2019). For example, selecting which lesions for RECIST measurements or identifying enhancing vs. nonenhancing tumor components in RANO can be subjective, leading to inconsistent results across different observers. Similarly, the choice of the "most FDG-avid" tumor lesion for metabolic assessment in PERCIST can also vary between observers.

Additionally, these guidelines rely on simplified metrics for response classification, which may lead to inaccurate response assessment that does not correlate well with real treatment benefits. RECIST and RANO rely on unidimensional or bidimensional measurements of tumor size. This size-based approach oversimplifies tumor biology, as many therapies, especially molecularly targeted treatments and immunotherapies, may not lead to significant changes in tumor size despite clinical benefits (Chiou and Burotto 2015; Nishino et al. 2012). On the other hand, PERCIST reduces the complex tumor glycolytic response to a single measure, which may not capture the multifactorial biological response of the tumor. The simplified measurements in these guidelines fail to capture tumor heterogeneity, where different parts of the tumor may respond differently to treatment. These can lead to inaccurate response assessment in the drug development process, affecting the reliability of clinical trial outcomes, regulatory approvals, and ultimately the availability of effective treatments for patients.

Lastly, all these guidelines rely on the acquisition of images after the initiation of treatment and often after completion of treatment to evaluate the response, which makes it impossible to predict treatment outcome prior to or early during the course of treatment. However, early treatment outcome prediction offers significant benefits by enabling personalized treatment that improves patient outcomes and optimizes resource use. Accurate prediction outcomes reduce the traditional "trial-and-error" approach, where multiple therapies are tried sequentially until one shows efficacy. By delivering the right treatment to the right patient at the right time, clinicians can avoid delays in effective treatment, sparing patients unnecessary side effects and progression of disease through ineffective treatments.

All these limitations highlight the need for developing advanced AI models to objectively and accurately predict treatment response and outcomes. Advanced AI models could extract high-level features from imaging and potentially provide a more accurate outcome prediction or a more comprehensive response assessment that is highly correlated with treatment outcome. These models could empower patients with support systems to make informed decisions that foster a shift toward precision medicine, reducing trial-and-error approaches and maximizing treatment success.

11.2 ASSESSMENT AND PREDICTION OF TREATMENT RESPONSE AND OUTCOME

Treatment response evaluation can take place at different time points, in which clinicians can make informed decisions during and after therapy, leading to adaptive interventions and improved patient management during follow-up. Response assessment can be performed at multiple spatial scales: at the patient level—encompassing long-term toxicity, disease control, and survival—and at the lesion level, assessing the response of individual lesions throughout treatment. Recently, image voxel-level response assessment has been explored, enabling clinicians to leverage spatial information to adjust therapeutic interventions.

Response prediction involves forecasting how a patient will respond to treatment before the actual response and outcome can be evaluated. This temporally predictive approach allows for clinical decision support based on the patient's specific condition at earlier stages in the dynamics of disease response, thereby enabling timely and prompt interventions. Response predictions can also be made at various time points for various future time horizons. When conducted prior to treatment initiation, predictions can help stratify patients into high- or low-risk categories for different treatment options or personalize treatment based on the patient's specific condition. Mid-treatment predictions can inform adaptive treatment strategies, including those detailed in Chapter 7 on Adaptive Radiation Therapy. Post-treatment predictions can improve long-term patient outcomes through better management during follow-up.

Response assessment and prediction will be summarized at key time points—pre-treatment, mid/during-treatment, post-treatment, and longitudinally. We will also address multi-scale treatment assessment and prediction. Beyond our primary focus on tumor response, we will briefly discuss normal tissue response assessment as part of Section 11.2.3 (Table 11.2).

TABLE 11.2

Tumor Response Assessment and Prediction Using Pre-, Mid/During-, Post-treatment, and Longitudinal Imaging

Imaging Modality	Method	Disease Site and Treatment	Response and Outcome
Pre-Treatment			
CT	CNN (resNet)	Squamous cell carcinoma (Xie et al. 2023)	Tumor response by RECIST 1.1
CT	Radiomics + MLP	NSCLC (Li et al. 2023)	Overall survival Progression-free survival
T2 MRI+ CT	Radiomics + mRMR	Prostate cancer (Wong et al. 2024)	1-month PSA-level post SBRT
T1 and T2 MRI	CNN (resNet)	Advanced cervical cancer (Jeong et al. 2024)	Tumor response by RECIST 1.1
FDG-PET/CT	Radiomics + cox regression	Early-stage NSCLC (Thor et al. 2024)	Progression-free survival
FDG-PET/CT	Radiomics + RF	Laryngeal cancer (Nakajo et al. 2023)	Progression-free survival
FDG-PET/CT	CNN (resNet18)	Early-stage NSCLC (Zhong et al. 2023)	Occult nodal metastasis post-surgery, lesion level
FDG-PET/CT	Statistical analysis	Squamous cell anal cancer (Sabbagh et al. 2019)	Voxel-level SUV uptake
FDG-PET/CT	CNN (encoder-decoder)	Oropharyngeal cancer (Ji et al. 2022)	Voxel-level SUV uptake
FDG-PET/CT	Multi-scale regression approach	NSCLC (Bowen et al. 2019)	Voxel-level SUV uptake
During/Mid-Treatment			
DWI-MRI	Radiomics + cox regression	Head-and-neck cancer (Mohamed et al. 2023)	Tumor response Local control Recurrence-free survival
FDG-PET/CT	Radiomics + cox regression	Diffuse large B-cell lymphoma (Lokre et al. 2024)	Overall survival
FDG-PET/CT	Statistical analysis	NSCLC (Bowen et al. 2021)	Tumor response
FMISO-PET/CT	Radiomics + cox regression	Head-and-neck cancer (Carles et al. 2021)	Local control
DWI-MRI + FDG-PET/CT	Statistical analysis	Head-and-neck cancer (Trada et al. 2023)	Local control

(*Continued*)

TABLE 11.2 (*Continued*)

Tumor Response Assessment and Prediction Using Pre-, Mid/During-, Post-treatment, and Longitudinal Imaging

Imaging Modality	Method	Disease Site and Treatment	Response and Outcome
		Pre-Treatment	
FDG-PET+ T1 and T2 MRI	Statistical analysis	Uterine cervical squamous cell carcinoma (Strandberg et al. 2024)	Tumor response by RECIST1.1 outcome relapse
		Post-Treatment	
T1 and T2 MRI	Gradient boost algorithm	Advanced rectal cancer (Wang et al. 2023)	Pathological tumor response
T1 and T2 MRI	LASSO+RF	Nasopharyngeal carcinoma (Sun et al. 2023)	Progression-free survival
PSMA PET/CT	Statistical analysis	Prostate cancer (Gafita et al. 2023)	Tumor response post 177Lu-PSMA treatment Overall survival
		Longitudinal Imaging	
A time series of MRI and contrast-enhanced CT	Statistical analysis	Rectal cell carcinoma (Schep et al. 2024)	Pattern of tumor response over time
A time series of MRI	Radiomics +LSTM	Prostate cancer (Sushentsev et al. 2023)	Tumor progression in active surveillance
A time series of CBCT	Statistical analysis	Locally advanced rectal cancer (Li et al. 2023)	Pathological complete response

11.2.1 Pre-treatment

At the pre-treatment stage, response cannot yet be assessed but can be predicted. In this subsection, we will review the use of various imaging modalities, including CT, MRI, and PET, to predict patient responses and outcomes. Additionally, we will discuss lesion- and voxel-level prediction using PET/CT imaging.

CT imaging is widely used to predict treatment response across various types of cancer. Given its widespread use as the primary imaging modality and standard of care, models based on pre-treatment CT scans have been validated externally and demonstrate their generalization. In advanced esophageal squamous cell carcinoma (Xie et al. 2023), deep neural networks (DNNs) have been applied to pre-treatment CT images to predict the response to radiation therapy. Notably, a pretrained ResNet model demonstrated superior performance compared to support vector machine (SVM) and random forest (RF) models in determining binary tumor treatment response in a multi-center study. Tumor response was quantified by the ratio of maximum tumor diameter between post-treatment and pre-treatment scans, following RECIST 1.1 criteria. This study offers valuable insights into identifying which advanced ESCC cases may benefit from radiation therapy and provides a pathway for selecting therapeutic choices upfront. In non-small cell lung cancer (NSCLC), pre-treatment contrast-enhanced CT images combined with clinicopathologic data were used to train a model that integrates MLP (multi-layer perceptron) and SurvivalNet to predict patient progression-free survival (PFS) and OS for risk stratification (Li et al. 2023). Radiomic features extracted from the tumor volume on CT scans, along with clinicopathologic data, were input into the MLP for predicting PFS and OS. The model has been externally validated, demonstrating its capability to stratify patients into high- and low-risk groups.

MR imaging is frequently used for diagnosing and treating genitourinary and abdominal cancers. Pre-treatment T2-weighted MRI, supplemented with CT imaging, has been shown to predict

1-month post-PSA levels in SBRT for prostate cancer patients (Wong et al. 2024). Radiomic features were extracted from both planning CT and MRI in MR-guided radiation therapy, with maximum relevance and minimum redundancy (mRMR) used to select the most important features. A combined MRI and CT approach demonstrated superior performance compared to single-modality models in a 3-fold cross-validation scheme. In another study, pre-treatment MRI was used to predict chemoradiotherapy response for locally advanced cervical cancer (Jeong et al. 2024). Tumor response was assessed 3 months post-treatment by pelvic MRI and biopsy using RECIST 1.1. Adopting the idea of transfer learning, a pretrained ResNet showed superior results than handcrafted radiomics features. Combined with clinical factors, they even further improve the prediction of tumor response.

PET/CT scans capture functional changes, revealing response heterogeneity and metabolic and physiological information that complement anatomic information from CT or MR images. In early-stage NSCLC treated with SBRT (Thor et al. 2024), two of the most frequently published features—tumor diameter and standardized uptake value (SUV) max from pre-treatment PET/CT—have been found to be associated with progression and OS. Pre-treatment PET/CT is also shown in predicting prognosis in laryngeal cancer (Nakajo et al. 2023). Clinical features and PET radiomics features were fed into RF and other classical machine learning (ML) methods for predicting PFS. At the lesion level, PET/CT shows promise in predicting occult nodal metastasis (ONM) in early-stage N0 NSCLC, aiding in the identification of candidates for adjuvant therapy post-surgery (Zhong et al. 2023). Deep learning (DL) features were developed using a large internal dataset of PET and CT images and validated across both prospective and external cohorts. Specifically, two ResNet18 backbone networks were used to extract features from PET and CT scans. These latent features were then concatenated and processed through a fully connected layer for ONM prediction. At the voxel level, in squamous cell anal cancer, baseline pre-treatment FDG-PET scans were found to be spatially consistent throughout the course of chemoradiotherapy. Subvolumes with 50% SUV overlap with regions of high SUV uptake during treatment are considered potential targets for dose escalation (Sabbagh et al. 2019). In oropharyngeal cancer, pre-treatment PET data, along with dose information, was used to generate voxel-level post-treatment PET images (Ji et al. 2022). A 3D CNN with encoder-decoder architecture was employed for this purpose. The mean SUV values in high-uptake regions and 2D gamma analysis were used to assess the similarity between the predicted and ground truth images. In NSCLC, a multi-scale regression approach (Bowen et al. 2019) was used to predict tumor voxel SUV on mid-treatment PET scans, utilizing baseline patient-level data (e.g., clinical characteristics and treatment factors) both with and without voxel-level covariates, such as pre-treatment voxel SUV, RT dose, and voxel distance from the tumor centroid. The combination of patient- and voxel-level information improved the prediction of spatially variant response on mid-treatment compared to using patient-level data alone. Pre-treatment voxel SUV emerged as the most important predictor of mid-treatment voxel SUV.

11.2.2 Mid/During-Treatment

During treatment, additional patient-specific information can be gathered through various imaging modalities, enabling a detailed evaluation of anatomical and physiological changes across multiple scales. This facilitates more precise adjustments to treatment plans, enhancing the immediate effectiveness of therapy and improving long-term outcomes by identifying candidates for further treatments or interventions when necessary.

Specifically, voxel-level spatial information from imaging is crucial for developing adaptive treatment strategies—whether anatomically or biologically based—that can optimize dose escalation for improved disease control or dose de-escalation to minimize normal tissue toxicity. In this section, our focus will be on assessing and predicting treatment response and outcomes to facilitate risk stratification and personalize treatment, rather than on implementing population-based adaptive strategies. Readers can find more information on adaptive radiation therapy in Chapter 7.

MRI has been utilized to assess mid-treatment response in head-and-neck cancer patients. Imaging features extracted from DWI-MRI were associated with tumor response and outcomes (Mohamed et al. 2023). Specifically, mean apparent diffusion coefficient (ADC) values were evaluated at both pre-treatment and mid-treatment stages. The delta ADC of the primary tumor was found to correlate with tumor response, local control (LC), and recurrence-free survival (RFS). A cox model was developed to compare clinical parameters alone versus a combination of clinical and imaging parameters. Additionally, a threshold for stratifying high- and low-risk patients was identified using recursive partitioning analysis (RPA).

PET/CT has been widely utilized to assess mid-treatment response in lymphoma, lung cancer, cervical cancer, etc. PET/CT images collected at baseline and during chemoradiation therapy for diffuse large B-cell lymphoma (DLBCL) and NSCLC were used to predict patient prognosis, demonstrating superior performance compared to RECIST and PERCIST in predicting OS (Lokre et al. 2024). A multivariable cox model was applied, incorporating various imaging features such as SUV mean, max, and peak, derived from all lesions, the five largest lesions, and the single hottest lesion. The analysis of all lesions provided the most accurate prognostication of survival. In unresectable NSCLC, mid-treatment FDG-PET and pre-treatment FDG-PET scans were evaluated to stratify patients into PET responders and non-responders as part of a personalized treatment strategy known as Functional Lung Avoidance and Response-adaptive Escalation Radiation Therapy (FLARE-RT) (Bowen et al. 2021). Specifically, PET responders were prospectively determined based on a metric combining FDG avidity and FDG volumetric extent. Patients classified as non-responders received biologically adaptive radiation dose escalation targeting the residual metabolic tumor burden, whereas responders received standard dosing regimens. FMISO-PET imaging (Carles et al. 2021) was used to evaluate treatment response to chemoradiation in head-and-neck cancer patients. Radiomic features were extracted at baseline, 2 weeks, and 5 weeks from the hypoxic subvolume within the tumor and used to predict outcomes, specifically local recurrence. The predictive model was validated using an internal validation cohort.

The combination of functional MRI and PET/CT is used to evaluate early responses to treatment and identify high-risk patients, enabling the development of additional strategies to improve outcomes. In a study of head-and-neck cancer patients undergoing radiation therapy, changes in the metrics of the mean ADC from DWI-MRI and metabolic tumor volume (MTV) from FDG-PET between week 3 and pre-treatment showed correlations with LC (Trada et al. 2023). These delta features were also associated with death, which was predominantly due to locoregional recurrence (LR) in most cases. In uterine cervical squamous cell carcinoma (CSCC), early response assessed by PET/MRI has been shown to correlate with patient outcomes (Strandberg et al. 2024). Specifically, changes in functional tumor volume (FTV) measured between pre-treatment and 1 week into mid-treatment were found to be predictive of relapse. Similarly, delta ADC values demonstrated a comparable correlation with relapse. In contrast, no such correlation was observed with response evaluation using RECIST 1.1 criteria, suggesting that early response, as indicated by FDG-PET/MRI functional imaging biomarkers, is more predictive of radiation therapy outcomes than standard tumor response assessments.

Voxel-level response evaluation at mid-treatment is valuable for anatomical adaptation based on CT/MRI across various cancers as well as biologically guided adaptation in lung (Kong et al. 2021; Bowen et al. 2021; Cooke et al. 2023) and head-and-neck cancers (Welz et al. 2022), etc. Anatomical adaptation involves assessing changes in organs-at-risk (OAR) and tumor contours to re-evaluate dosimetric metrics, with the potential to trigger re-planning if needed. Biologically adaptive approaches, on the other hand, deliver a boost dose to the target based on spatial variations in tumor response, aiming to enhance treatment efficacy. For more detailed information on biologically adaptive radiation therapy, please refer to Chapter 7.

11.2.3 Post-Treatment

After treatment, short-term responses can be evaluated, while predicting long-term treatment outcomes at both the patient and lesion level is also valuable. In this subsection, we will first discuss tumor response evaluation and prediction post-treatment, followed by a discussion of long-term toxicity prediction in normal tissues using the combination of dose and imaging information.

MR-based pre-treatment and delta-radiomics features are predictive of treatment response in locally advanced rectal cancer (LARC) to neoadjuvant chemoradiotherapy. MRI radiomics features were extracted from T1- and T2-weighted MRI scans at baseline and post-treatment, and a gradient boosting algorithm was applied to predict tumor response. The results were assessed using multiple cross-validation schemes and an independent dataset (Wang et al. 2023). MR-based radiomics features, including both pre-treatment and post-treatment, were proposed to predict PFS in patients with nasopharyngeal carcinoma who underwent chemoradiation. ML techniques, including recursive feature elimination, RF, and mRMR, were employed to identify key radiomics features. LASSO was then used to develop a comprehensive model that integrated clinical and imaging features (Sun et al. 2023).

Theranostic approaches to response assessment continue to expand and accelerate toward clinical translation in the era of radiopharmaceutical therapies. For example, PSMA PET/CT shows significant potential for assessing response in patients with metastatic castration-resistant prostate cancer undergoing 177Lu-PSMA therapy (Gafita et al. 2023). Both quantitative imaging features and qualitative assessments by clinicians at baseline and 12 weeks post-treatment demonstrate strong correlations with OS and response outcomes. These findings were observed in a multi-center patient cohort.

So far, we have focused on imaging-based prediction of tumor response. For normal tissue, dosimetric information is usually combined with or without imaging to predict toxicity. Whereas tumors typically have less variable external beam radiation dose distributions at both the patient and voxel levels, normal tissue usually exhibits a highly heterogeneous dose distribution. This variability provides additional or even primary insights into toxicity events, offering opportunities for dose-response modeling. Traditional NTCP models often consider only specific dosimetric variables and overlook the spatial dose distribution. Recently, more studies have begun combining 3D imaging with 3D dose distribution for patient-level toxicity prediction, where spatial information is crucial for accurate results. In addition, many studies have explored the dose-response relationship of normal tissue at the voxel level (Schaub et al. 2018; Hmt et al. 2019; Price et al. 2018; H. J. Lee et al. 2018), aiming to identify associations between voxel-level dose and voxel-level response as assessed through imaging. In lung cancer, a DL framework (Zhang et al. 2023) that combines 3D dose distribution with 3D CT imaging was used to predict radiation pneumonitis (RP) in patients who received radical chemoradiation. A 3D ResNet architecture was employed to extract high-level features from the 3D inputs. Fully connected layers, applied after average pooling, were used to compute the probability of RP. The training dataset consisted of 314 institutional cases, with three test datasets: one from a prospectively collected institutional cohort and two from external datasets with different fractionation schemes. The model demonstrated strong performance on the institutional test set and reasonable performance on the two external test sets. In nasopharyngeal carcinoma, a CNN (OuYang et al. 2023) was used to predict radiation-induced temporal lobe injury (TLI). Inputs included planning CT, dose distribution, and the shape of the temporal lobe, which were inputs of a 3D ResNet to extract imaging features. Clinical variables were also concatenated with imaging features in the fully connected layer for the prediction of TLI. The study utilized a multi-center dataset of 5,100 patients, testing the model on an internal cohort of 1,000 patients and over 1,300 external cases from three different institutions. At the voxel level, the relationship between lung parenchyma dose and changes in CT density (Defraene et al. 2018) was investigated in patients with locally advanced NSCLC. A deformable registration was applied to align the 3-month follow-up CT with the planning CT. The change in Hounsfield units (ΔHU) was then correlated with lung dose and plotted as a lung dose-density curve, showing a saturation of ΔHU above 60 Gy. Additionally, ΔHU was analyzed in relation to distance from the tumor and angular dependence. These and other voxel-based analyses (Monti et al. 2022; Palma et al. 2021) require deforming dose and images onto common grids, enabling permutation testing at every voxel to correlate spatial locations with changes on imaging and future toxicity events.

11.2.4 Longitudinal Evaluation

Rather than relying solely on a single snapshot at various time points (pre-, mid-, post-treatment), integrating information from various time points provides a richer and more detailed trajectory of the disease response or progression to a treatment. These longitudinal images provide prognostic and predictive data on individual disease dynamics, tumor evolution, and regional resistance patterns as part of an iterative process to personalize therapies over time.

Long-term longitudinal monitoring of tumors was conducted on patients with renal cell carcinoma (RCC) treated with stereotactic ablative radiotherapy (SABR) (Schep et al. 2024). Tumors were contoured on all follow-up scans, with imaging collected every 3 months during the first year and every 6 months thereafter. Both tumor linear dimensions and volumetric measurements were extracted for analysis. The pattern of tumor size and HU changes was evaluated, with separate analyses for T1a and T1b stage tumors. Although transient increases in tumor volume post-treatment were common, volumetric response assessment demonstrated earlier changes compared to linear measurements. This suggests that volumetric analysis may offer a more sensitive method for assessing treatment response in RCC patients undergoing SABR, providing earlier insight into therapeutic efficacy.

Serial MRI is critical for monitoring prostate cancer patients on active surveillance (AS). A DL model, utilizing long short-term memory (LSTM) networks (Sushentsev et al. 2023), was developed to predict histopathological progression based on serial MRI data. This model, which combines tumor-to-stroma ratio (TSR) and serial PSA density, outperformed traditional models that rely on delta-radiomics and delta-PSA density. The LSTM-based approach offers a more viable and unbiased framework for tracking longitudinal changes in tumor imaging features throughout AS. The model's performance was evaluated using multiple iterations of leave-one-out cross-validation, demonstrating its robustness.

In LARC, a time series of cone-beam CT (CBCT) images can be leveraged to predict pathological complete response (Li et al. 2023). The study employs an automated workflow, where daily CBCT images are automatically registered to the planning CT, and tumor features are extracted for detailed analysis after normalization. Longitudinal trends in these features are analyzed and used to predict tumor response post-treatment. The model's performance was assessed using leave-one-out cross-validation. It has the potential to automate systematic monitoring, enhance response prediction, and support more informed clinical decision-making.

11.3 AI MODELING FOR RESPONSE AND OUTCOME PREDICTION

Data-driven models are the most common method for response and outcome prediction (Cui et al. 2022; Niraula et al. 2022). They are the type of models which are trained and developed based on data. Both radiomics models and DL-based models fall into this category. One can refer to Chapter 4 on Radiomics and Chapter 5 on AI for Medical Image Analysis for a more thorough discussion of this topic.

11.3.1 Radiomics Approach

In radiomics models, pre-defined quantitative features are extracted from medical images. These can range from simple first-order statistics such as the mean of SUV or HU to second-order and higher-order texture features, which provide richer information about the tumor's characteristics.

For example, radiomics features can offer detailed insights into tumor heterogeneity by identifying distinct tumor habitats—subregions within the tumor that exhibit similar characteristics. This granular level of detail is especially valuable for assessing treatment response. Imaging habitats can be inferred through clustering at either the patch (Cherezov et al. 2019) or voxel level (Duan et al. 2020; Bernatowicz et al. 2021), allowing for a more nuanced understanding of the spatial variation within the tumor.

Simple radiomics features are generally easier to interpret, making them more straightforward for clinical applications in terms of model development and interpretability. The examples include such metrics as tumor size, tumor sphericity, and MTV. However, more abstract texture features, such as those derived from gray-level co-occurrence matrix (GLCM), gray-level run-length matrix (GLRLM), gray-level dependence matrix (GLDM), gray-level size zone matrix (GLSZM), and neighborhood gray-tone difference matrix (NGTDM), capture additional aspects of the patients' anatomical or physiological information. However, these more complex features can be challenging to intuitively interpret, though they still offer a degree of interpretability compared to the black-box nature of DL approaches.

When developing ML-based radiomics models, two key elements are essential: feature selection and the predictive model (Cui et al. 2019). Feature selection serves as a method for dimensionality reduction, learning an abstract representation that maximizes relevant information for the given predictive problem while minimizing redundant information. There are several categories of feature selection methods. Filter methods are typically pre-selection techniques that operate independently of ML algorithms, evaluating features based on statistical measures such as correlation and mutual information. In contrast, wrapper methods utilize ML algorithms to select a subset of important features by assessing the performance of different subsets of features through model training and evaluation. Embedded methods, on the other hand, integrate feature selection with model development, often incorporating L1 (Lasso) regularization, L2 (Ridge) regularization, or combined L1 and L2 (elastic net) regularization terms into the loss function during training. This approach helps identify the most relevant features while simultaneously developing the model.

A major challenge in developing radiomics models lies in the numerous features generated from various parameters during image acquisition and reconstruction that can greatly inflate both dimensionality and non-biologic variability in the extracted data. These sources of variability include parameters in scanning protocols, reconstruction settings, and the intrinsic properties of the radiomics features themselves. As a result, a carefully designed validation scheme of models is crucial, particularly in partitioning datasets to ensure an independent test set is held out, thereby minimizing bias. Additionally, to ensure the generalizability and robustness of the model, it is critical to standardize the imaging acquisition, reconstruction, and radiomics feature processing. Harmonization of radiomics data across multiple institutions is necessary when standardization is not achievable.

11.3.2 Deep Learning Approach

In recent years, DL models have gained significant attention due to their superior predictive power across various applications. Beyond just accuracy, DL offers several advantages. For supervised learning, one notable benefit is its end-to-end approach, which streamlines the process by eliminating the need for separate stages of feature extraction and predictive model development. Instead, DL methods automatically extract relevant information from raw data, progressively learning meaningful representations through multiple layers of neural networks. In the context of unsupervised learning, DL techniques excel at extracting representations from large datasets of unlabeled data, enabling the automatic discovery of intrinsic patterns and the identification of new insights. Although treatment response prediction is inherently a supervised problem that can be effectively addressed using an end-to-end DL approach, unsupervised representation learning can be helpful for extracting latent features, which can enhance the performance of downstream prediction tasks.

DL has notable advantages over classical ML methods in treatment response prediction. Its flexible neural network structures can easily incorporate spatial and longitudinal series (Cui et al. 2019) of imaging data. CNNs and their variants are widely used in imaging tasks. ResNet (Zhong et al. 2023; Çiçek et al. 2016), for example, addresses the vanishing gradient problem by using skip connections, allowing for deeper networks without loss of information. U-Net (Çiçek et al. 2016), with its encoder-decoder structure, is highly effective in medical imaging tasks such as segmentation. DenseNet (Fu, Singhrao, Qi, et al. 2021), which enhances information flow between layers by connecting each layer to every other layer, and Inception networks (e.g., Inception-v3), which combine multiple filter sizes to capture features at different scales within a single layer. Additionally, recurrent neural networks (RNNs), such as LSTM and GRU, are effective in capturing temporal dependencies in longitudinal data. One may develop a customized architecture that combines CNNs for spatial feature extraction with RNNs for temporal modeling in tasks involving both spatial and sequential data. Meanwhile, other recent architectures, such as vision transformers, have shown promise in imaging tasks by leveraging self-attention mechanisms for better feature extraction. Generative models like GANs (Shi et al. 2024; Tseng et al. 2017), VAEs (Cui et al. 2019), and diffusion models have the capability to generate 3D outputs, which can be directly applied to voxel or region-level predictions. In short, these DL models offer remarkable flexibility in handling diverse input dimensions, making them adaptable and easy to implement across a wide range of applications.

However, there are several caveats to DL. It typically requires large datasets for effective training and often benefits from techniques such as pretraining and transfer learning. Additionally, DL models can lack interpretability, making it challenging to explain what the model has learned. These and other challenges, with potential mitigating solutions, are discussed in the following section.

11.4 CHALLENGES AND SOLUTIONS IN CLINICAL TRANSLATION OF AI-BASED RESPONSE AND OUTCOME PREDICTION MODELS

Despite the promising potential of AI models for predicting treatment response and outcome, translating these models into clinical practice presents several significant challenges that hinder their widespread adoption. One major challenge arises from data scarcity. Acquiring large and high-quality clinical datasets is often difficult due to factors like patient privacy regulations and the cost required for data collection and labeling. These limitations lead to several issues, most notably overfitting, where AI models capture patterns specific to the training set but fail to generalize to unseen data. Furthermore, limited datasets often lack diversity, resulting in models that may be biased and unable to perform reliably across diverse patient populations, which is critical for safe and effective clinical application.

Another challenge is the lack of interpretability and transparency in many AI models, especially those utilizing DL techniques. Clinicians are generally cautious about integrating tools into their practice that function as "black boxes," offering predictions without clear explanations. In healthcare, understanding the rationale behind a prognosis is essential for informed decision-making and for maintaining trust with patients. Without transparent reasoning, clinicians may be reluctant to rely on AI predictions, fearing they cannot adequately justify treatment decisions based on opaque algorithms.

Additionally, many AI models only provide point estimates without conveying the associated uncertainty or confidence levels. Neglecting these uncertainties in AI models can lead to overconfidence in the model's predictions and potentially put patient safety at risk. Uncertainty quantification allows clinicians to assess the reliability of the predictions when making clinical decisions and identify the "difficult-to-predict" cases that need to be examined cautiously.

In the following section, we will review solutions to address these challenges, including strategies such as transfer learning for improving model performance and generalizability, explainable AI for improving model transparency, and uncertainty quantification to ensure safe and reliable predictions.

11.4.1 Transfer Learning

Transfer learning is an ML technique where a model trained to perform one task in the source domain is adapted to perform the same or a different task in the target domain (Zhuang et al. 2021). Instead of training a model from scratch, transfer learning leverages the knowledge gained from a large source dataset and applies it to a small target dataset, often leading to better model performance with less training data and time. This approach is especially useful in healthcare, where high-quality data is expensive to obtain. An alternative solution to address limited high-quality data is federated learning (Pati et al. 2022; Niraula et al. 2022; Jochems et al. 2017), which differs from traditional centralized learning. Unlike centralized models that require data to be stored in one location, federated learning allows data to remain within its original institution, preserving privacy and adhering to regulatory requirements. We will not delve into federated learning here, as it is primarily an infrastructural approach rather than a technical modeling method.

Several methods could be used to perform transfer learning. Each is tailored to the characteristics of the target task and dataset. One common method is feature extraction, where pretrained DL models are used to extract radiomic features from medical images. Extracted features can be fed into ML models to predict treatment response and outcome. For example, studies have shown that compared with conventional handcrafted radiomic features, transfer learning features, extracted from MR images using the VGG19 pretrained on ImageNet, helped achieve better performance in predicting treatment response in LARC and OS in glioblastoma (Fu et al. 2020; Fu, Singhrao, Zhong, et al. 2021). Additionally, transfer learning features extracted from CT using the pretrained CNNs achieved promising performance in predicting OS in patients with pancreatic ductal adenocarcinoma and recurrence risk in NSCLC patients (Zhang et al. 2020; Bove et al. 2023).

Another common approach is fine-tuning, which involves retraining some or all of the model's layers on the new dataset. Fine-tuning is beneficial when the target task is more complex or different from the original task, as it allows the model to adapt its learned representations more specifically to the new domain. For instance, Xu et al. finetuned a ResNet, which was pretrained on ImageNet for natural object recognition tasks, along with RNN to predict 2-year OS status (dead vs alive) from baseline and follow-up CT images in stage III NSCLA patients (Xu et al. 2019). The model achieved a mean AUC of 0.74 and could be used to stratify the patients into two risk groups that were significantly associated with OS.

A combination of fine-tuning and feature extraction could be used for transfer learning. Lu *et al.* proposed a DL network, consisting of GoogleNets and a bi-LSTM, to predict tumor response to targeted therapy in metastatic colorectal cancer based on serial CT images (Lu et al. 2021). The authors first finetuned a pretrained GoogleNet to distinguish lesion images from normal tissue images in the training dataset. The finetuned classification model was then used to extract image features from CT acquired at each time point. These features were fed into the bi-LSTM to predict 1-year OS status. The integration of the DL-generated probability score and size-based measurements achieved a higher mean concordance index for OS compared with size/DL-based-only models.

Moreover, domain adaptation, a specialized type of transfer learning, can be employed to tackle challenges arising from domain shifts where the data distribution in the target domain differs from that of the source domain. Domain shifts could result from variations in patient populations, imaging equipment, or clinical protocols across different clinical centers, leading to poor model generalizability. Common domain adaptation approaches include feature alignment methods, which aim to learn domain-invariant features across domains through specially designed CNNs. A survey of domain adaptation methods for medical imaging analysis can be found in this review article (Guan and Liu 2022).

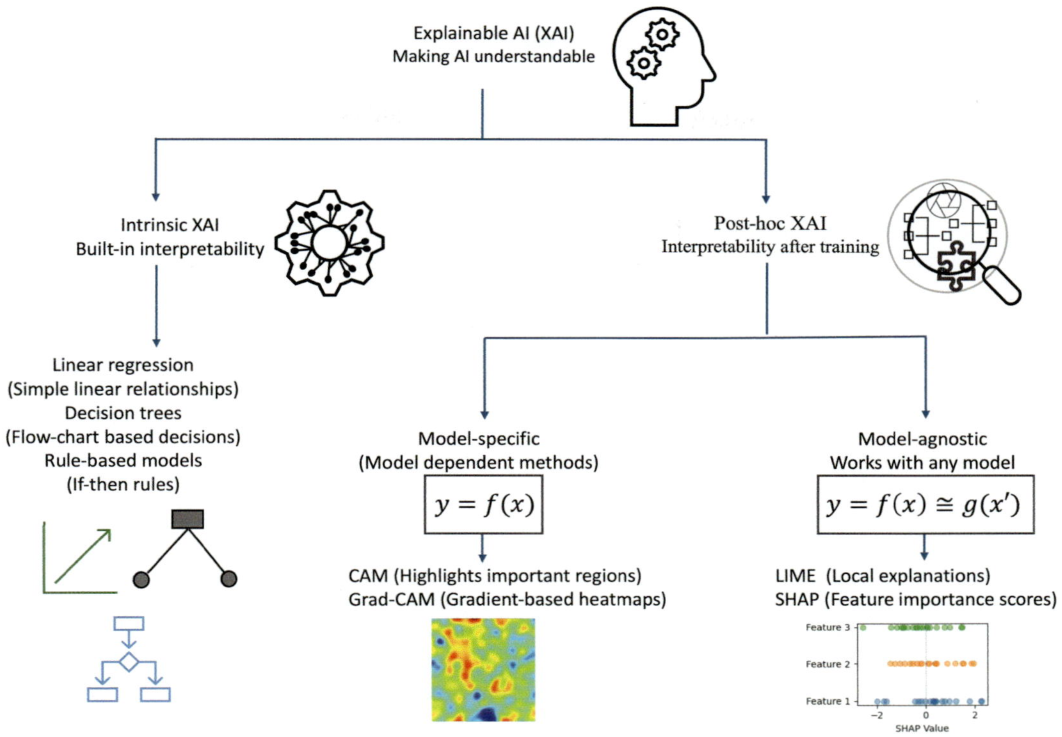

FIGURE 11.1 A diagram illustrating the key categories and methods of post-hoc XAI techniques.

11.4.2 Explainable AI

Explainable AI (XAI) refers to methods and models that allow humans to understand and trust the AI model outputs (Hassija et al. 2024). The decision-making process of many ML models, especially DL models, is often seen as a "black box" due to model complexity and non-transparency. XAI provides transparency and trust in high-stakes decision-making, where patient lives and outcomes are directly impacted (Saraswat et al. 2022). Clinicians need to understand and justify AI-driven predictions to ensure patient safety and ethical care. By offering clear explanations, XAI could help prevent errors, support compliance with regulatory standards, and promote the responsible use of AI in healthcare.

There are two types of XAI approaches: intrinsic XAI and post-hoc XAI. Intrinsic XAI involves using inherently interpretable models, such as decision trees, linear regression, or rule-based models (Duan et al. 2024), where the decision-making process is naturally transparent and easy to follow. On the other hand, post-hoc XAI provides explanations for complex models like DNNs and is applied after the model is trained. Post-hoc methods can be further categorized into model-specific and model-agnostic methods. In the following discussion, we will present a few methods from each category and illustrate their applications in treatment outcome prediction. A detailed list of post-hoc XAI methods can be found in these review articles (Cui et al. 2023) (Figure 11.1)

11.4.2.1 Model-Specific

Model-specific methods are particularly designed for specific models that take advantage of the model's internal structure and properties to provide insights. For example, class activation mapping (CAM) was proposed for the classification-trained CNN to highlight the regions of an image that contribute to the classification result (Zhou et al. 2016). It works by computing a feature vector from the activations of the final activation layers and projecting the output layers' weights onto these maps to visualize important areas. It provides insights only at the final layer, offering no interpretability at earlier stages of the network, and requires the neural network to have a very specific structure in the final layer.

Gradient-weighted CAM (Grad-CAM) is a gradient-based and generalized version of CAM used for visualization of any CNN, regardless of its architecture (Selvaraju et al. 2020). Grad-CAM creates coarse localization maps of important regions in the image by using class-specific gradient information. Despite an improved version of CAM, Grad-CAM struggles with localizing multiple object occurrences, accurately determining class-region coverage, and potential signal loss due to upsampling and downsampling. Grad-CAM ++ is an extension of Grad-CAM that provides better visual explanations of CNN model predictions in terms of better object localization as well as explaining occurrences of multiple object instances in a single image (Chattopadhay et al. 2018). Grad-CAM ++ generates visual explanations for class labels by using a weighted combination of positive partial derivatives of the last convolutional layer feature maps with respect to a specific class score.

CAM-based methods have been extensively investigated in healthcare applications such as medical imaging segmentation and disease classification (Xiao et al. 2021; Jiang et al. 2020; Zhang et al. 2021). Also, many studies have utilized Grad-CAM to explain AI models in the application of cancer treatment response and outcome prediction. In a recent study conducted by Peng et al., a 3D ResNet50 model was developed to predict tumor response (responder: complete response and partial response; non-responder: progressive disease and stable disease) to concurrent chemoradiotherapy in NSCLC patients based on pre-treatment contrast-enhanced CT images (Peng et al. 2024). Grad-CAM was used to highlight the CT regions that have more contributions to the prediction results. The authors found that patients who responded to treatment exhibited high activation regions within the tumor, while this pattern was absent in non-responders. Additionally, several DL models were proposed to predict survival status (dead versus alive) at certain time points based on pre-treatment CT for NSCLC patients, and Grad-CAM highlighted the importance of tumor-surrounding tissue for model predictions (Hosny et al. 2018; H. Kim et al. 2020).

11.4.2.2 Model-Agnostic

Model-agnostic techniques can be applied to any ML algorithm regardless of its underlying structure. They provide a way to understand and explain the model predictions with any internal knowledge of the model. For example, local interpretable model-agnostic explanations (LIME) explain individual predictions of any AI model by locally approximating the model's decision boundary around the instance being explained (Ribeiro, Singh, and Guestrin 2016). It does so by creating perturbed versions of the input data, getting predictions for those perturbed instances from the original model, and then training a simpler, interpretable model, such as a linear model, on this local data to explain the original model's behavior in that specific region. Astley *et al.* investigated several ML models, including DeepSurV, to predict OS after radiotherapy in patients with stage I-IV NSCLC based on pre-treatment clinical features (Astley et al. 2024). LIME values were computed for each model to provide feature explanations for the trained survival models and select the three most important features.

Although LIME is easy and relatively fast to implement, it only provides local explanations and can also be unstable, as small changes in data points or perturbations can lead to different explanations for similar predictions. Shapley additive explanations (SHAP) is another model-agnostic explanation method based on a more rigorous theoretical foundation from cooperative game theory (Lundberg, Allen, and Lee, n.d.). SHAP assigns each feature a Shapley value that represents its contribution to the prediction, ensuring that the feature attributions are consistent, fair, and globally interpretable. SHAP is often preferred in high-stakes healthcare applications due to its stability and ability to provide both local and global explanations. Lee et al. trained various types of AI models based on DVH features of cardiopulmonary substructures to predict OS in patients with locally advanced NSCLC enrolled in the RTOG 0617 clinical trial (Lee et al. 2023). SHAP values were computed for each model to select important features that are associated with OS. A binary change point detection algorithm was applied to the SHAP values to identify potential dose-volume constraints for improving OS.

11.4.3 Uncertainty Quantification

Uncertainty quantification (UQ) in AI models is vital for improving clinical decision-making when assessing and predicting response (Seoni et al. 2023). There are two types of uncertainty that affect AI models: aleatoric and epistemic uncertainties (Hüllermeier and Waegeman 2021). Aleatoric uncertainty, also known as data uncertainty, is caused by inherent randomness in the data. Example causes include variable responses to treatment from one patient to another due to biological differences, noisy measurements, and stochastic processes in the data. Aleatoric uncertainty cannot be reduced by collecting more data, as it is a property of the system being modeled. Epistemic uncertainty, also known as model uncertainty, occurs due to a lack of knowledge during the modeling process. For example, models trained with limited data or inherent biases could have poor generalizability and high epistemic uncertainty. Also, wrong choices of models (e.g., a linear model for non-linear data) or training strategies can lead to high uncertainty. Epistemic uncertainty can be reduced by gathering more training data, choosing a better model structure, and adopting better training strategies.

Clinicians can better understand the confidence in expected treatment outcomes and identify cases where the model is less certain by quantifying uncertainties in model predictions. For example, when a model predicts tumor response with high uncertainty, it signals the need for closer monitoring or alternative treatment strategies. In critical cancer care decisions, where over- or under-treatment can have severe consequences, UQ provides an additional layer of safety by allowing clinicians to factor in the risks associated with prediction uncertainties, leading to better-tailored treatments and improved patient outcomes.

Many methods have been proposed for UQ in AI models. Bayesian neural networks (BNN) introduce uncertainty by placing probability distributions over the weights of the neural network, as opposed to deterministic weights in standard neural networks (Olivier, Shields, and Graham-Brady 2021). It estimates posterior distributions over model parameters, typically using methods like the Markov Chain Monte Carlo algorithm or variational inference (Neal 1992; Graves 2011). However, it is computationally expensive and often hard to scale to large networks. Monte Carlo dropout is a practical and scalable approximation to BNN that uses dropout during both training and inference to simulate stochastic forward passes. A distribution over the model's predictions can be obtained by sampling multiple forward passes through a neural network with dropout. The variance in these predictions gives an estimate of uncertainty (Gal and Ghahramani 2016). Additionally, deep ensembles involve training multiple DNNs independently and then combining their predictions to estimate the model uncertainty (Lakshminarayanan, Pritzel, and Deepmind, n.d.).

Conformal prediction (CP) is a relatively new ML framework that uses past experience to determine the precise level of confidence in new predictions (Shafer and Vovk 2008). For example, it evaluates the AI models' predictions for a new patient's response by comparing them to predictions for a group of similar patients whose outcomes are already known. This is done by adjusting the model's predictive accuracy based on its confidence levels across all potential responses. This approach shifts the model's output from the most likely single response to a list of possible outcomes, providing a more comprehensive view of possible treatment effects. CP can be applied to any ML algorithm as long as the data exchangeability assumption is met (Shafer and Vovk 2008). It provides prediction sets instead of a single prediction for classification tasks and prediction intervals instead of a point prediction for regression tasks. If the model is not confident about its predictions, then prediction sets will be larger for classification, and prediction intervals will be wider for regression.

CP has been widely used in various fields, including finance, NLP, computer vision, and climate science. In recent years, CP has also been used in healthcare. In a study (Alnemer, Rajab, and Aljarah 2016), researchers predicted the breast cancer survivability using four different ML algorithms and applied CP to assess the reliability of individual predictions. They showed that applying a confidence measure for each classification result reduces the false predictions. In another study (Lu et al. 2022), researchers investigated the application of CP in clinical settings by conducting interviews with radiologists and identifying two use cases for skin lesion classification. Their research focused on modifying CP to account for subgroup differences in patient skin tones, ensuring fair and adaptive coverage. Their results showed CP can enhance clinicians trust in AI models by providing reliable uncertainty measures across diverse patient groups.

11.5 FUTURE PERSPECTIVES

11.5.1 Integration of Multi-Modal Data

Traditionally, treatment response has been primarily assessed using imaging data. However, with the increasing availability of patient-specific data, we are entering an era of precision oncology. Rich data sources such as electronic medical records (EMRs), cancer knowledge bases, and multi-omics data (genomics, proteomics, metabolomics, transcriptomics, microbiomics, etc.) offer immense potential to provide a more comprehensive understanding of disease progression and treatment response. By integrating this diverse data, we can gain a holistic view of a patient's physiological and biological state alongside cancer biology, creating a more complete picture than imaging alone can provide.

EMR data include both structured information, such as billing codes, demographics, and medication records, as well as unstructured data, including progress notes, radiology reports, lab results, and claims. EMRs offer a wealth of information about a patient's medical history (Lee et al. 2019; Cui et al. 2022). Additionally, scientific resources like PubMed and clinical guidelines provide valuable, up-to-date insights that are crucial for informed cancer care. Incorporating biological data, such as single-nucleotide polymorphisms (SNPs) (Conte et al. 2023; Valter et al. 2023; Cui, Ten Haken, and El Naqa 2021) and copy number variations (CNVs) (Martell et al. 2024; Masood et al. 2024), can enhance our ability to predict tumor responses to therapy and patient outcomes. Similarly, epigenomics data, including DNA methylation patterns (Sturm et al. 2023) and non-coding RNA (e.g., miRNA), can reveal regulatory changes associated with disease progression. Cytokines (Takeuchi and Gotoh 2023) can reflect immune responses and inflammation within the tumor microenvironment, offering insights into cancer progression and treatment response.

By going beyond imaging and leveraging multi-modal data, we can significantly improve treatment response prediction and move toward truly personalized treatment strategies.

11.5.2 Combined Biophysical and Data-Driven Models

Data-driven models are typically built purely on data, identifying patterns and associations without incorporating domain knowledge or underlying mechanisms. While they excel at discovering new, previously unknown patterns, they often lack interpretability and fail to integrate expert insights. In contrast, biophysical models are grounded in established rules, relationships, and domain-specific knowledge, making them easier to understand and interpret. However, they may rely on simplified assumptions, limiting their ability to handle real-world complexity, and their accuracy may fall short compared to data-driven models. Each approach has its strengths; combining both could yield a more accurate, robust, interpretable, and translational tool that harnesses the advantages of both methods.

There are several ways to leverage the strengths of both data-driven and biophysical models when analyzing imaging data for outcome and response prediction. One approach is to integrate physical rules or regularization terms into the loss function of data-driven models to enforce practical constraints and incorporate known scientific principles. Examples of this include physics-informed DL networks, which have been applied in areas like brain hemodynamics (Sarabian, Babaee, and Laksari 2022) and intravoxel incoherent motion modeling for pancreatic cancer patients (Kaandorp et al. 2021).

Another approach involves using patient-specific imaging to enhance biophysical models with individualized data. This can help in determining key parameters for biophysical models or contribute domain-specific insights to numerical methods. An example of this is the use of partial differential equations (PDE) for modeling GBM progression, where personalized imaging data is used to model tumor characteristics and better capture patient heterogeneity (Meaney et al. 2023; Jackson et al. 2015). Additionally, agent-based models (ABMs) can be fitted to tumor imaging, refining the parameters within the ABM to reflect the specific tumor characteristics (Cess and Finley 2023).

11.5.3 Multi-Task Learning

Multi-task learning (MTL) is a ML technique designed to train models on multiple tasks simultaneously, exploiting the shared feature representations learned across different tasks to enhance overall model performance (Caruana 1997; Zhang and Yang 2022). By learning related tasks together, the model can generalize better, as the shared information across tasks helps to prevent overfitting to any single task.

MTL is very useful when the tasks share the underlying features and patterns. For example, tumor segmentation could allow the model to extract the tumor characteristics that are useful for other related tasks. Many studies have demonstrated the benefits of using MTL in joint tumor segmentation and classification tasks compared with single-task learning (Zhou et al. 2021; Schacky et al. 2021; Ling et al. 2024). Additionally, other studies have shown that integrating tumor segmentation using MTL helped achieve more accurate treatment response and outcome prediction (Jin et al. 2021; Meng, Gu, et al. 2022; Meng, Peng, et al. 2022). Specifically, Jin et al. proposed two Siamese subnetworks to simultaneously delineate tumor on pre- and post-treatment MR images and predict treatment response (pathologic complete response vs non-response) after neoadjuvant chemoradiotherapy in patients with rectal cancer (Jin et al. 2021). The authors found that MTL improved the mean AUC by 0.08 compared with single-task learning in the external validation dataset.

Several studies (Forouzannezhad et al. 2022; Y. Liu et al. 2022; Asaoka et al. 2021) have been conducted, and more are underway, that investigate the training of multi-task models to simultaneously predict clinical outcomes such as tumor response, normal tissue toxicity, and OS based on multi-omics data. These outcomes are often biologically intertwined, as processes influencing one may impact others. The joint learning approach may allow the model to not only learn about how the tumor and surrounding tissue respond to radiation but also identify factors that might contribute to long-term patient survival. By using MTL, these complex, interdependent outcomes can be modeled in a more holistic manner, ultimately leading to better clinical decision-making and personalized treatment strategies.

11.5.4 The Emerging Role of Foundation Models

Foundation models (Bommasani et al. 2021) are large AI models pretrained on vast unlabeled datasets, allowing them to learn useful data representations from various modalities such as texts, images, or videos. Unlike traditional models that are trained for specific tasks, foundation models can be adapted to numerous downstream tasks with little or no task-specific training data by leveraging the knowledge gained from extensive pretraining. Examples of foundation models include language models such as generative pretrained transformer (GPT) (Radford and Narasimhan 2018) and bidirectional encoder representations from transformers (BERT) (Devlin et al. 2018), vision models like self-distillation with no labels (DINO) (Caron et al. 2021) and masked autoencoders (MAE) (He et al. 2022), multi-modal models including contrastive language-image pretraining (CLIP) (Radford et al. 2021) and LLaVA (large language and vision assistant) (Liu et al. 2023). These models have demonstrated state-of-the-art performance across diverse fields, ranging from natural language understanding to computer vision. Foundation models could drive a paradigm shift in healthcare AI by handling diverse clinical tasks after being finetuned with small task-specific datasets (Moor et al. 2023). Their adaptability makes them ideal for applications in healthcare where shortage of labeled data presents significant challenges.

These models are emerging as powerful tools for treatment response and outcome prediction, thanks to their ability to interpret diverse data types such as medical images, EMRs, and genomics. For instance, the clinical histopathology imaging evaluation foundation (CHIEF) model trained using about 60K whole-slide image was finetuned for survival prediction in various cancer types, achieving a higher mean C-index compared with the state-of-the-art baseline models (Wang et al. 2024). In a study conducted by Pai et al., a foundation model trained using 11K annotated CT lesions was used to extract imaging features for various downstream tasks, including NSCLC prognostication (Pai et al. 2024). It outperformed conventional supervised models and other pretrained implementations, demonstrating the potential of using the foundation model in discovering more prognostic imaging biomarkers. Additionally, foundation models for EMR (FEMRs) can ingest a patients' medical history consisting of structured and unstructured EMR data and generate a patient embedding that can be used as input to downstream prediction tasks (Wornow et al. 2023).

Looking ahead, foundation models represent a transformative advancement in precision oncology. Their capacity to generalize across diverse data types allows them to offer a unified approach to handle complex multi-modal healthcare datasets and improve accuracy in predicting treatment response and outcome. By overcoming the limitations of traditional models that require extensive task-specific data, foundation models enable more efficient and scalable AI solutions, potentially reducing costs and accelerating the implementation of AI in clinical decision-making. As ongoing research continues to enhance their robustness and adaptability, foundation models are poised to become integral to precision oncology, supporting clinicians in making data-driven, individualized cancer treatment decisions that improve patient outcomes (Figure 11.2).

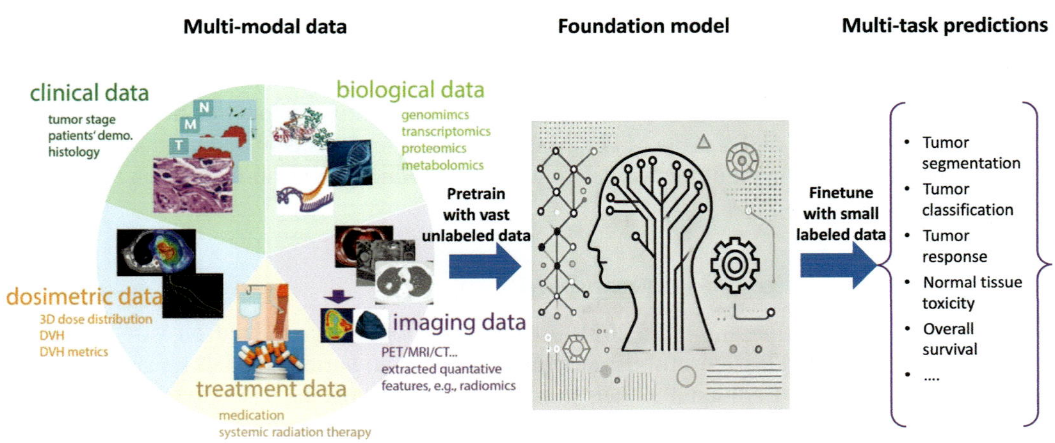

FIGURE 11.2 Future perspective on applying foundation models to multi-modal data, followed by multi-task downstream fine-tuning.

11.5.5 Digital Twins of Treatment Response

Digital twins of cancer response are multi-scale and multi-modal representations of each unique patient that are continuously updated with new information over time, synthesizing all prior information and predicting a dynamic spatial-temporal trajectory at future time horizons (Hernandez-Boussard et al. 2021; Stahlberg et al. 2022; Abdollahi et al. 2024). They bring together data-driven and mechanistic models to refine the digital twin representation of complex cancer response, fueling increasing computational demands. They enable the simulation of cost-effective virtual clinical trials to inform treatment selection, dosing, sequencing, and adaptation in each patient prior to expensive testing in randomized trial settings. This area of investigation into holistic response assessment and prediction has been identified as a priority by the NIH, NSF, and FDA under their Foundations for Digital Twins as Catalyzers of Biomedical Technological Innovation program ('Foundations for Digital Twins as Catalyzers of Biomedical Technological Innovation', n.d.), which will continue to experience rapid progress over the next decade.

11.6 SUMMARY

We have reviewed the assessment of treatment response with imaging at varying temporal and spatial scales. We have compared and contrasted data-driven approaches to response prediction, emphasizing the need for explainable AI and UQ. The future resides in big multi-omics data, multi-task and multi-modal frameworks, flexible foundational models, and synthesis of information into increasingly precise digital twin representations of individual cancer biological response to combinations of external beam radiation, radiopharmaceutical radiation, molecularly targeted therapies, and immune modulating therapies. AI-assisted treatment response prediction will power next-generation oncologic decision support platforms, requiring both technical innovation and regulatory oversight to realize its full potential.

REFERENCES

Abdollahi, Hamid, Fereshteh Yousefirizi, Isaac Shiri, Julia Brosch-Lenz, Elahe Mollaheydar, Ali Fele-Paranj, Kuangyu Shi, et al. 2024. 'Theranostic Digital Twins: Concept, Framework and Roadmap towards Personalized Radiopharmaceutical Therapies'. *Theranostics*. Ivyspring International Publisher. https://doi.org/10.7150/thno.93973.

Alnemer, Loai, Lama Rajab, and Ibrahim Aljarah. 2016. 'Conformal Prediction Technique to Predict Breast Cancer Survivability'. *International Journal of Advanced Science and Technology* 96 (November):1–10. https://doi.org/10.14257/ijast.2016.96.01.

Asaoka, Ryo, Linchuan Xu, Hiroshi Murata, Taichi Kiwaki, Masato Matsuura, Yuri Fujino, Masaki Tanito, et al. 2021. 'A Joint Multitask Learning Model for Cross-Sectional and Longitudinal Predictions of Visual Field Using OCT'. *Ophthalmology Science* 1 (4): 100055. https://doi.org/10.1016/j.xops.2021.100055.

Astley, Joshua R., James M. Reilly, Stephen Robinson, Jim M. Wild, Matthew Q. Hatton, and Bilal A. Tahir. 2024. 'Explainable Deep Learning-Based Survival Prediction for Non-Small Cell Lung Cancer Patients Undergoing Radical Radiotherapy'. *Radiotherapy and Oncology* 193 (April):110084. https://doi.org/10.1016/j.radonc.2024.110084.

Bent, M. J. Van den, J. S. Wefel, D. Schiff, M. J.B. Taphoorn, K. Jaeckle, L. Junck, T. Armstrong, et al. 2011. 'Response Assessment in Neuro-Oncology (a Report of the RANO Group): Assessment of Outcome in Trials of Diffuse Low-Grade Gliomas'. *The Lancet. Oncology* 12 (6): 583–93. https://doi.org/10.1016/S1470-2045(11)70057-2.

Bernatowicz, Kinga, Francesco Grussu, Marta Ligero, Alonso Garcia, Eric Delgado, and Raquel Perez-Lopez. 2021. 'Robust Imaging Habitat Computation Using Voxel-Wise Radiomics Features'. *Scientific Reports* 11 (1): 20133. https://doi.org/10.1038/s41598-021-99701-2.

Bhatia, Aashim, Noah D. Sabin, Michael J. Fisher, and Tina Young Poussaint. 2023. 'Review of Imaging Recommendations from Response Assessment in Pediatric Neuro-Oncology (RAPNO)'. *Pediatric Radiology* 53 (13): 2723–41. https://doi.org/10.1007/S00247-023-05780-W.

Bommasani, Rishi, Drew A. Hudson, Ehsan Adeli, Russ Altman, Simran Arora, Sydney von Arx, Michael S. Bernstein, et al. 2021. 'On the Opportunities and Risks of Foundation Models', August. https://arxiv.org/abs/2108.07258v3.

Bove, Samantha, Annarita Fanizzi, Federico Fadda, Maria Colomba Comes, Annamaria Catino, Angelo Cirillo, Cristian Cristofaro, et al. 2023. 'A CT-Based Transfer Learning Approach to Predict NSCLC Recurrence: The Added-Value of Peritumoral Region'. *Plos One* 18 (5): e0285188. https://doi.org/10.1371/JOURNAL.PONE.0285188.

Bowen, Stephen R., Daniel S. Hippe, W. Art Chaovalitwongse, Chunyan Duan, Phawis Thammasorn, Xiao Liu, Robert S. Miyaoka, et al. 2019. 'Voxel Forecast for Precision Oncology: Predicting Spatially Variant and Multiscale Cancer Therapy Response on Longitudinal Quantitative Molecular Imaging'. *Clinical Cancer Research* 25 (16): 5027–37. https://doi.org/10.1158/1078-0432.CCR-18-3908.

Bowen, Stephen R., Daniel S. Hippe, Hannah M. Thomas, Balukrishna Sasidharan, Paul D. Lampe, Christina S. Baik, Keith D. Eaton, et al. 2021. 'Prognostic Value of Early Fluorodeoxyglucose-Positron Emission Tomography Response Imaging and Peripheral Immunologic Biomarkers: Substudy of a Phase II Trial of Risk-Adaptive Chemoradiation for Unresectable Non-Small Cell Lung Cancer'. *Advances in Radiation Oncology* 7: 100857. http://doi.org/10.1016/j.adro.2021.100857.

Carles, Montserrat, Tobias Fechter, Anca L. Grosu, Arnd Sörensen, Benedikt Thomann, Raluca G. Stoian, Nicole Wiedenmann, et al. 2021. '18 F-Fmiso-Pet Hypoxia Monitoring for Head-and-Neck Cancer Patients: Radiomics Analyses Predict the Outcome of Chemo-Radiotherapy'. *Cancers* 13 (14). https://doi.org/10.3390/cancers13143449.

Caron, Mathilde, Hugo Touvron, Ishan Misra, Hervé Jegou, Julien Mairal, Piotr Bojanowski, and Armand Joulin. 2021. 'Emerging Properties in Self-Supervised Vision Transformers'. *2021 IEEE/CVF International Conference on Computer Vision (ICCV)*, Montreal, QC, Canada, April, 2021, 9630–9640. https://doi.org/10.1109/ICCV48922.2021.00951.

Caruana, Rich. 1997. 'Multitask Learning'. *Machine Learning* 28 (1): 41–75. https://doi.org/10.1023/A:1007379606734.

Cess, Colin G., and Stacey D. Finley. 2023. 'Calibrating Agent-Based Models to Tumor Images Using Representation Learning'. *PLoS Computational Biology* 19 (4). https://doi.org/10.1371/journal.pcbi.1011070.

Chamberlain, Marc, Larry Junck, Dieta Brandsma, Riccardo Soffietti, Roberta Rudà, Jeffrey Raizer, Willem Boogerd, et al. 2017. 'Leptomeningeal Metastases: A RANO Proposal for Response Criteria'. *Neuro-Oncology* 19 (4): 484–92. https://doi.org/10.1093/NEUONC/NOW183.

Chattopadhay, Aditya, Anirban Sarkar, Prantik Howlader, and Vineeth N. Balasubramanian. 2018. 'Grad-CAM++: Generalized Gradient-Based Visual Explanations for Deep Convolutional Networks'. *Proceedings – 2018 IEEE Winter Conference on Applications of Computer Vision, WACV 2018,* 2018-January (May), 839–47. https://doi.org/10.1109/WACV.2018.00097.

Cherezov, Dmitry, Dmitry Goldgof, Lawrence Hall, Robert Gillies, Matthew Schabath, Henning Müller, and Adrien Depeursinge. 2019. 'Revealing Tumor Habitats from Texture Heterogeneity Analysis for Classification of Lung Cancer Malignancy and Aggressiveness'. *Scientific Reports* 9 (1): 4500. https://doi.org/10.1038/s41598-019-38831-0.

Chiou, Victoria L., and Mauricio Burotto. 2015. 'Pseudoprogression and Immune-Related Response in Solid Tumors'. *Journal of Clinical Oncology* 33 (31): 3541. https://doi.org/10.1200/JCO.2015.61.6870.

Choi, Haesun, Chuslip Charnsangavej, Silvana C. Faria, Homer A. Macapinlac, Michael A. Burgess, Shreyaskumar R. Patel, Lei L. Chen, Donald A. Podoloff, and Robert S. Benjamin. 2007. 'Correlation of Computed Tomography and Positron Emission Tomography in Patients with Metastatic Gastrointestinal Stromal Tumor Treated at a Single Institution with Imatinib Mesylate: Proposal of New Computed Tomography Response Criteria'. *Journal of Clinical Oncology* 25 (13): 1753–59. http://doi.org/10.1200/JCO.2006.07.3049.

Chukwueke, Ugonma N., and Patrick Y. Wen. 2019. 'Use of the Response Assessment in Neuro-Oncology (RANO) Criteria in Clinical Trials and Clinical Practice'. *CNS Oncology* 8 (1): 28. https://doi.org/10.2217/CNS-2018-0007.

Çiçek, Özgün, Ahmed Abdulkadir, Soeren S. Lienkamp, Thomas Brox, and Olaf Ronneberger. 2016. '3D U-Net: Learning Dense Volumetric Segmentation from Sparse Annotation'. In Ourselin, S., Joskowicz, L., Sabuncu, M., Unal, G., Wells, W. (eds), *Medical Image Computing and Computer-Assisted Intervention – MICCAI 2016*. Athens, Greece, October 17-21, MICCAI 2016. Lecture Notes in Computer Science 9901.

Conte, Benedetta, Luca Boni, Giancarlo Bisagni, Antonio Durando, Giovanni Sanna, Stefania Gori, Ornella Garrone, et al. 2023. 'SNP of Aromatase Predict Long-Term Survival and Aromatase Inhibitor Toxicity in Patients with Early Breast Cancer: A Biomarker Analysis of the GIM4 and GIM5 Trials'. *Clinical Cancer Research* 29 (24): 5217–26. https://doi.org/10.1158/1078-0432.CCR-23-1568.

Cooke, Saskia A., Dirk de Ruysscher, Bart Reymen, Maarten Lambrecht, Gitte Fredberg Persson, Corinne Faivre-Finn, Edith M.T. Dieleman, et al. 2023. '18F-FDG-PET Guided vs Whole Tumour Radiotherapy Dose Escalation in Patients with Locally Advanced Non-Small Cell Lung Cancer (PET-Boost): Results from a Randomised Clinical Trial'. *Radiotherapy and Oncology* 181 (April). https://doi.org/10.1016/j.radonc.2023.109492.

Cui, Sunan, Yi Luo, Huan-Hsin Tseng, Randall K. Ten Haken, and Issam El Naqa. 2019. 'Artificial Neural Network With Composite Architectures for Prediction of Local Control in Radiotherapy'. *IEEE Transactions on Radiation and Plasma Medical Sciences* 3 (2): 242–49. https://doi.org/10.1109/TRPMS.2018.2884134.

Cui, Sunan, Randall K. Ten Haken, and Issam El Naqa. 2021. 'Integrating Multiomics Information in Deep Learning Architectures for Joint Actuarial Outcome Prediction in Non-Small Cell Lung Cancer Patients after Radiation Therapy'. *International Journal of Radiation Oncology, Biology, Physics* 110 (3): 893–904. https://doi.org/10.1016/j.ijrobp.2021.01.042.

Cui, Sunan, Andrew Hope, Thomas J. Dilling, Laura A. Dawson, Randall Ten Haken, and Issam El Naqa. 2022. 'Artificial Intelligence for Outcome Modeling in Radiotherapy'. *Seminars in Radiation Oncology* 32 (4): 351–64. https://doi.org/10.1016/j.semradonc.2022.06.005.

Cui, Sunan, Alberto Traverso, Dipesh Niraula, Jiaren Zou, Yi Luo, Dawn Owen, Issam El Naqa, and Lise Wei. 2023. 'Interpretable Artificial Intelligence in Radiology and Radiation Oncology'. *British Journal of Radiology* 96 (1150): 20230142. https://doi.org/10.1259/bjr.20230142.

Cui, Sunan, Yi Luo, Huan-Hsin Tseng, Randall K. Ten Haken, and Issam El Naqa. 2019. 'Combining Handcrafted Features with Latent Variables in Machine Learning for Prediction of Radiation-Induced Lung Damage'. *Medical Physics* 46 (5): 2497–511. https://doi.org/10.1002/mp.13497.

Defraene, Gilles, Matthew La Fontaine, Simon van Kranen, Bart Reymen, José Belderbos, Jan-Jakob Sonke, and Dirk De Ruysscher. 2018. 'Radiation-Induced Lung Density Changes on CT Scan for NSCLC: No Impact of Dose-Escalation Level or Volume'. *International Journal of Radiation Oncology, Biology, Physics* 102 (3): 642–50. https://doi.org/10.1016/j.ijrobp.2018.06.038.

Delgado, Amanda, and Achuta Kumar Guddati. 2021. 'Clinical Endpoints in Oncology - a Primer'. *American Journal of Cancer Research* 11 (4): 1121. /pmc/articles/PMC8085844/.

Devlin, Jacob, Ming Wei Chang, Kenton Lee, and Kristina Toutanova. 2018. 'BERT: Pre-Training of Deep Bidirectional Transformers for Language Understanding'. *NAACL HLT 2019 – 2019 Conference of the North American Chapter of the Association for Computational Linguistics: Human Language Technologies – Proceedings of the Conference*, Minneapolis, Minnesota, 1 (October), 4171–86. https://arxiv.org/abs/1810.04805v2.

Driscoll, James J., and Oliver Rixe. 2009. 'Overall Survival: Still the Gold Standard: Why Overall Survival Remains the Definitive End Point in Cancer Clinical Trials'. *Cancer Journal* 15 (5): 401–5. https://doi.org/10.1097/PPO.0B013E3181BDC2E0.

Duan, Chunyan, Qiantuo Liu, Jiajie Wang, Qianqian Tong, Fangyun Bai, Jie Han, Shouyi Wang, Daniel S. Hippe, Jing Zeng, and Stephen R. Bowen. 2024. 'GWO+RuleFit: Rule-Based Explainable Machine-Learning Combined with Heuristics to Predict Mid-Treatment FDG PET Response to Chemoradiation for Locally Advanced Non-Small Cell Lung Cancer'. *Physics in Medicine & Biology* 69 (15): 155018. https://doi.org/10.1088/1361-6560/ad6118.

Duan, Chunyan, W. Art Chaovalitwongse, Fangyun Bai, Daniel S. Hippe, Shouyi Wang, Phawis Thammasorn, Larry A. Pierce, et al. 2020. 'Sensitivity Analysis of FDG PET Tumor Voxel Cluster Radiomics and Dosimetry for Predicting Mid-Chemoradiation Regional Response of Locally Advanced Lung Cancer'. *Physics in Medicine & Biology* 65 (20): 205007. https://doi.org/10.1088/1361-6560/abb0c7.

Eisenhauer, E. A., P. Therasse, J. Bogaerts, L. H. Schwartz, D. Sargent, R. Ford, J. Dancey, et al. 2009. 'New Response Evaluation Criteria in Solid Tumours: Revised RECIST Guideline (Version 1.1)'. *European Journal of Cancer* 45 (2): 228–47. https://doi.org/10.1016/J.EJCA.2008.10.026.

Ellingson, Benjamin M., Patrick Y. Wen, and Timothy F. Cloughesy. 2017. 'Modified Criteria for Radiographic Response Assessment in Glioblastoma Clinical Trials'. *Neurotherapeutics: The Journal of the American Society for Experimental NeuroTherapeutics* 14 (2): 307–20. https://doi.org/10.1007/S13311-016-0507-6.

Forouzannezhad, Parisa, Dominic Maes, Daniel S. Hippe, Phawis Thammasorn, Reza Iranzad, Jie Han, Chunyan Duan, et al. 2022. 'Multitask Learning Radiomics on Longitudinal Imaging to Predict Survival Outcomes Following Risk-Adaptive Chemoradiation for Non-Small Cell Lung Cancer'. *Cancers* 14 (5). https://doi.org/10.3390/cancers14051228.

'Foundations for Digital Twins as Catalyzers of Biomedical Technological Innovation'. n.d. Accessed 3 November 2024. https://datascience.nih.gov/tools-and-analytics/digital-twins.

Fu, Jie, Kamal Singhrao, X. Sharon Qi, Yingli Yang, Dan Ruan, and John H. Lewis. 2021. 'Three-Dimensional Multipath DenseNet for Improving Automatic Segmentation of Glioblastoma on Pre-Operative Multimodal MR Images'. *Medical Physics* 48 (6): 2859–66. https://doi.org/10.1002/MP.14800.

Fu, Jie, Kamal Singhrao, Xinran Zhong, Yu Gao, Sharon X. Qi, Yingli Yang, Dan Ruan, and John H. Lewis. 2021. 'An Automatic Deep Learning–Based Workflow for Glioblastoma Survival Prediction Using Preoperative Multimodal MR Images: A Feasibility Study'. *Advances in Radiation Oncology* 6 (5). https://doi.org/10.1016/j.adro.2021.100746.

Fu, Jie, Xinran Zhong, Ning Li, Ritchell Van Dams, John Lewis, Kyunghyun Sung, Ann C Raldow, Jing Jin, and X Sharon Qi. 2020. 'Deep Learning-Based Radiomic Features for Improving Neoadjuvant Chemoradiation Response Prediction in Locally Advanced Rectal Cancer.' *Physics in Medicine and Biology* 65 (7): 075001. https://doi.org/10.1088/1361-6560/ab7970.

Gafita, Andrei, Loïc Djaileb, Isabel Rauscher, Wolfgang P. Fendler, Boris Hadaschik, Steven P. Rowe, Ken Herrmann, et al. 2023. 'Response Evaluation Criteria in PSMA PET/CT (RECIP 1.0) in Metastatic Castration-Resistant Prostate Cancer'. *Radiology* 308 (1). https://doi.org/10.1148/radiol.222148.

Gal, Yarin, and Zoubin Ghahramani. 2016. 'Dropout as a Bayesian Approximation: Representing Model Uncertainty in Deep Learning'. PMLR. https://proceedings.mlr.press/v48/gal16.html.

Gallamini, Andrea, Sally F. Barrington, Alberto Biggi, Stephane Chauvie, Lale Kostakoglu, Michele Gregianin, Michel Meignan, et al. 2014. 'The Predictive Role of Interim Positron Emission Tomography for Hodgkin Lymphoma Treatment Outcome Is Confirmed Using the Interpretation Criteria of the Deauville Five-Point Scale'. *Haematologica* 99 (6): 1107–13. https://doi.org/10.3324/haematol.2013.103218.

Graves, Alex. 2011. 'Practical Variational Inference for Neural Networks'. . In *Proceedings of the 25th International Conference on Neural Information Processing Systems (NIPS'11)*, Granada, Spain.

Guan, Hao, and Mingxia Liu. 2022. 'Domain Adaptation for Medical Image Analysis: A Survey'. *IEEE Transactions on Bio-Medical Engineering* 69 (3): 1173. https://doi.org/10.1109/TBME.2021.3117407.

Hassija, Vikas, Vinay Chamola, Atmesh Mahapatra, Abhinandan Singal, Divyansh Goel, Kaizhu Huang, Simone Scardapane, Indro Spinelli, Mufti Mahmud, and Amir Hussain. 2024. 'Interpreting Black-Box Models: A Review on Explainable Artificial Intelligence'. *Cognitive Computation* 16 (1): 45–74. https://doi.org/10.1007/s12559-023-10179-8.

He, Kaiming, Xinlei Chen, Saining Xie, Yanghao Li, Piotr Dollar, and Ross Girshick. 2022. 'Masked Autoencoders Are Scalable Vision Learners'. *2022 IEEE/CVF Conference on Computer Vision and Pattern Recognition (CVPR)*, New Orleans, LA, USA, 2022-June, 15979–88. https://doi.org/10.1109/CVPR52688.2022.01553.

Hernandez-Boussard, Tina, Paul Macklin, Emily J. Greenspan, Amy L. Gryshuk, Eric Stahlberg, Tanveer Syeda-Mahmood, and Ilya Shmulevich. 2021. 'Digital Twins for Predictive Oncology Will Be a Paradigm Shift for Precision Cancer Care'. *Nature Medicine*. Nature Research. https://doi.org/10.1038/s41591-021-01558-5.

Hmt, Thomas, Hannah T. Mary Thomas, Jing Zeng, Howard J. lee, Balu Krishna Sasidharan, Paul Kinahan, Robert S. Miyaoka, Hubert J. Vesselle, Ramesh Rengan, and Stephen Bowen. 2019. 'Comparison of Regional Lung Perfusion Response on Longitudinal Maa SPeCT/CT in Lung Cancer Patients Treated with and without Functional Tissue-Avoidance Radiation Therapy'. *British Journal of Radiology*. 2019 Nov;92(1103): 20190174. doi: 10.1259/bjr.20190174. Epub 2019 Aug 12. PMID: 31364397; PMCID: PMC6849661

Hosny, Ahmed, Chintan Parmar, Thibaud P. Coroller, Patrick Grossmann, Roman Zeleznik, Avnish Kumar, Johan Bussink, Robert J. Gillies, Raymond H. Mak, and Hugo J.W.L. Aerts. 2018. 'Deep Learning for Lung Cancer Prognostication: A Retrospective Multi-Cohort Radiomics Study'. *PLOS Medicine* 15 (11): e1002711. https://doi.org/10.1371/JOURNAL.PMED.1002711.

Hüllermeier, Eyke, and Willem Waegeman. 2021. 'Aleatoric and Epistemic Uncertainty in Machine Learning: An Introduction to Concepts and Methods'. *Machine Learning* 110 (3): 457–506. https://doi.org/10.1007/s10994-021-05946-3.

Jackson, Pamela R., Joseph Juliano, Andrea Hawkins-Daarud, Russell C. Rockne, and Kristin R. Swanson. 2015. 'Patient-Specific Mathematical Neuro-Oncology: Using a Simple Proliferation and Invasion Tumor Model to Inform Clinical Practice'. *Bulletin of Mathematical Biology* 77 (5): 846–56. https://doi.org/10.1007/s11538-015-0067-7.

Jeong, Sungmoon, Hosang Yu, Shin Hyung Park, Dongwon Woo, Seoung Jun Lee, Gun Oh Chong, Hyung Soo Han, and Jae Chul Kim. 2024. 'Comparing Deep Learning and Handcrafted Radiomics to Predict Chemoradiotherapy Response for Locally Advanced Cervical Cancer Using Pretreatment MRI'. *Scientific Reports* 14 (1). https://doi.org/10.1038/s41598-024-51742-z.

Ji, Hangjie, Kyle Lafata, Yvonne Mowery, David Brizel, Andrea L. Bertozzi, Fang Fang Yin, and Chunhao Wang. 2022. 'Post-Radiotherapy PET Image Outcome Prediction by Deep Learning under Biological Model Guidance: A Feasibility Study of Oropharyngeal Cancer Application'. *Frontiers in Oncology* 12 (May). https://doi.org/10.3389/fonc.2022.895544.

Jiang, Hongyang, Jie Xu, Rongjie Shi, Kang Yang, Dongdong Zhang, Mengdi Gao, He Ma, and Wei Qian. 2020. 'A Multi-Label Deep Learning Model with Interpretable Grad-CAM for Diabetic Retinopathy Classification'. *2020 42nd Annual International Conference of the IEEE Engineering in Medicine & Biology Society (EMBC)*, Montreal, QC, Canada, 2020-July, 1560–63. https://doi.org/10.1109/EMBC44109.2020.9175884.

Jin, Cheng, Heng Yu, Jia Ke, Peirong Ding, Yongju Yi, Xiaofeng Jiang, Xin Duan, et al. 2021. 'Predicting Treatment Response from Longitudinal Images Using Multi-Task Deep Learning'. *Nature Communications* 12 (1): 1–11. https://doi.org/10.1038/s41467-021-22188-y.

Jochems, Arthur, Timo M Deist, Issam El Naqa, Marc Kessler, Chuck Mayo, Jackson Reeves, Shruti Jolly, et al. 2017. 'Developing and Validating a Survival Prediction Model for NSCLC Patients Through Distributed Learning Across 3 Countries'. *International Journal of Radiation Oncology, Biology, Physics* 99 (2): 344–52. https://doi.org/10.1016/j.ijrobp.2017.04.021.

Kaandorp, Misha P. T., Sebastiano Barbieri, Remy Klaassen, Hanneke W. M. van Laarhoven, Hans Crezee, Peter T. While, Aart J. Nederveen, and Oliver J. Gurney-Champion. 2021. 'Improved Unsupervised Physics-Informed Deep Learning for Intravoxel Incoherent Motion Modeling and Evaluation in Pancreatic Cancer Patients'. *Magnetic Resonance in Medicine* 86 (4): 2250–65. https://doi.org/10.1002/mrm.28852.

Kim, Hyungjin, Jin Mo Goo, Kyung Hee Lee, Young Tae Kim, and Chang Min Park. 2020. 'Preoperative Ct-Based Deep Learning Model for Predicting Disease-Free Survival in Patients with Lung Adenocarcinomas'. *Radiology* 296 (1): 216–24. http://doi.org/10.1148/radiol.2020192764.

Kim, Jung Han, Bum Jun Kim, Hyun Joo Jang, and Hyeong Su Kim. 2017. 'Comparison of the RECIST and EORTC PET Criteria in the Tumor Response Assessment: A Pooled Analysis and Review'. *Cancer Chemotherapy and Pharmacology* 80 (4): 729–35. https://doi.org/10.1007/s00280-017-3411-9.

Kong, Feng-Ming Spring, Chen Hu, Randall Ten Haken, Ying Xiao, Martha Matuszak, Vera Hirsh, Daniel A Pryma, et al. 2021. 'NRG-RTOG 1106/ACRIN 6697: A Phase IIR Trial of Standard versus Adaptive (Mid-Treatment PET-Based) Chemoradiotherapy for Stage III NSCLC—Results and Comparison to NRG-RTOG 0617 (Non-Personalized RT Dose Escalation).' *Journal of Clinical Oncology* 39 (15_suppl): 8548. https://doi.org/10.1200/JCO.2021.39.15_suppl.8548.

Lakshminarayanan, Balaji, Alexander Pritzel, and Charles Blundell Deepmind. n.d. 'Simple and Scalable Predictive Uncertainty Estimation Using Deep Ensembles'. Accessed 22 October 2024. https://doi.org/10.48550/arXiv.1612.01474.

Lee, Howard J., Jing Zeng, Hubert J. Vesselle, Shilpen A. Patel, Ramesh Rengan, and Stephen R. Bowen. 2018. 'Correlation of Functional Lung Heterogeneity and Dosimetry to Radiation Pneumonitis Using Perfusion SPECT/CT and FDG PET/CT Imaging'. *International Journal of Radiation Oncology, Biology, Physics* 102 (4): 1255–64. https://doi.org/10.1016/j.ijrobp.2018.05.051.

Lee, Jeong Won, Dongryul Oh, Keun-Yong Eom, Jin Hee Kim, Woo Chul Kim, Mi Joo Chung, and Jong Hoon Lee. 2020. 'The Prognostic Value of PET/CT Evaluation with Deauville Score on the Recurrence and Survival in Diffuse Large B-Cell Lymphoma: A Multi-Institutional Study of KROG 17-02'. *Clinical & Experimental Metastasis* 37 (1): 125–31. https://doi.org/10.1007/s10585-019-09992-z.

Lee, Jinhyuk, Wonjin Yoon, Sungdong Kim, Donghyeon Kim, Sunkyu Kim, Chan Ho So, and Jaewoo Kang. 2019. 'BioBERT: A Pre-Trained Biomedical Language Representation Model for biomedical Text Mining'. *CoRR* abs/1901.08746. https://arxiv.org/abs/1901.08746.

Lee, Sang Ho, Huaizhi Geng, Jacinta Arnold, Richard Caruana, Yong Fan, Mark A. Rosen, Aditya P. Apte, Joseph O. Deasy, Jeffrey D. Bradley, and Ying Xiao. 2023. 'Interpretable Machine Learning for Choosing Radiation Dose-Volume Constraints on Cardio-Pulmonary Substructures Associated with Overall Survival in NRG Oncology RTOG 0617'. *International Journal of Radiation Oncology, Biology, Physics* 117 (5): 1270–86. https://doi.org/10.1016/J.IJROBP.2023.06.009.

Li, Butuo, Linlin Yang, Chao Jiang, Yueyuan Yao, Haoqian Li, Shuping Cheng, Bing Zou, Bingjie Fan, and Linlin Wang. 2023. 'Integrated Multi-Dimensional Deep Neural Network Model Improves Prognosis Prediction of Advanced NSCLC Patients Receiving Bevacizumab'. *Frontiers in Oncology* 13. https://doi.org/10.3389/fonc.2023.1052147.

Li, Zirong, Ann C. Raldow, Joanne B. Weidhaas, Qichao Zhou, and X. Sharon Qi. 2023. 'Prediction of Radiation Treatment Response for Locally Advanced Rectal Cancer via a Longitudinal Trend Analysis Framework on Cone-Beam CT'. *Cancers* 15 (21). https://doi.org/10.3390/cancers15215142.

Lin, Nancy U., Eudocia Q. Lee, Hidefumi Aoyama, Igor J. Barani, Daniel P. Barboriak, Brigitta G. Baumert, Martin Bendszus, et al. 2015. 'Response Assessment Criteria for Brain Metastases: Proposal from the RANO Group'. *The Lancet. Oncology* 16 (6): e270–78. https://doi.org/10.1016/S1470-2045(15)70057-4.

Ling, Yating, Yuling Wang, Wenli Dai, Jie Yu, Ping Liang, and Dexing Kong. 2024. 'MTANet: Multi-Task Attention Network for Automatic Medical Image Segmentation and Classification'. *IEEE Transactions on Medical Imaging* 43 (2): 674–85. https://doi.org/10.1109/TMI.2023.3317088.

Liu, Haotian, Chunyuan Li, Qingyang Wu, and Yong Jae Lee. 2023. 'Visual Instruction Tuning'. *Advances in Neural Information Processing Systems* 36 (April). https://arxiv.org/abs/2304.08485v2.

Liu, Yu, Ying Wang, Yuxiang Wang, Yu Xie, Yanfen Cui, Senwen Feng, Mengxia Yao, et al. 2022. 'Early Prediction of Treatment Response to Neoadjuvant Chemotherapy Based on Longitudinal Ultrasound Images of HER2-Positive Breast Cancer Patients by Siamese Multi-Task Network: A Multicentre, Retrospective Cohort Study'. *EClinicalMedicine* 52 (October). https://doi.org/10.1016/j.eclinm.2022.101562.

Lokre, Ojaswita, Timothy G. Perk, Amy J. Weisman, Rajkumar Munian Govindan, Song Chen, Meijie Chen, Jens Eickhoff, Glenn Liu, and Robert Jeraj. 2024. 'Quantitative Evaluation of Lesion Response Heterogeneity for Superior Prognostication of Clinical Outcome'. *European Journal of Nuclear Medicine and Molecular Imaging*. https://doi.org/10.1007/s00259-024-06764-0.

Lu, Charles, Andreanne Lemay, Ken Chang, Katharina Hoebel, and Jayashree Kalpathy-Cramer. 2022. 'Fair Conformal Predictors for Applications in Medical Imaging'. *Proceedings of the AAAI Conference on Artificial Intelligence* 36 (June):12008–16. https://doi.org/10.1609/aaai.v36i11.21459.

Lu, Lin, Laurent Dercle, Binsheng Zhao, and Lawrence H. Schwartz. 2021. 'Deep Learning for the Prediction of Early On-Treatment Response in Metastatic Colorectal Cancer from Serial Medical Imaging'. *Nature Communications* 12 (1): 1–11. https://doi.org/10.1038/s41467-021-26990-6.

Lundberg, Scott M., Paul G. Allen, and Su-In Lee. n.d. 'A Unified Approach to Interpreting Model Predictions'. Accessed 19 October 2024. https://doi.org/10.48550/arXiv.1705.07874.

Martell, Kevin, John B. McIntyre, Tasnima Abedin, Elizabeth N. Kornaga, Angela M. Y. Chan, Emeka Enwere, Martin Köbel, et al. 2024. 'Prevalence and Prognostic Significance of PIK3CA Mutation and CNV Status and Phosphorylated AKT Expression in Patients with Cervical Cancer Treated with Primary Surgery'. *International Journal of Gynecological Pathology* 43 (2). https://journals.lww.com/intjgynpathology/fulltext/2024/03000/prevalence_and_prognostic_significance_of_pik3ca.8.aspx.

Masood, Daniall, Luyao Ren, Cu Nguyen, Francesco G. Brundu, Lily Zheng, Yongmei Zhao, Erich Jaeger, et al. 2024. 'Evaluation of Somatic Copy Number Variation Detection by NGS Technologies and Bioinformatics Tools on a Hyper-Diploid Cancer Genome'. *Genome Biology* 25 (1). https://doi.org/10.1186/s13059-024-03294-8.

Meaney, Cameron, Sunit Das, Errol Colak, and Mohammad Kohandel. 2023. 'Deep Learning Characterization of Brain Tumours with Diffusion Weighted Imaging'. *Journal of Theoretical Biology* 557: 111342. https://doi.org/10.1016/j.jtbi.2022.111342.

Meng, Mingyuan, Bingxin Gu, Lei Bi, Shaoli Song, David Dagan Feng, and Jinman Kim. 2022. 'DeepMTS: Deep Multi-Task Learning for Survival Prediction in Patients with Advanced Nasopharyngeal Carcinoma Using Pretreatment PET/CT'. *IEEE Journal of Biomedical and Health Informatics* 26 (9): 4497–4507. https://doi.org/10.1109/JBHI.2022.3181791.

Meng, Mingyuan, Yige Peng, Lei Bi, and Jinman Kim. 2022. 'Multi-Task Deep Learning for Joint Tumor Segmentation and Outcome Prediction in Head and Neck Cancer'. In *Head and Neck Tumor Segmentation and Outcome Prediction: Second Challenge, HECKTOR 2021*, Held in Conjunction with MICCAI 2021, Strasbourg, France, September 27, 2021, Proceedings. Springer-Verlag, Berlin, Heidelberg, 160–167. https://doi.org/10.1007/978-3-030-98253-9_15.

Mohamed, Abdallah S.R., Abdelrahman Abusaif, Renjie He, Kareem A. Wahid, Vivian Salama, Sara Youssef, Brigid A. McDonald, et al. 2023. 'Prospective Validation of Diffusion-Weighted MRI as a Biomarker of Tumor Response and Oncologic Outcomes in Head and Neck Cancer: Results from an Observational Biomarker Pre-Qualification Study'. *Radiotherapy and Oncology* 183 (June). https://doi.org/10.1016/j.radonc.2023.109641.

Monti, Serena, Ting Xu, Radhe Mohan, Zhongxing Liao, Giuseppe Palma, and Laura Cella. 2022. 'Radiation-Induced Esophagitis in Non-Small-Cell Lung Cancer Patients: Voxel-Based Analysis and NTCP Modeling'. *Cancers* 14 (7). https://doi.org/10.3390/cancers14071833.

Moor, Michael, Oishi Banerjee, Zahra Shakeri Hossein Abad, Harlan M. Krumholz, Jure Leskovec, Eric J. Topol, and Pranav Rajpurkar. 2023. 'Foundation Models for Generalist Medical Artificial Intelligence'. *Nature 2023* 616:7956 616 (7956): 259–65. https://doi.org/10.1038/s41586-023-05881-4.

Nakajo, Masatoyo, Hiromi Nagano, Megumi Jinguji, Yoshiki Kamimura, Keiko Masuda, Koji Takumi, Atsushi Tani, et al. 2023. 'The Usefulness of Machine-Learning-Based Evaluation of Clinical and Pretreatment18F-FDG-PET/CT Radiomic Features for Predicting Prognosis in Patients with Laryngeal Cancer'. *British Journal of Radiology* 96 (1149). https://doi.org/10.1259/bjr.20220772.

Nayak, Lakshmi, Lisa M. Deangelis, Alba A. Brandes, David M. Peereboom, Evanthia Galanis, Nancy U. Lin, Riccardo Soffietti, et al. 2017. 'The Neurologic Assessment in Neuro-Oncology (NANO) Scale: A Tool to Assess Neurologic Function for Integration into the Response Assessment in Neuro-Oncology (RANO) Criteria'. *Neuro-Oncology* 19 (5): 625–35. https://doi.org/10.1093/NEUONC/NOX029.

Neal, Radford M. 1992. 'Bayesian Learning via Stochastic Dynamics'. *Advances in Neural Information Processing Systems* 5 [NIPS Conference]. Morgan Kaufmann Publishers Inc., San Francisco, CA, USA, 475–482.

Niraula, Dipesh, Sunan Cui, Julia Pakela, Lise Wei, Yi Luo, Randall K Ten Haken, and Issam El Naqa. 2022. 'Current Status and Future Developments in Predicting Outcomes in Radiation Oncology'. *British Journal of Radiology* 95 (1139): 20220239. https://doi.org/10.1259/bjr.20220239.

Nishino, Mizuki, Jyothi P. Jagannathan, Katherine M. Krajewski, Kevin O'Regan, Hiroto Hatabu, Geoffrey Shapiro, and Nikhil H. Ramaiya. 2012. 'Personalized Tumor Response Assessment in the Era of Molecular Medicine: Cancer-Specific and Therapy-Specific Response Criteria to Complement Pitfalls of RECIST'. *American Journal of Roentgenology* 198 (4): 737. https://doi.org/10.2214/AJR.11.7483.

Okada, Hideho, Michael Weller, Raymond Huang, Gaetano Finocchiaro, Mark R. Gilbert, Wolfgang Wick, Benjamin M. Ellingson, et al. 2015. 'Immunotherapy Response Assessment in Neuro-Oncology: A Report of the RANO Working Group'. *The Lancet. Oncology* 16 (15): e534–42. https://doi.org/10.1016/S1470-2045(15)00088-1.

Olivier, Audrey, Michael D. Shields, and Lori Graham-Brady. 2021. 'Bayesian Neural Networks for Uncertainty Quantification in Data-Driven Materials Modeling'. *Computer Methods in Applied Mechanics and Engineering* 386 (December):114079. https://doi.org/10.1016/J.CMA.2021.114079.

OuYang, Pu-Yun, Bao-Yu Zhang, Jian-Gui Guo, Jia-Ni Liu, Jiajian Li, Qing-He Peng, Shan-Shan Yang, et al. 2023. 'Deep Learning-Based Precise Prediction and Early Detection of Radiation-Induced Temporal Lobe Injury for Nasopharyngeal Carcinoma'. *EClinicalMedicine* 58 (April). https://doi.org/10.1016/j.eclinm.2023.101930.

Pai, Suraj, Dennis Bontempi, Ibrahim Hadzic, Vasco Prudente, Mateo Sokač, Tafadzwa L. Chaunzwa, Simon Bernatz, et al. 2024. 'Foundation Model for Cancer Imaging Biomarkers'. *Nature Machine Intelligence* 6 (3): 354–67. https://doi.org/10.1038/s42256-024-00807-9.

Palma, Giuseppe, Serena Monti, Roberto Pacelli, Zhongxing Liao, Joseph O Deasy, Radhe Mohan, and Laura Cella. 2021. 'Radiation Pneumonitis in Thoracic Cancer Patients: Multi-Center Voxel-Based Analysis'. *Cancers* 13 (14). https://doi.org/10.3390/cancers13143553.

Pati, Sarthak, Ujjwal Baid, Brandon Edwards, Micah Sheller, Shih Han Wang, G. Anthony Reina, Patrick Foley, et al. 2022. 'Federated Learning Enables Big Data for Rare Cancer Boundary Detection'. *Nature Communications* 13 (1): 1–17. https://doi.org/10.1038/s41467-022-33407-5.

Peng, Jie, Xudong Zhang, Yong Hu, Tianchu He, Jun Huang, Mingdan Zhao, and Jimei Meng. 2024. 'Deep Learning to Estimate Response of Concurrent Chemoradiotherapy in Non-Small-Cell Lung Carcinoma'. *Journal of Translational Medicine* 22 (1): 896. https://doi.org/10.1186/s12967-024-05708-4.

Price, Ryan G., Smith Apisarnthanarax, Stephanie K. Schaub, Matthew J. Nyflot, Tobias R. Chapman, Manuela Matesan, Hubert J. Vesselle, and Stephen R. Bowen. 2018. 'Regional Radiation Dose-Response Modeling of Functional Liver in Hepatocellular Carcinoma Patients with Longitudinal Sulfur Colloid SPECT/CT: A Proof of Concept'. *International Journal of Radiation Oncology*Biology*Physics* 102 (4): 1349–56. https://doi.org/10.1016/j.ijrobp.2018.06.017.

Provenzale, James M., Claro Ison, and David DeLong. 2009. 'Bidimensional Measurements in Brain Tumors: Assessment of Interobserver Variability'. *American Journal of Roentgenology* 193 (6). https://doi.org/10.2214/AJR.09.2615.

Provenzale, James M., and Michael C. Mancini. 2012. 'Assessment of Intra-Observer Variability in Measurement of High-Grade Brain Tumors'. *Journal of Neuro-Oncology* 108 (3): 477–83. https://doi.org/10.1007/s11060-012-0843-2.

Radford, Alec, Jong Wook Kim, Chris Hallacy, Aditya Ramesh, Gabriel Goh, Sandhini Agarwal, Girish Sastry, et al. 2021. 'Learning Transferable Visual Models from Natural Language Supervision'. *Proceedings of Machine Learning Research* 139 (February): 8748–63. https://arxiv.org/abs/2103.00020v1.

Radford, Alec, and Karthik Narasimhan. 2018. 'Improving Language Understanding by Generative Pre-Training'. https://cdn.openai.com/research-covers/language-unsupervised/language_understanding_paper.pdf

Ribeiro, Marco Tulio, Sameer Singh, and Carlos Guestrin. 2016. '"Why Should i Trust You?" Explaining the Predictions of Any Classifier'. *Proceedings of the ACM SIGKDD International Conference on Knowledge Discovery and Data Mining*, San Francisco, California, USA, 13–17-August-2016 (August), 1135–44. https://doi.org/10.48550/arXiv.1602.04938.

Riedl, Christopher C., Katja Pinker, Gary A. Ulaner, Leonard T. Ong, Pascal Baltzer, Maxine S. Jochelson, Heather L. McArthur, Mithat Gönen, Maura Dickler, and Wolfgang A. Weber. 2017. 'Comparison of FDG-PET/CT and Contrast-Enhanced CT for Monitoring Therapy Response in Patients with Metastatic Breast Cancer'. *European Journal of Nuclear Medicine and Molecular Imaging* 44 (9): 1428–37. https://doi.org/10.1007/s00259-017-3703-7.

Ruchalski, Kathleen, Marta Braschi-Amirfarzan, Michael Douek, Victor Sai, Antonio Gutierrez, Rohit Dewan, and Jonathan Goldin. 2021. 'A Primer on RECIST 1.1 for Oncologic Imaging in Clinical Drug Trials'. *Radiology. Imaging Cancer* 3 (3). https://doi.org/10.1148/RYCAN.2021210008.

Sabbagh, A., C. Jacobs, R. Cooke, K. Y. Chu, S. M. Ng, V. Y. Strauss, P. S. Virdee, M. A. Hawkins, M. C. Aznar, and R. Muirhead. 2019. 'Is There a Role for an 18F-Fluorodeoxyglucose-Derived Biological Boost in Squamous Cell Anal Cancer?' *Clinical Oncology* 31 (2): 72–80. https://doi.org/10.1016/j.clon.2018.11.034.

Sarabian, Mohammad, Hessam Babaee, and Kaveh Laksari. 2022. 'Physics-Informed Neural Networks for Brain Hemodynamic Predictions Using Medical Imaging'. *IEEE Transactions on Medical Imaging* 41 (9): 2285–2303. https://doi.org/10.1109/TMI.2022.3161653.

Saraswat, Deepti, Pronaya Bhattacharya, Ashwin Verma, Vivek Kumar Prasad, Sudeep Tanwar, Gulshan Sharma, Pitshou N. Bokoro, and Ravi Sharma. 2022. 'Explainable AI for Healthcare 5.0: Opportunities and Challenges'. *IEEE Access* 10: 84486–517. https://doi.org/10.1109/ACCESS.2022.3197671.

Schacky, Claudio E. von, Nikolas J. Wilhelm, Valerie S. Schäfer, Yannik Leonhardt, Felix G. Gassert, Sarah C. Foreman, Florian T. Gassert, et al. 2021. 'Multitask Deep Learning for Segmentation and Classification of Primary Bone Tumors on Radiographs'. *Radiology* 301 (2): 398–406. https://doi.org/10.1148/radiol.2021204531.

Schaub, Stephanie K., Smith Apisarnthanarax, Ryan G. Price, Matthew J. Nyflot, Tobias R. Chapman, Manuela Matesan, Hubert J. Vesselle, and Stephen R. Bowen. 2018. 'Functional Liver Imaging and Dosimetry to Predict Hepatotoxicity Risk in Cirrhotic Patients with Primary Liver Cancer'. *International Journal of Radiation Oncology*Biology*Physics* 102 (4): 1339–48. https://doi.org/10.1016/j.ijrobp.2018.08.029.

Schep, Daniel G., Jasmin Vansantvoort, Ian Dayes, Himanshu Lukka, Kimmen Quan, Anil Kapoor, Tom Chow, William Chu, and Anand Swaminath. 2024. 'Evaluation of Volumetric Response Assessment from SABR for Renal Cell Carcinoma'. *International Journal of Radiation Oncology Biology Physics* 119 (3): 832–37. https://doi.org/10.1016/j.ijrobp.2023.12.005.

Selvaraju, Ramprasaath R., Michael Cogswell, Abhishek Das, Ramakrishna Vedantam, Devi Parikh, and Dhruv Batra. 2020. 'Grad-CAM: Visual Explanations from Deep Networks via Gradient-Based Localization'. *International Journal of Computer Vision* 128 (2): 336–59. https://doi.org/10.1007/s11263-019-01228-7.

Seoni, Silvia, Vicnesh Jahmunah, Massimo Salvi, Prabal Datta Barua, Filippo Molinari, and U. Rajendra Acharya. 2023. 'Application of Uncertainty Quantification to Artificial Intelligence in Healthcare: A Review of Last Decade (2013–2023)'. *Computers in Biology and Medicine* 165 (October): 107441. https://doi.org/10.1016/j.compbiomed.2023.107441.

Seymour, Lesley, Jan Bogaerts, Andrea Perrone, Robert Ford, Lawrence H. Schwartz, Sumithra Mandrekar, Nancy U. Lin, et al. 2017. 'IRECIST: Guidelines for Response Criteria for Use in Trials Testing Immunotherapeutics'. *The Lancet. Oncology* 18 (3): e143–52. https://doi.org/10.1016/S1470-2045(17)30074-8.

Shafer, Glenn, and Vladimir Vovk. 2008. 'A Tutorial on Conformal Prediction'. *Journal of Machine Learning Research* 9: 371–421.

Shi, Mengying, Sunan Cui, Cynthia Chuang, Oluwaseyi Oderinde, Nataliya Kovalchuk, Murat Surucu, Lei Xing, and Bin Han. 2024. 'A Time- and Space-Saving Monte Carlo Simulation Method Using Post-Collimation Generative Adversarial Network for Dose Calculation of an O-Ring Gantry Linac'. *Physica Medica* 119: 103318. https://doi.org/10.1016/j.ejmp.2024.103318.

Sorace, Anna G., Asser A. Elkassem, Samuel J. Galgano, Suzanne E. Lapi, Benjamin M. Larimer, Savannah C. Partridge, C. Chad Quarles, et al. 2020. 'Imaging for Response Assessment in Cancer Clinical Trials: Seminars in Nuclear Medicine'. *Seminars in Nuclear Medicine* 50 (6): 488. https://doi.org/10.1053/J.SEMNUCLMED.2020.05.001.

Stahlberg, Eric A., Mohamed Abdel-Rahman, Boris Aguilar, Alireza Asadpoure, Robert A. Beckman, Lynn L. Borkon, Jeffrey N. Bryan, et al. 2022. 'Exploring Approaches for Predictive Cancer Patient Digital Twins: Opportunities for Collaboration and Innovation'. *Frontiers in Digital Health* 4 (October). https://doi.org/10.3389/fdgth.2022.1007784.

Strandberg, Sara, Joakim Jonsson, Maryam Zarei, Kristina Aglund, Lennart Blomqvist, and Karin Söderkvist. 2024. 'Baseline and Early Response 2-[18F]FDG-PET/MRI for Prediction of Radiotherapy Outcome in Uterine Cervical Squamous Cell Carcinoma: A Prospective Single-Center Observational Cohort Study'. *EJNMMI Reports* 8 (1). https://doi.org/10.1186/s41824-024-00188-7.

Sturm, Dominik, David Capper, Felipe Andreiuolo, Marco Gessi, Christian Kölsche, Annekathrin Reinhardt, Philipp Sievers, et al. 2023. 'Multiomic Neuropathology Improves Diagnostic Accuracy in Pediatric Neuro-Oncology'. *Nature Medicine* 29 (4): 917–26. https://doi.org/10.1038/s41591-023-02255-1.

Sun, Mi Xue, Meng Jing Zhao, Li Hao Zhao, Hao Ran Jiang, Yu Xia Duan, and Gang Li. 2023. 'A Nomogram Model Based on Pre-Treatment and Post-Treatment MR Imaging Radiomics Signatures: Application to Predict Progression-Free Survival for Nasopharyngeal Carcinoma'. *Radiation Oncology* 18 (1). https://doi.org/10.1186/s13014-023-02257-w.

Sushentsev, Nikita, Leonardo Rundo, Luis Abrego, Zonglun Li, Tatiana Nazarenko, Anne Y. Warren, Vincent J. Gnanapragasam, et al. 2023. 'Time Series Radiomics for the Prediction of Prostate Cancer Progression in Patients on Active Surveillance'. *European Radiology* 33 (6): 3792–3800. https://doi.org/10.1007/s00330-023-09438-x.

Takeuchi, Yasuto, and Noriko Gotoh. 2023. 'Inflammatory Cytokine-Enriched Microenvironment Plays Key Roles in the Development of Breast Cancers'. *Cancer Science* 114 (5): 1792–99. https://doi.org/10.1111/cas.15734.

Therasse, Patrick, Susan G. Arbuck, Elizabeth A. Eisenhauer, Jantien Wanders, Richard S. Kaplan, Larry Rubinstein, Jaap Verweij, et al. 2000. 'New Guidelines to Evaluate the Response to Treatment in Solid Tumors'. *JNCI: Journal of the National Cancer Institute* 92 (3): 205–16. https://doi.org/10.1093/JNCI/92.3.205.

Thor, Maria, Kelly Fitzgerald, Aditya Apte, Jung Hun Oh, Aditi Iyer, Otasowie Odiase, Saad Nadeem, et al. 2024. 'Exploring Published and Novel Pre-Treatment CT and PET Radiomics to Stratify Risk of Progression among Early-Stage Non-Small Cell Lung Cancer Patients Treated with Stereotactic Radiation'. *Radiotherapy and Oncology* 190 (January). https://doi.org/10.1016/j.radonc.2023.109983.

Tirkes, Temel, Margaret A. Hollar, Mark Tann, Marc D. Kohli, Fatih Akisik, and Kumaresan Sandrasegaran. 2013. 'Response Criteria in Oncologic Imaging: Review of Traditional and New Criteria'. *Multisystem Radiology* 33 (5): 1323–41. https://doi.org/10.1148/RG.335125214.

Trada, Yuvnik, Paul Keall, Michael Jameson, Daniel Moses, Peter Lin, Phillip Chlap, Lois Holloway, et al. 2023. 'Changes in Serial Multiparametric MRI and FDG-PET/CT Functional Imaging during Radiation Therapy Can Predict Treatment Response in Patients with Head and Neck Cancer'. *European Radiology* 33 (12): 8788–99. https://doi.org/10.1007/s00330-023-09843-2.

Tseng, Huan-Hsin, Yi Luo, Sunan Cui, Jen-Tzung Chien, Randall K. Ten Haken, and Issam El Naqa. 2017. 'Deep Reinforcement Learning for Automated Radiation Adaptation in Lung Cancer'. *Medical Physics* 44 (12): 6690–6705. https://doi.org/10.1002/mp.12625.

Turgeon, Guy Anne, Amir Iravani, Tim Akhurst, Alexis Beaulieu, Jason W. Callahan, Mathias Bressel, Aidan J. Cole, et al. 2019. 'What 18F-FDG PET Response-Assessment Method Best Predicts Survival After Curative-Intent Chemoradiation in Non-Small Cell Lung Cancer: EORTC, PERCIST, Peter Mac Criteria, or Deauville Criteria?' *Journal of Nuclear Medicine: Official Publication, Society of Nuclear Medicine* 60 (3): 328–34. https://doi.org/10.2967/JNUMED.118.214148.

Valter, A., L. Luhari, H. Pisarev, B. Truumees, A. Planken, O. P. Smolander, and K. Oselin. 2023. 'Genomic Alterations as Independent Prognostic Factors to Predict the Type of Lung Cancer Recurrence'. *Gene* 885: 147690. https://doi.org/10.1016/j.gene.2023.147690.

Velez, Erik M., Bhushan Desai, Lingyun Ji, David I. Quinn, Patrick M. Colletti, and Hossein Jadvar. 2020. 'Comparative Prognostic Implication of Treatment Response Assessments in MCRPC: PERCIST 1.0, RECIST 1.1, and PSA Response Criteria'. *Theranostics* 10 (7): 3254–62. https://doi.org/10.7150/thno.39838.

Wang, Likun, Xueliang Wu, Ruoxi Tian, Hongqing Ma, Zekun Jiang, Weixin Zhao, Guoqing Cui, et al. 2023. 'MRI-Based Pre-Radiomics and Delta-Radiomics Models Accurately Predict the Post-Treatment Response of Rectal Adenocarcinoma to Neoadjuvant Chemoradiotherapy'. *Frontiers in Oncology* 13. https://doi.org/10.3389/fonc.2023.1133008.

Wang, Xiyue, Junhan Zhao, Eliana Marostica, Wei Yuan, Jietian Jin, Jiayu Zhang, Ruijiang Li, et al. 2024. 'A Pathology Foundation Model for Cancer Diagnosis and Prognosis Prediction'. *Nature* 634 (8035): 970–78. https://doi.org/10.1038/s41586-024-07894-z.

Welz, Stefan, Frank Paulsen, Christina Pfannenberg, Matthias Reimold, Gerald Reischl, Konstantin Nikolaou, Christian La Fougère, et al. 2022. 'Dose Escalation to Hypoxic Subvolumes in Head and Neck Cancer: A Randomized Phase II Study Using Dynamic [18F]FMISO PET/CT: Hypoxia Dose Escalation in HNC'. *Radiotherapy and Oncology* 171 (June): 30–36. https://doi.org/10.1016/j.radonc.2022.03.021.

Wen, Patrick Y., Martin Van Den Bent, Gilbert Youssef, Timothy F. Cloughesy, Benjamin M. Ellingson, Michael Weller, Evanthia Galanis, et al. 2023. 'RANO 2.0: Update to the Response Assessment in Neuro-Oncology Criteria for High- and Low-Grade Gliomas in Adults'. *Journal of Clinical Oncology* 41 (33): 5187–99. https://doi.org/10.1200/JCO.23.01059.

Wen, Patrick Y., Susan M. Chang, Martin J. Van Den Bent, Michael A. Vogelbaum, David R. Macdonald, and Eudocia Q. Lee. 2017. 'Response Assessment in Neuro-Oncology Clinical Trials'. *Journal of Clinical Oncology: Official Journal of the American Society of Clinical Oncology* 35 (21): 2439–49. https://doi.org/10.1200/JCO.2017.72.7511.

Wen, Patrick Y., David R. Macdonald, David A. Reardon, Timothy F. Cloughesy, A. Gregory Sorensen, Evanthia Galanis, John DeGroot, et al. 2010. 'Updated Response Assessment Criteria for High-Grade Gliomas: Response Assessment in Neuro-Oncology Working Group'. *Journal of Clinical Oncology: Official Journal of the American Society of Clinical Oncology* 28 (11): 1963–72. https://doi.org/10.1200/JCO.2009.26.3541.

Wong, Tsz Lung Jacky, Xinzhi Teng, Wilson Leung, and Jing Cai. 2024. 'MULTI-Modal Radiomics to Predict Early Treatment Response from PSA (Prostate Specific Antigen) Decline in Prostate Cancer Patients under Stereotactic Body Radiotherapy in MR-Linac'. *Journal of Radiation Research and Applied Sciences* 17 (2): 100841. https://doi.org/10.1016/j.jrras.2024.100841.

Wornow, Michael, Yizhe Xu, Rahul Thapa, Birju Patel, Ethan Steinberg, Scott Fleming, Michael A. Pfeffer, Jason Fries, and Nigam H. Shah. 2023. 'The Shaky Foundations of Large Language Models and Foundation Models for Electronic Health Records'. *Npj Digital Medicine* 6 (1): 1–10. https://doi.org/10.1038/s41746-023-00879-8.

Xiao, Mengying, Liyuan Zhang, Weili Shi, Jianhua Liu, Wei He, and Zhengang Jiang. 2021. 'A Visualization Method Based on the Grad-CAM for Medical Image Segmentation Model'. *2021 International Conference on Electronic Information Engineering and Computer Science, EIECS 2021*, Changchun, China, September, 242–47. https://doi.org/10.1109/EIECS53707.2021.9587953.

Xie, Yuchen, Qiang Liu, Chao Ji, Yuchen Sun, Shuliang Zhang, Mingyu Hua, Xueting Liu, et al. 2023. 'An Artificial Neural Network-Based Radiomics Model for Predicting the Radiotherapy Response of Advanced Esophageal Squamous Cell Carcinoma Patients: A Multicenter Study'. *Scientific Reports* 13 (1). https://doi.org/10.1038/s41598-023-35556-z.

Xu, Yiwen, Ahmed Hosny, Roman Zeleznik, Chintan Parmar, Thibaud Coroller, Idalid Franco, Raymond H. Mak, and Hugo J.W.L. Aerts. 2019. 'Deep Learning Predicts Lung Cancer Treatment Response from Serial Medical Imaging'. *Clinical Cancer Research* 25 (11): 3266–75. https://doi.org/10.1158/1078-0432.CCR-18-2495.

Yoon, Soon Ho, Kyung Won Kim, Jin Mo Goo, Dong Wan Kim, and Seokyung Hahn. 2016. 'Observer Variability in RECIST-Based Tumour Burden Measurements: A Meta-Analysis'. *European Journal of Cancer* 53 (January): 5–15. https://doi.org/10.1016/J.EJCA.2015.10.014.

Zhang, Yu, and Qiang Yang. 2022. 'A Survey on Multi-Task Learning'. *IEEE Transactions on Knowledge and Data Engineering* 34 (12): 5586–5609. https://doi.org/10.1109/TKDE.2021.3070203.

Zhang, Yucheng, Edrise M. Lobo-Mueller, Paul Karanicolas, Steven Gallinger, Masoom A. Haider, and Farzad Khalvati. 2020. 'Prognostic Value of Transfer Learning Based Features in Resectable Pancreatic Ductal Adenocarcinoma'. *Frontiers in Artificial Intelligence* 3 (October):550890. https://doi.org/10.3389/frai.2020.550890.

Zhang, Yunyan, Daphne Hong, Daniel McClement, Olayinka Oladosu, Glen Pridham, and Garth Slaney. 2021. 'Grad-CAM Helps Interpret the Deep Learning Models Trained to Classify Multiple Sclerosis Types Using Clinical Brain Magnetic Resonance Imaging'. *Journal of Neuroscience Methods* 353 (April):109098. https://doi.org/10.1016/J.JNEUMETH.2021.109098.

Zhang, Zhen, Zhixiang Wang, Tianchen Luo, Meng Yan, Andre Dekker, Dirk De Ruysscher, Alberto Traverso, Leonard Wee, and Lujun Zhao. 2023. 'Computed Tomography and Radiation Dose Images-Based Deep-Learning Model for Predicting Radiation Pneumonitis in Lung Cancer Patients after Radiation Therapy'. *Radiotherapy and Oncology* 182:109581. https://doi.org/10.1016/j.radonc.2023.109581.

Zhong, Yifan, Chuang Cai, Tao Chen, Hao Gui, Jiajun Deng, Minglei Yang, Bentong Yu, et al. 2023. 'PET/CT Based Cross-Modal Deep Learning Signature to Predict Occult Nodal Metastasis in Lung Cancer'. *Nature Communications* 14 (1). https://doi.org/10.1038/s41467-023-42811-4.

Zhou, Bolei, Aditya Khosla, Agata Lapedriza, Aude Oliva, and Antonio Torralba. 2016. 'Learning Deep Features for Discriminative Localization'. *Proceedings of the IEEE Computer Society Conference on Computer Vision and Pattern Recognition* 2016-December (December):2921–29. https://doi.org/10.1109/CVPR.2016.319.

Zhou, Yue, Houjin Chen, Yanfeng Li, Qin Liu, Xuanang Xu, Shu Wang, Pew Thian Yap, and Dinggang Shen. 2021. 'Multi-Task Learning for Segmentation and Classification of Tumors in 3D Automated Breast Ultrasound Images'. *Medical Image Analysis* 70 (May):101918. https://doi.org/10.1016/J.MEDIA.2020.101918.

Zhuang, Fuzhen, Zhiyuan Qi, Keyu Duan, Dongbo Xi, Yongchun Zhu, Hengshu Zhu, Hui Xiong, and Qing He. 2021. 'A Comprehensive Survey on Transfer Learning'. *Proceedings of the IEEE* 109 (1): 43–76. https://doi.org/10.1109/JPROC.2020.3004555.

12 The Promise and Peril of AI in Clinical Practice

Jacob Wynne

Recent advances in computing technology have spurred unprecedented growth in the fields of machine learning (ML) and artificial intelligence (AI). Improvements in automatic segmentation, natural language processing, and generative AI have transformed the ways in which we interact with each other and the world. These exciting innovations have prompted new challenges, requiring careful investigations into safety, interpretability, equity, and sustainability. Medical image analysis has been transformed by these burgeoning technologies, and their application in precision radiation therapy holds great promise. Image quality improvement, target segmentation, plan generation, quality assurance, clinical decision support, and patient education all stand to benefit from the careful implementation of these new tools in the radiation therapy clinic.

Image analysis is among the most active areas of investigation of imaging in medical physics today. Quality imaging and its accurate interpretation are central to the radiation oncology workflow. However, due to physical hardware limitations, image contrast and resolution, from treatment planning to delivery verification, remain inferior to that achieved in the diagnostic setting. Methods adapted from natural image super-resolution interpolation, natural image generation, and even natural language processing have all been used with great success in overcoming these limitations.

Among the first requisites of a quality treatment plan is a quality planning image. Diagnostic fan-beam computed tomography (CT), magnetic resonance (MR), and positron-emission tomography/computed tomography (PET/CT) are all frequently used in conjunction with a fan-beam CT planning image. While diagnostic CT, MR, and PET/CT images are typically employed, CT planning images in the radiation oncology clinic are acquired for the purpose of target localization, utilize a flat couch, and may use acquisition parameters that degrade overall image quality relative to diagnostic imaging, such as greater slice thickness.

At most centers, image-guided radiation therapy (IGRT) utilizes kilovoltage CT (kVCT) or megavoltage CT (MVCT) on-board imaging on the treatment machine for the purpose of treatment delivery verification. These imaging modalities are used to prioritize efficiency, allowing image acquisition and interpretation while the patient remains on the treatment table. However, due to the temporal and physical limitations on their deployment, image quality remains poor, even when compared to planning CT images. While recent hardware advances have allowed for the integration of PET and MR on-board imaging, kVCT and MVCT remain in widespread use.

Numerous AI solutions for these problems have been proposed, most leveraging the benefits of deep learning strategies to enhance image quality. U-Nets,[1] generative adversarial networks (GANs),[2] and transformers[3] have all been reported. While early studies focused on reporting small improvements in relatively obscure imaging metrics, recent works have focused much more frequently on demonstrating the resultant translational improvements in physician target identification and delineation and dosimetry. Continued emphasis on clinically meaningful advances remains critical to proving value and ultimately sustaining innovation.

Proving clinical utility can be challenging. One strategy is to directly compare AI-assisted workflow management with traditional human-led efforts. This approach is commonly applied in the evaluation of segmentation models. Segmentation of tumor targets and surrounding healthy organs-at-risk is a time-consuming and labor-intensive task in the radiation oncology clinic.

DOI: 10.1201/9781003480365-13

Technologies developed for object identification in natural images and video are readily adapted to solve this problem. However, challenges unique to the medical image domain, including limited dataset sizes and datasets without complete annotations, must be overcome. Various solutions to these problems, including unsupervised learning, have been explored, and direct comparisons between human expert segmentations and their AI-generated counterparts can readily demonstrate clinical utility.

The increasing availability of ever more powerful computing devices has allowed for new applications of AI with immediately apparent clinical value. The interpretation and generation of natural language was previously limited by the availability of computing resources and appropriately large datasets from which to draw inferences. These limitations have been recently overcome, primarily due to investment from private sector research and development, owing to the significant commercial value of these technologies.[4] With the public release of related application programming interfaces (APIs) and the broad availability of cloud computing resources, more investigators are now able to begin seeking solutions to increasingly complex clinical problems.

Among these is the interpretation of multi-modality clinical data. In clinical practice, data from different modalities often provide complementary insights into a patient's health. The interpretation of multi-modality clinical data is one of the most complex and critical challenges in modern medicine. Physicians are tasked with integrating a wide range of data sources, including physical examination findings, medical imaging results, laboratory tests, and written clinical notes, to arrive at an accurate diagnosis and devise an appropriate treatment plan. The challenge lies not only in the volume of data but also in the complexity of interpreting the relationships between different types of information. Physicians must identify patterns, trends, and potential discordance across data sources, a task that is cognitively demanding and error-prone. Multi-modal AI tools may permit streamlining of clinical workflows, improvements in accuracy, and reduction in the incidence of medical errors.

AI tools are now being developed to assist in the integration of multi-modality data, aiming to alleviate the cognitive burden on physicians and improve diagnostic accuracy. These tools leverage advancements in ML, natural language processing (NLP), and computer vision to analyze large volumes of clinical data from different modalities simultaneously, identifying patterns and correlations that may not be immediately apparent to physicians.

One of the advantages of AI in this context is its ability to process and synthesize diverse forms of data quickly and accurately. Deep learning models can be trained to interpret medical images and assess laboratory results or genetic data, while NLP algorithms can analyze clinical notes. By combining these capabilities, AI tools can synthesize a complete view of a patient's health, allowing for more precise diagnoses and possibly even personalized treatment recommendations.

A crucial component of AI-driven multi-modal data integration is the ability to translate imaging data into natural language. Traditionally, radiologists manually interpret imaging studies and generate written reports summarizing their findings. AI models can now be trained to generate natural language summaries directly from medical imaging data. These models use computer vision techniques to analyze the images, identify relevant anatomical structures, abnormalities, and disease patterns, and then use NLP algorithms to construct human-readable reports.[5] This not only saves time but also ensures that critical findings are consistently highlighted in the report, reducing the risk of important details being overlooked.

The ability of AI to translate imaging data into natural language also has the potential to improve communication with patients. Medical reports are complex and often filled with unfamiliar language and phrasing that has developed in response to regulatory and legal pressures on the medical profession. The rapid availability of these reports following passage of the Cures Act[6] has increased patient access and transparency but has also resulted in confusion and anxiety when patients misinterpret them in the absence of their physician. AI-generated reports can be tailored to different audiences, producing both detailed technical summaries for physicians and simplified explanations for patients. This could enhance patient engagement by ensuring that individuals fully understand their diagnoses and treatment options.

Multi-modal data translation is increasingly possible with the advent of transformer-based imaging models. Because transformers were initially developed for accurate encoding of long-range relationships in natural language, their outputs are uniquely well suited for integration with those of language models. From automatic tumor detection and interpretation of medical imaging results to natural language agents capable of reporting results to patients in an interactive manner, transformers have made AI useful in the patient-facing setting:

> … machines can be constructed which will simulate the behaviour of the human mind very closely. They will make mistakes at times, and at times they may make new and very interesting statements, and on the whole the output of them will be worth attention to the same sort of extent as the output of a human mind.
>
> *—Alan Turing, "Intelligent Machinery, A Heretical Theory," Philosophia Mathematica, 4(3), pp. 256–260.*

AI stands to transform the practice of medicine in the coming decade, but as with any nascent technology, great advances bring with them a host of important technical, social, and philosophical questions that must be considered.

Many argue that AI in the form of large language models has passed the Turing test, a benchmark attributed to computer science pioneer Alan Turing describing the inability of a human observer to differentiate AI from a sentient being. In the clinical setting, it will be critical to apply safeguards to ensure easy differentiation of human versus machine outputs. In this way, results can be interpreted critically, and trust can be established and maintained.

Trust in technology within the radiation oncology clinic is maintained through quality assurance. How will quality assurance be addressed for AI? Quality assurance in radiation oncology in the United States has primarily been led by the American Association of Physicists in Medicine (AAPM), which publishes process-specific task group reports as technology advances and standards are established. Because formal guidance on quality assurance of AI models is lacking in the clinic, practices are expected to vary widely in the early stages of deployment.

The data on which models in AI are trained are inherently biased, shaped by the biases present in both the datasets and the individuals who design and curate them. Biases in AI training data often stem from two primary sources: the historical and cultural context embedded in the data itself and the implicit biases of the people who create and select the data. For instance, medical datasets are frequently drawn from populations that are predominantly white, male, and from higher socioeconomic backgrounds.[7] These biases reflect long-standing structural inequalities in access to healthcare and medical research, where historically marginalized groups, such as people of color and women, have been underrepresented. As a result, AI models trained on these datasets may make accurate predictions or provide more effective recommendations for the majority population while performing less well for minority groups.

This reality has significant implications for AI applications, particularly in sensitive domains like healthcare, where biased outcomes may have life-altering consequences. Biases in AI training data are often subtle but pervasive, leading to a disproportionate representation of majority groups while underrepresenting minority populations based on race, gender, sexual orientation, and other demographic or socioeconomic factors. This imbalance exacerbates existing social disparities, perpetuating inequality in healthcare outcomes and treatment quality. In the healthcare setting, these biases can contribute to disparities in diagnosis, treatment recommendations, and ultimately treatment outcomes.

Bias can be overcome through a thoughtful and proactive approach to dataset curation and AI model design. Datasets that are inclusive and balanced are more likely to yield equitable outcomes when the resultant models are placed into production. In healthcare, this may involve careful recruitment of participants in medical research and clinical trials from which these datasets are often derived.

Another approach is to build models that are robust to bias. Techniques such as fairness-aware ML[8] can be employed to ensure that models do not disproportionately impact certain groups. These methods involve adjusting the model's decision-making process to account for known biases or even explicitly penalizing the model when it makes biased predictions. In addition, algorithmic transparency is essential for detecting and addressing bias.[9] By making AI models more interpretable, it becomes easier for clinicians and researchers to identify when and how bias is influencing the model's outputs. Finally, continuous monitoring and evaluation of AI models in clinical settings are crucial for ensuring that they perform equitably across all patient groups. This requires healthcare institutions to regularly audit the performance of AI models. Bias detection would prompt model re-training.

The rise of AI has revolutionized industries across the globe, enabling unprecedented advancements in healthcare, finance, and communication. However, this technology comes at a significant cost. The enterprise servers fueling the AI revolution are housed in large liquid-cooled data centers which consume enormous amounts of both energy and water. As the world experiences the consequences of climate change and moves away from fossil fuels, the increasing demand for energy by AI systems places additional strain on already burdened infrastructure. This growing reliance on data centers raises critical questions about sustainability, resource allocation, and the potential for exploitation in underregulated regions.

AI models, particularly those involved in deep learning and neural networks, require extensive computational power. Training a single large AI model can consume vast amounts of energy, as it involves processing massive datasets over extended periods. For example, training of GPT-3 at 175B parameters is estimated to have consumed 1287 MWh—equivalent to the combined energy consumption of 120 average American households over the course of a year.[10] Once deployed, AI models continue to consume significant energy during inference. It's estimated that a single generative AI query consumes ten times the energy of an internet search.[11]

The AI boom is occurring during a global shift toward renewable energy sources, driven by the urgent need to mitigate climate change. Governments, businesses, and international organizations are prioritizing the transition away from fossil fuels such as coal, oil, and natural gas and toward alternatives like wind, solar, nuclear, and hydropower. However, the pace of this energy transition has not kept up with the rapidly increasing energy. The growing energy needs of AI pose a unique challenge: how can society ensure that the power requirements of emerging technologies do not undermine efforts to reduce carbon emissions?

One potential solution is for data center operators to invest in renewable energy sources to power their operations. However, as AI-driven data centers continue to grow in size and number, the demand for electricity and water places an increasing burden on local infrastructure. In some cases, datacenters have been criticized for overtaxing local energy grids, leading to blackouts or power shortages for nearby communities.[12] In regions that already experience energy shortages or are struggling to modernize their infrastructure, the rapid growth of data centers can exacerbate these problems, diverting resources away from critical public services.

Moreover, the unequal distribution of AI's energy demands raises questions about just resource allocation. While tech companies profit from AI applications, the environmental and infrastructural costs are often borne by the communities in which their data centers are located. These data centers are frequently situated in remote or rural areas where land and resources are more abundant but where local populations may have limited political or economic power. In such cases, the benefits of AI may not be shared equitably, and communities may suffer from depleted resources, environmental degradation, or other negative consequences without receiving proportional benefits.

This issue is particularly concerning in regions with undeveloped or weak public policy frameworks, where regulation may be insufficient to protect local communities from exploitation. In the pursuit of cheap land, water, and energy, companies may be tempted to establish data centers in areas with lax environmental regulations, poor labor protections, or limited oversight. In these regions, the lack of robust public policy can allow bad actors to subvert strict environmental standards or ethical business practices, leading to long-term harm for local ecosystems and populations.

Without adequate public policy safeguards, remote communities with abundant energy or water resources could find themselves exploited by multinational corporations looking to cut costs. This exploitation could take various forms, from environmental degradation due to excessive water use, to the overuse of local energy grids, leaving little power for the local population. Additionally, such regions might see little economic benefit from the presence of datacenters, as many of these facilities are highly automated and require only a small workforce to maintain operations.

Radiation therapy, medicine, and society at large stand to benefit from the adoption and integration of AI technology. As AI continues to pervade every aspect of modern life, it is crucial to confront important questions about safety, interpretability, equity, and sustainability. Addressing these issues requires thoughtful public policy that encourages and incentivizes investment in equitable research practices, conscientious allocation of natural resources, and careful regulatory monitoring. Ensuring the benefits of this exciting technology are shared equally while minimizing its environmental impact will be one of the most important challenges of this decade.

REFERENCES

1. Ronneberger, O., Fischer, P. & Brox, T. U-Net: Convolutional Networks for Biomedical Image Segmentation. Preprint at https://doi.org/10.48550/arXiv.1505.04597 (2015).
2. Goodfellow, I. J., Pouget-Abadie, J., Mirza, M., Xu, B., Warde-Farley, D., Ozair, S., Courville, A., Bengio, Y. Generative Adversarial Networks. Preprint at https://doi.org/10.48550/arXiv.1406.2661 (2014).
3. Vaswani, A. Shazeer, N., Parmar, N., Uszkoreit, J., Jones, L., Gomez, A. N., Kaiser, L., Polosukhin, I. Attention Is All You Need. Preprint at https://doi.org/10.48550/arXiv.1706.03762 (2023).
4. Brown, T. B., Mann, B., Ryder, N., Subbiah, M., Kaplan, J., Dhariwal, J., Neelakantan, A., Shyam, P., Sastry, G., Askell, A., Agarwal, S., Herbert-Voss, A., Krueger, G., Henighan, T., Child, R., Ramesh, A., Ziegler, D. M., Wu, J., Winter, C., Hesse, C., Chen, M., Sigler, E., Litwin, M., Gray, S., Chess, B., Clark, J., Berner, C., McCandlish, S., Radford, A., Sutskever, I., Amodei, D. Language Models are Few-Shot Learners. Preprint at https://doi.org/10.48550/arXiv.2005.14165 (2020).
5. Hosny, A., Parmar, C., Quackenbush, J., Schwartz, L. H. & Aerts, H. J. W. L. Artificial Intelligence in Radiology. *Nature Reviews. Cancer* **18**, 500 (2018).
6. H.R.34–114th Congress (2015–2016): 21st Century Cures Act | Congress.gov | Library of Congress. https://www.congress.gov/bill/114th-congress/house-bill/34/text.
7. Celi, L. A., Cellini, J., Charpignon, M. L., Dee, E. C., Dernoncourt, F., Eber, R., Mitchell, W. G., Moukheiber, L., Schirmer, J., Situ, J., Paguio, J., Park, J., Wawira, J. G., Yao, G. Sources of Bias in Artificial Intelligence that Perpetuate Healthcare Disparities—A Global Review. *PLOS Digital Health* **1**, e0000022 (2022).
8. A Survey on Datasets for Fairness-Aware Machine Learning – Le Quy -2022- WIREs Data Mining and Knowledge Discovery – Wiley Online Library. https://wires.onlinelibrary.wiley.com/doi/10.1002/widm.1452.
9. Meng, C., Trinh, L., Xu, N., Enouen, J. & Liu, Y. Interpretability and Fairness Evaluation of Deep Learning Models on MIMIC-IV Dataset. *Scientific Reports* **12**, 7166 (2022).
10. Luccioni, A. S., Viguier, S. & Ligozat, A.-L. Estimating the Carbon Footprint of BLOOM, a 176B Parameter Language Model. Preprint at https://doi.org/10.48550/arXiv.2211.02001 (2022).
11. Powering Intelligence: Analyzing Artificial Intelligence and Data Center Energy Consumption. Paper published by Electric Power Research Institute. https://www.epri.com/research/products/000000003002028905.
12. O'Donovan, C. Data Centers Strain Power Grids. Should Tech Firms Pay for Upgrades? – *The Washington Post*. https://www.washingtonpost.com/technology/2024/09/13/data-centers-power-grid-ohio/.

Perspectives

This book has highlighted the remarkable advancement artificial intelligence (AI) has made in medical image analysis and its growing integration across multiple aspects of radiation oncology. From image synthesis and segmentation to real-time guidance, adaptive planning, and treatment response assessment, AI has demonstrated the potential to enhance accuracy, efficiency, and personalization in cancer care. Yet, the journey from innovation to routine clinical adoption remains complex, requiring sustained collaboration among clinicians, researchers, and engineers.

Looking forward, the next phase of progress relies on several key developments. First, the generation and curation of large, high-quality, and diverse datasets can be a priority. Current AI models are often trained and validated on single-institution datasets with limited generalizability. To achieve robust, reproducible performance across diverse clinical environments, multi-institutional collaborations and open data initiatives are essential. Establishing standardized data formats, labeling protocols, and benchmark datasets will further accelerate algorithm development and comparative validation.

Second, the emergence of foundation models and self-supervised learning represents a new shift in how AI can learn from medical imaging data. These models, trained on massive, heterogeneous datasets, show promise in generalizing across tasks and modalities with minimal fine-tuning. In radiation oncology, their use could enable versatile systems capable of supporting a wide range of applications, from image reconstruction to outcome prediction, with improved efficiency and reduced annotation burden. However, these large models require rigorous evaluation to ensure their reliability, fairness, and interpretability in clinical contexts.

In addition to foundation models, vision-language models (VLMs) have emerged as powerful tools for bridging medical images and clinical text. These models, trained on paired image-text datasets, are capable of interpreting visual data in the context of language prompts—enabling tasks such as automated report generation, image captioning, and even zero-shot segmentation. In radiation oncology, VLMs could facilitate seamless communication between imaging findings and clinical decision-making, support automated contour verification against clinical guidelines, and enable more intuitive interactions with AI systems through natural language. While still in their early stages, VLMs such as MedCLIP and BioViL represent a new frontier for multimodal intelligence, with the potential to unify disparate sources of clinical information into coherent, explainable, and clinically useful insights.

The integration of AI into clinical workflows must be accompanied by advances in human–AI collaboration. Rather than replacing clinicians, AI should serve as an intelligent assistant—augmenting human expertise, reducing cognitive load, and supporting decision-making. This requires the design of intuitive user interfaces, transparent reasoning mechanisms, and training programs that encourage clinician trust and competence in AI-assisted tools. Interdisciplinary education will be crucial, enabling a new generation of radiation oncologists and medical physicists to work together effectively.

Finally, ongoing clinical validation and prospective trials are needed to move AI from proof of concept to standard of care. Despite promising retrospective studies, there is a relative scarcity of large-scale, prospective evaluations of AI systems in radiation oncology. Demonstrating improved clinical outcomes, workflow efficiency, or cost-effectiveness through randomized trials will be a decisive step toward broader adoption. Partnerships between academic institutions, industry, and health care systems will be vital in designing and executing these studies.

In conclusion, AI offers transformative possibilities for radiation oncology, but its full impact will depend on how thoughtfully and collaboratively we pursue its development. As AI continues to mature, our collective responsibility is to ensure that it enhances—not replaces—the human connection at the heart of cancer care. Through shared commitment to innovation, validation, and equity, we can shape a future where AI empowers clinicians, supports patients, and elevates the standard of care in precision radiation therapy.

Index

Note: **Bold** page numbers refer to tables; *italic* page numbers refer to figures.

D

E

F

G

H

I

J

K

L

M

N

O

P

R

S

For Product Safety Concerns and Information please contact our EU representative GPSR@taylorandfrancis.com Taylor & Francis Verlag GmbH, Kaufingerstraße 24, 80331 München, Germany